Clinical Laboratory Tests
Significance and Implications for Nursing

Kathleen Morrison Treseler, R.N., M.S.N.

Associate Professor, School of Nursing, Seattle University

PRENTICE-HALL, INC., Englewood Cliffs, New Jersey 07632

Library of Congress Cataloging in Publication Data

Treseler, Kathleen Morrison.
Clinical laboratory tests.

Bibliography: p.
Includes index.
1. Nursing. 2. Diagnosis, Laboratory. I. Title.
[DNLM: 1. Diagnosis, Laboratory–Nursing texts. QY 4 T796c]
RT48.T73 616.07'56 81-21091
ISBN 0-13-137760-4 (pbk.) AACR2

Editorial production supervision by Leslie Nadell and Zita de Schauensee
Internal design by Leslie Nadell
Cover design by Judith A. Matz
Manufacturing buyer: John Hall

Printed in the United States of America

10 9 8 7 6 5 4

ISBN 0-13-137760-4

Prentice-Hall International, Inc., *London*
Prentice-Hall of Australia Pty. Limited, *Sydney*
Prentice-Hall of Canada, Ltd., *Toronto*
Prentice-Hall of India Private Limited, *New Delhi*
Prentice-Hall of Japan, Inc., *Tokyo*
Prentice-Hall of Southeast Asia Pte. Ltd., *Singapore*
Whitehall Books Limited, *Wellington, New Zealand*

Dedicated to

Elizabeth McDermott Morrison

A role model

Summary Contents

Complete Contents

Foreword

In the setting of today's modern hospital, it is essential that all members of the health care team have an understanding of the functions and abilities of the various support services to insure the proper and efficient use of these services for the patient's benefit. This is especially important in the relationship between nursing service and the clinical laboratory. The modern clinical nurse has a pivotal role in the ongoing care of a patient and is often relied on to detect changes in a patient's clinical condition. In this setting a nurse who can also detect and understand significant changes in a patient's laboratory values will be more effective in carrying out that role. Also, an understanding of specimen requirements for various tests will improve the quality of specimens obtained and allow the laboratory to deliver more clinically relevant results.

My involvement with this book was undertaken with the hope and expectation that it would serve as an instrument to improve and maintain better patient care. I believe it will be useful in not only the training of members of the health care team, but as an ongoing resource in both the inpatient and outpatient settings. The author has brought to the book a rich clinical nursing experience and a commitment to improve the nurse's ability to interpret laboratory data. I believe she has succeeded admirably in this effort. Although technologic advances in the laboratory will change the way many constituents are analyzed, the basic pathophysiologic mechanisms will remain valid, as will the majority of the interpretative statements in the book.

I am grateful for the opportunity to have played a small part in the production of this book and look forward to the results of its contribution to better patient care.

David D. Nordin, M.D.
Pathology Associates of Everett, Washington
Instructor, Department of Pathology,
University of Washington, Seattle, Washington

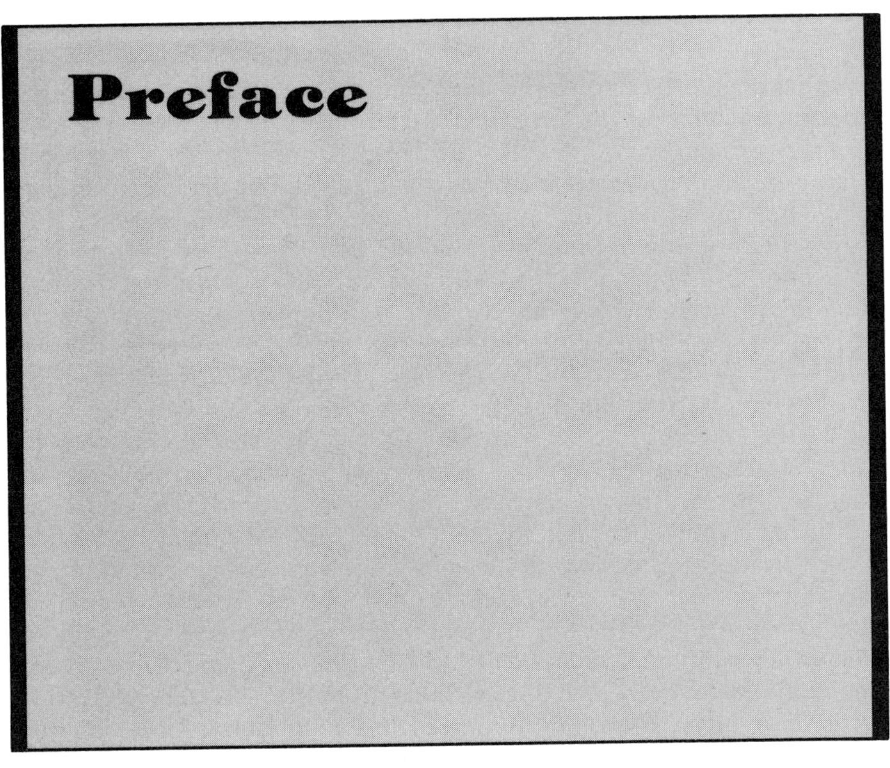

Preface

This book focuses on the implications of laboratory tests for individuals studying or practicing health care delivery. The stress is on using the *results* of laboratory testing to better plan and evaluate health care. By understanding the physiologic and pathophysiologic mechanisms that brought about a test result, the reader should be better able to act in the identification and implementation of preventative or supportive measures.

The book was written for baccalaureate nursing students in a medical-surgical setting. However, it will be of value to any student in any aspect of health care delivery, from vocational nursing students to medical students, since the book functions as a composite resource. It is hoped and expected that it will be of ready-reference value to the practicing professional as well, as it is designed to serve both as a teaching and reference tool.

The book was written out of frustration—frustration on the part of my students and myself as we were consistently unable to find information about variations in reference ranges of patients' laboratory test results. Gathering such information alone required a major search of literature. To synthesize the applicable patient care needs and potential problems, and to provide accurate rationale for intervention, necessitated an even broader search, requiring more time and more resources than were usually available. Consequently, data from laboratory findings were infrequently utilized. As a medical-surgical nursing instructor of many years experience, I have synthesized a fund of information about the significance of laboratory findings and their implications for nursing which I shared verbally with my students as the need arose. But this method resulted in haphazard and inadequate learning at best, and inaccurate recall, therefore inaccurate understanding and use by the student at worst. Other books available for use on laboratory testing did not adequately address the reasons for variations in test results, the interrelationships between abnormal tests' results, and certainly gave no clues as to what actions might be undertaken by the health care worker to prevent abnormalities, or to deal with them as they occurred. My colleagues expressed similar frustration, as well as concern about the effects of inaccurate understanding of laboratory findings on the patient care of health care providers. The book was written with the encouragement of my peers and guidance from experts in many areas of health care delivery. It is the result of a long and thorough search of available literature on clinical testing. Certainly, whenever conflicts appeared in the literature, I used my own experience and judgment to select the more commonly agreed upon methods of testing, values, or results, but the book is primarily objective in scope. It represents a collection of most of what is known or thought to be good technique in testing.

The book is organized to benefit both students and practicing professionals. Some of the major features include:

1. *Outline format* to provide quick retrieval of specific information about specific tests.
2. *Implications for nursing* to help the reader know what to do with the information available from test results, whether the reader is a nurse or not.
3. *Extensive use of lists and tables* to help the reader find material rapidly and to enable the student to memorize, and the working professional to consult quickly, the details of any particular test.
4. *Current information* on tests in use, providing an evaluation of the current usefulness of a given test.
5. *Reference range of normal variation in tests' results for different age groups* when available (e.g., senior adult, adult, and specified age levels for pediatric patients).
6. *Causes of variation from normal range* are extensively covered, including physiologic variation.

7. *Usefulness as a teaching tool.* If introduced early in the nursing curriculum, the book will help students understand the relationship of the test to the patients' medical problems. The overview of physiology for each screening test will reinforce learning from courses in anatomy and physiology. It will serve as a supplementary reference text in almost all nursing courses. The implications for nursing *are* medical-surgical nursing concepts, and consist of extensive instruction in general patient care in the disease conditions related most frequently to the test under discussion.
8. *Usefulness as a reference tool.* The book is envisioned as a guide for employed health care professionals that can be quickly consulted whenever needed on the job. It can serve as an aid at the hospital nursing station, in doctors' offices, in out-patient clinics, in the health professionals' personal library, and certainly in hospital and school of nursing libraries.
9. *Provision of rationale* for physiologic or pathophysiologic occurrences, and for suggested interventions.
10. *Definition of terms* which may be unfamiliar to a new health care worker. For the most part such terms are defined in the body of the text where they first occur. Because the book will probably not be read in a consecutive order, the definitions may not always appear in the area being read. Thus, a few basic terms are defined in Appendix E.
11. *Supplementary information* about subjects of interest, but not essential to understanding the material in the book, is given in the appendixes.
12. *Extensive cross referencing* within the body of the text. Material such as the anion gap is explained for the reader's use.

The book is divided into three parts. Part 1, "Multisystem Screening Tests," includes the more commonly used screening tests for blood chemistry, hematology, coagulation, urinalysis, as well as special pediatric screening tests. The tests in this portion of the book are covered in the greatest depth. Each section is devoted to one test, and contains the procedure and purpose of the tests, underlying physiology and pathophysiology, lists of those conditions in which test results are altered (which includes a statement as to the usual mechanisms), and implications for nursing related to the patient problems usually evident with abnormalities in the tests. These implications are focused strongly on preventive measures. The in-depth information given with these tests transfers readily to specific physiologic systems, covered in Part 3 (e.g., serum creatinine; section 1.5 material applies to the renal system, Chapter 9).

Part 2, "Diagnosis of Infectious Disease," covers very broad areas of testing, describing general approaches to laboratory methods. Specific implications for nursing are interspersed throughout, including areas in some of the many tables, and are found as well at the end of the section. This latter coverage focuses on both prevention and management of infectious disease. Prevention is considered as a major responsibility for health care persons.

Part 3, "Laboratory Tests of Specific Body Systems," is more in the genre of what has become an expectation in a laboratory book, that is, a listing of tests by physiologic systems with normal reference ranges and a brief description of the test. Management suggestions for the health care worker are limited to patient preparation. It is a strength of the book that material contained in implications for nursing sections in Part 1 may be transferred for use here. A very complete listing of conditions that will alter test results is given, an addition not routinely found in other texts. Unique to this book is the inclusion, at the beginning of each chapter, or prior to discussion of a discrete functional area of a system, of a listing of "clues" that indicate need for in-depth evaluation of the system or function. These "clues" are made up of findings from screening tests and clinical signs and symptoms. This list provides the reader with a ready-made set of necessary and important observations to be made of any person with a suspected, or already diagnosed, disorder of the given system.

It is the author's belief that the use of this text will enhance the knowledgeable application of laboratory findings to the data base on which patient care is planned.

ACKNOWLEDGMENTS

The author would like to acknowledge with thanks and gratitude the remarkable amount of help and guidance received—so freely and generously given, and "without which this book would never have been written": or, if written, would not have been anywhere nearly as accurate, or as well done. Although this large group of people have no part in any errors or lack of style the book may possess, they are responsible for most of that which may be good. Space, unfortunately, does not allow listing each and every person, but some must receive specific recognition.

A deeply appreciative thank you is extended to:

Dave Nordin, M.D., for his careful, tireless reading of rough drafts of the total text, his guidance in revising, his generosity in sharing an impressive fund of knowledge, and his obvious interest in the nursing profession and its education;

Patricia Harris, M.S., SM (AAM) for volunteering to read and critique the unit on infectious disease, for preparation of the most useful and unique chart of normal and abnormal body flora for the book, and for opening the author's eyes to another source of mutual support and sharing for nurses involved in patient care;

Lynn Ballo Treseler, B.S., MT (ASCP), for the hundreds of hours spent reading, editing, correcting and indexing the complete text; her knowledge of laboratory procedures, of microbiology, of blood banking, and her remarkable memory for detail were all gifts beyond price;

The family, the major basis of moral support:

Don, for moral *and* financial support and for his role as an effective devil's advocate;

Mike, whose support included the loss of his typewriter and many hours of his wife Lynn's company;

Maureen, who was able to provide the noncritical and ever available listening ear, now known as an essential for an author;

Patrick, whose interest was whetted *after* he had read part of the manuscript, a compliment not soon forgotten;

Dr. Dolly Ito and Wanda Roberts who provided the necessary self-confidence to allow the author to begin, to continue, and to complete the work, as well as acting as reviewers;

The Dean and Faculty of Seattle University School of Nursing who provided a ready resource for the many questions, and a constant well of positive reinforcement;

Joan who turned a sow's ear into a silk purse with neat, clear typing;

Diane who supplied the student's point of view; and most of all to the many students over the years who identified the need and supplied the first enthusiasm.

To all these and to all whose names should appear on this page but do not, THANK YOU.

Seattle, Washington Kathleen M. Treseler

Note to the Reader

To help the reader of this book get maximum benefit from it, the following "caveats" are supplied.

1. The "normal range" for any given test varies with the method used for testing and with many specific characteristics of the laboratory itself, such as distance from sea level and the ambient temperature routinely present during testing. Therefore, *all the reference ranges given are examples only,* and can be expected to differ from the local laboratory's reference range. The reader is *strongly encouraged* to use the "normals" from the laboratory that has performed the test rather than those given herein. Normals for this text have been acquired from many sources—all accurate in their own setting, but perhaps not as accurate for the reader's setting.

2. Where data were available, the normal range has been separated into normals for given age groups. The age spans used are defined as follows:

Premature	birth to 1 month of age
Newborn	birth to 1 week of age
Neonatal	1 week to 1 month of age
Infant	1 month to 2 years of age

Child	2 years to puberty
Adolescent	puberty to 18 years of age
Adult	18 years to 69 years
Senior adult	70 years and thereafter

3. The terms "serum" and "plasma," although not synonymous (see Appendix E for definitions), are often used interchangeably—and are so used to a degree in this text. When either serum or plasma can be used for a given test, both terms may be used, although "serum" is used more frequently. When only one is preferred in a given test, it is so indicated in the text and so used.

4. Units of measurement are generally abbreviated. For the less common units, the term is spelled out the first time it is used. Definitions, as well as some conversions, for many of the measurement units are given in Appendix D.

Multisystem Screening Tests

PART 1

Screening tests increase the reliability and precision of the diagnostic process, often provide an indication of the initial severity of a disease process, and are one of the more reliable indicators that treatment is effecting desirable change.

At one time, with the appearance of automated analyzers, screening tests were expanded to large batteries of tests (multiphasic screening) because automation provided multiple determinations at low cost. Because of the cost of the subsequent follow-up on false, or non-pathologic, positive or negative findings, however, and the increasing reluctance of insurance carriers to cover such costs, this wholesale approach is much less in evidence today (Harvey et al, 1976).

The term *screening test* still implies to many the idea of a large group of tests done together to investigate a full system, or total body function. Such a group of tests is perhaps better termed a *profile*—an in-depth investigation. As used here, "screening test" means just that—a singular test that can give information about a fairly broad area of body function.

Through visual, tactile, auditory, and verbal investigation of an individual a diagnostician can frequently, but not always, gather sufficient clues to make suspect a specific disease process. If there are several possible causes, the diagnostician must seek specific data for each possible diagnosis from clinical laboratory tests, or the other diagnostic testing tools available (e.g., x-ray, CAT scan, echogram, ultrasound scan, exercise testing, pulmonary function tests). This process works well when there are overt signs or symptoms evident in the initial observations. However, in many pathologic states no overt clues are present until the condition is fairly well established or advanced. Because of this, screening tests are used to assist the diagnostician in determining the state of health, supporting the presence of a disorder, or ruling it out. Screening tests make it possible to decrease risks. For example, the person undergoing surgery will face fewer chances of having a heretofore unknown disorder cause serious complications when met with the stress of surgery. Screening tests also guide the practitioner in the provision of preventative measures, or teaching, which can keep the disorder from further development. Still another use of such tests is the reinforcement of the diagnostician's initial, considered hunch as to the presence of a physiologic dysfunction.

Just as a person's blood pressure is taken routinely on a visit to a physician, or during a stay in the hospital—in the absence of hypertension or even a family history of increased blood pressure—screening tests can be done without clinical indication to detect abnormalities having a high incidence in the general population. It is evident then that screening tests will vary with the population served. Not all hospitals or physicians, even in the same given area, will use the same tests for screening purposes. The information gathered from screening tests forms part of the "data base" for problem-oriented medical and nursing practice.

According to Collins (1975), a test must meet five criteria to qualify as a screening test. It must be:

1. Simple to perform and inexpensive.
2. An accurate procedure with few false positives or negatives.
3. Capable of being performed completely by laboratory or nursing personnel.
4. Harmless and relatively painless.
5. Used for the purpose of uncovering a serious or common disease that is treatable.

An additional criterion, directed at the diagnostician—whether a physician, a nurse, a laboratory technologist, or other member of the health care team—should be presence of the necessary knowledge and understanding of human physiology, and of the test in question, to interpret the results in relation to what is known of the history and present status of the person tested. This implies, as well, an understanding of the interrelationships among the screening tests, and common, nonpathologic variations in the results. Fundamental to this criterion is the diagnostician's knowledge and understanding of the scope of his own discipline's practice in the management of abnormalities, and the scope of practice of other members of the health care team, so that collaboration and cooperation will exist among those members in management. The focus of this text is to help the nurse to meet this criterion.

Blood Chemistry Screen

chapter 1

1.1 PLASMA SODIUM

Synonym: serum sodium

Normal Ranges

Adult	136–145 mEq/L
Senior adult	
Male	134–147 mEq/L
Female	135–145 mEq/L
Pediatric	
Premature	
(cord)	116–140 mEq/L
Newborn	
(cord)	126–166 mEq/L
Infant	139–146 mEq/L
Child	138–145 mEq/L

This test is a measurement of the major cation (electrolyte, positive charge) in the vascular space, part of the extracellular fluid

(ECF). Plasma is preferred for sodium determination, as there are platelet factors released during clotting which can interfere with some methods of sodium determination.

It should be considered as a ratio measurement, the ratio between sodium and water, rather than a direct measure of the total body sodium. Plasma sodium levels reflect the balance of water to sodium. There is no laboratory test that can measure the sodium concentration of the total body. However, one can look at the size of the extracellular space (by looking at postural blood pressure, edema, and neck vein distension, for example) and gain an estimation of the total body sodium, because water and sodium imbalances coexist.

The sodium bicarbonate buffer system is one of the major renal controls of hydrogen levels, which makes sodium an important cation in maintaining the body's acid-base balance as well as in maintaining fluid distribution in the body.

1.1.1 Hypernatremia

Hypernatremia (increased plasma sodium) often, but not necessarily, coexists with hyperosmolality (increased total number of osmotically active molecules in the solution tested). Other terms often used interchangeably are sodium excess of ECF, salt excess, and hypertonic dehydration. Hypernatremia is a fairly rare occurrence but is seen most often in the elderly, in critical care, or in neurological populations. An increase in the plasma sodium level above normal limits suggests loss of body water in excess of sodium loss, or an increase in sodium in excess of water. True sodium excess (also called absolute sodium excess) is almost always accompanied by edema because of the corresponding excess of body water. Sodium is osmotically active and water follows it. Therefore, all body compartments will be involved, given time. The dilution within the intravascular space may be the cause of a normal serum sodium reading when in fact the total body sodium is elevated.

Physiology. Increased concentrations of sodium in the ECF, whether due to water loss or sodium gain, lead to an increase in extracellular osmolality. Water then leaves the cell via osmosis in an attempt to achieve iso-osmolality, which, in turn, causes water depletion within the cell. The causes the cell to shrink, with the potential result of cellular dysfunction. The *specific* compensatory mechanism to the increase in vascular sodium is suppression of aldosterone secretion by the adrenal gland and an increase in sodium excretion in urine. Antidiuretic hormone (ADH) is released by the pituitary in response to the increased osmolality of the ECF.

PLASMA SODIUM INCREASED IN:

1. *Conditions causing water loss:*

   a. Severe, prolonged vomiting due to any cause, but especially pyloric obstruction.
   b. Nasogastric suctioning, which removes more water and chloride than sodium.
   c. Some infectious diseases, such as tracheobronchitis, in which more water is lost than electrolytes, due to deep, rapid respirations and to fever. (The rate of insensible water loss is greatly increased with fever.)
   d. Profuse, watery diarrhea from any cause, when electrolyte replacement is absent or is inadequate. Diarrhea in infants and the elderly is most likely to lead to a hyperosmolar state than in adults. The thirst stimulus may not be intact in the elderly, or they may be confused and unaware of thirst, or unable to respond to it appropriately. Therefore, lost fluids would not be replaced adequately. Infants, having higher metabolic rates than adults, require more water. The greater relative skin surface area, which includes the gastrointestinal membranes as they are essentially an extension of body surface area until the age of three, results in greater relative fluid losses from both the gastrointestinal tract and the outer skin surfaces, especially if fever is present (Metheny and Snively, 1979).
   e. Diabetes insipidus, due to decreased secretion or the total absence of secretion of ADH, leading to a decrease in reabsorption of water by the distal and collecting kidney tubules. Sodium continues to be reabsorbed as the aldosterone mechanism still functions. An extremely low urine specific gravity will be noted (Sabiston, 1977).
   f. Primary aldosteronism, although debated in the literature, is felt by many to involve consistent reabsorption of more sodium than water, due to the increased reabsorption of sodium in exchange for potassium and hydrogen in the kidney. Serum concentrations are "virtually always above 140 mEq/L and often above 144 mEq/L" (Streeten, 1971) despite water reabsorption. This may be due to the polyuria accompanying the disease (Sodeman and Sodeman, 1974).

2. *Conditions causing sodium increase:*

   a. Inadequate intake of free water, probably the most frequent cause of hypernatremia. This may be due to an inability to perceive thirst, or an inability to respond to thirst. Such problems can be found in the unconscious person, the person with clouded sensorium (stroke, cerebral edema, or the elderly) (see item 1d above), the person with food or water restriction (NPO) for prolonged periods in preparation for diagnostic tests and/or surgery, and the infant whose needs are misinterpreted.

b. High-solute feedings, such as high-protein tube feedings or formula with a high salt content (rare now with commercial formula preparation). Infants are at particular risk because of their immature renal function. The high solute load acts as an osmotic diuretic, removing water from the body in a dilute urine.

3. There are many conditions in which total body sodium is increased but the increase is not reflected in the sodium value because of *water retention*, which follows salt retention, and which produces serum levels within normal limits (see Table 1.1).

TABLE 1.1 *Comparison of plasma sodium levels with total body sodium*[a]

Condition	Plasma sodium	Total body sodium
Edema (cardiac, renal, hepatic disease)	Low (hyponatremia)	High
Prolonged sweating	Low	Low
Diuretics and low-sodium diets	Low	Low
Addison's disease	Low	Low
Edema (cardiac, renal, hepatic disease)	Normal	High
Excretion of dilute urine, early stages of GI sodium loss	Normal	Low
Excess oral or intravenous sodium intake	High (hypernatremia)	High
Water and sodium loss with water loss greater than sodium loss	High	Low

[a]Note that a low or high serum level does not necessarily correspond with the total body sodium.

Source: Barbara Soltis, "Fluid and Electrolyte Imbalance," in Wilma J. Phipps, Barbara C. Long, and Nancy F. Woods, eds., *Medical-Surgical Nursing: Concepts and Clinical Practice* (St. Louis, Mo.: The C.V. Mosby Co., 1979).

1.1.2 Hyponatremia

Hyponatremia (decreased plasma sodium), except when it is the result of an excess of another extracellular solute such as glucose, is associated with low serum osmolality. Other terms used with the state of sodium loss or fluid excess include low-sodium syndrome and hypotonic dehydration. A plasma sodium level of less than 136 mEq/L is defined as hyponatremia. The plasma concentration is not a true indicator of the total body sodium in this instance, as it was also not a true indicator in *hyper*osmolality. Low plasma levels can coexist with a normal, an increased, or an actually diminished total body sodium concentration (see Table 1.1).

Physiology. Decreased concentration of sodium due to an increase in water or a loss of sodium in the intravascular space causes diffusion of water into the interstitial and the intracellular spaces until the osmolality is equalized between all compartments. In response to this, potassium—the major intracellular cation—moves out of the cell and is ultimately eliminated in the urine. The compensatory mechanism in response to increased secretion of aldosterone is an increased reabsorption of sodium by the kidney, a decrease in the sodium content of sweat, a decrease in the ability to produce perspiration, and an increase in the absorption of sodium from the gut. Aldosterone secretion is stimulated by the complex renin-angiotensin mechanism in response to a decrease in renal arterial pressure. When ECF hypoosmolality occurs, cells swell, which is thought to be the mechanism in the hypothalamic receptors that causes inhibition of ADH secretion. Thirst is inhibited and water is excreted.

PLASMA SODIUM DECREASED IN:

1. *Conditions causing sodium loss:*
   a. Diarrhea or vomiting may be the cause of sodium loss in excess of water, as well as water loss in excess of sodium (see "Plasma Sodium Increased in," item 1). Isotonic loss can occur as well, depleting both sodium and water equally. Sodium loss in excess of water loss is more likely to occur in:
      (1) Diarrhea occurring in an ileostomate.
      (2) Prolonged vomiting involving loss of intestinal as well as gastric fluids.
      (3) Infants, who are at particular risk for sodium loss as well as fluid loss, because they tend to lose large amounts of sodium through their skins even when well, and their kidneys do not concentrate urine well (Phipps et al., 1979).
   b. Draining intestinal fistulas.
   c. Prolonged use of diuretics, with inadequate electrolyte replacement or replacement with water only.
   d. Addison's disease, due to loss of secretion of mineral corticoids (aldosterone) with subsequent loss of the reabsorptive mechanism for sodium in the kidney.
   e. Chronic renal insufficiency with acidosis, the so-called "salt wasting" disease, due to an inability of the kidney to conserve sodium and the excretion of maximal amounts of salt.

2. *Conditions causing water excess:*
   a. Secondary to abnormal water retention:
      (1) Liver disease with ascites, due to consistently reduced excretion of both water and sodium coupled with renal failure that causes poor water excretion, even of that diminished amount in the glomerular filtrate.
      (2) Congestive heart failure with edema (dependent or pulmonary), due to decreased cardiac output, which decreases the glomerular filtration rate (GFR).
      (3) Renal insufficiency with urinary suppression.
      (4) Increased serum glucose, due to increased osmotic pull of glucose.
   b. Secondary to excess water intake and inadequate salt replacement:
      (1) Overheating of the body, due to strenuous exercise, high fever, or sudden increases in ambient temperature.
      (2) Individuals on diuretics, or who are vomiting.
      (3) Some mental aberrations characterized by excessive intake of water.
      (4) Some elderly persons whose thirst satisfaction requires excess water (Metheny and Snively, 1979).
3. *Conditions causing both water excess and sodium loss.* Only the syndrome of inappropriate ADH (SIADH) has been found to cause both water excess and sodium loss. SIADH occurs as a complication of many conditions and should be considered when low sodium levels are reported with cancer of the lung, head trauma, myxedema, tuberculosis, or meningitis. The water excess is secondary to inappropriate release of ADH, irrespective of the usual mechanisms of release through the osmoreceptors in the hypothalamus. A decrease in aldosterone secretion occurs secondary to the plasma dilution and increased GFR, and sodium is excreted. In this condition, therefore, the serum sodium level is decreased by two mechanisms: dilution by water retention and excessive urinary sodium losses (Sodeman and Sodeman, 1974).

IMPLICATIONS FOR NURSING IN IMBALANCES OF WATER: HYPER- AND HYPO-OSMOLALITY

1. *Determine patients at risk* for water imbalances by:
   a. Noting the written medical history, or by interviewing the

individual. Check for conditions that may lead to, or enhance, water imbalance (e.g., heart disease, inadequate liver function; see previous pages for others).

b. Expecting a change in plasma sodium level immediately after most surgery. This change is generally due to rapid administration of intravenous fluids (a plasma sodium decrease) or to the tendency of the body to conserve extracellular fluid postoperatively (an increase). Serum sodium levels usually return to normal limits in 24 to 72 hr. IVs generally contain sodium, which fosters sodium excretion. Care must be taken not to swamp the postoperative patient with sodium and water loads which are hypotonic at a time when ADH is high. Fluid overload can cause dilutional hypoprotenemia, leading to tissue edema of the lungs, brain, and peripheral areas particularly (Sabiston, 1977).

2. Prior to working with an individual at risk, *increase your own knowledge of sodium concentrations in the diet* in order to help the person adapt his or her dietary selections to prevent the occurrence of imbalance. Collaboration with the physician and dietician is encouraged in order to facilitate and reinforce each's plan of care.

3. *General implicatons for persons with a water imbalance:*

   a. All individuals with actual or potential water imbalances should be placed on strict intake and output measurement and daily weight checks as independent nursing actions.
   b. All persons with actual or potential water imbalances should have urine specific gravity tested at least once daily, or more often, as an independent nursing measure. If the ability of the kidney to concentrate is of particular concern, the first voiding in the morning should be tested.
   c. In the presence of a water imbalance of unknown origin, check for present use, and possible abuse, of diuretics. Early physiologic response to diuretics is the loss of extracellular water primarily. With prolonged use and replacement of the water loss, only actual plasma sodium depletion can occur.
   d. Be aware of how long a patient has been kept with nothing by mouth (NPO), especially those persons at risk for water imbalance. Monitor baseline data (items a and b above) and inform the physician when the data indicate a developing water imbalance.
   e. Any patient who is dehydrated, whatever the imbalance causing the problem, should receive mouth care for comfort and to prevent tissue damage. The nurse should also consult

with the physician to provide adequate hydration consistent with the patient's physical problems. Hydration must be undertaken with caution to prevent fluid overload, particularly in persons with cardiac or renal dysfunction.

4. *Nursing implications with saline imbalance* (loss of proportional amounts of water and sodium–isotonic dehydration–isotonic saline loss):

   a. Baseline laboratory data to be monitored include red blood cell count (RBC) and hematocrit. Urinary sodium levels are of value as well (see Chapter 4). Serum protein and lipid levels are affected by too many variables to be useful as baseline data for evaluation. If a recent RBC and hematocrit are not available, an order might be requested from the physician.

      Compare the RBC and hematocrit with the serum sodium. If the serum sodium is within normal limits and the RBC and hematocrit are elevated, isotonic saline loss–saline imbalance–probably exists, a state of true sodium and water deficit. (Patients with polycythemia will show this without saline depletion.)

   b. Monitor patients with, or at risk for, saline imbalance for signs of circulatory overload or collapse.
      (1) Check vital signs at least every 4 hr during the day, noting especially changes in blood pressure and pulse.
      (2) Inspect neck veins in both supine position and with the head of the bed elevated at 45 degrees.
      (3) Note the quality and rate of vein filling of the hands. Normal filling rate is 3 to 5 sec.
      (4) Weigh daily, same time, same clothing.
      (5) Listen to the lungs for rales.
      (6) Check for dependent edema: the ankles in ambulatory persons or those up in a chair; the sacrum in the person on bedrest. Measure the ankle circumference for baseline data and record.
      (7) Take blood pressure lying, sitting, and standing for postural changes.

5. *Nursing implications related to decreased plasma sodium due to excess water:*

   a. Confirmation of excess water (dilutional hyponatremia) can be done by the nurse by checking characteristic laboratory evidence and comparing with data from the patient history and physical. Laboratory data suggesting or confirming the presence of excess water is as follows:

(1) Serum osmolality decreased to less than 274 mOsm (milliosmols) / kg of plasma water. If a serum osmolality test has not been done, serum sodium concentration can be used as a fairly accurate estimation. Use the following equation (Groer and Shekleton, 1979) to get a rough, but adequate measurement of serum osmolality:

$$\text{plasma sodium } [Na^+] \times 2 = \text{serum osmolality}$$

(2) Plasma sodium decreased to less than 130 mEq/L. (This can be decreased to less than 115 mEq/L.)
(3) Plasma potassium decreased or within normal limits.
(4) Serum urea nitrogen (BUN) decreased or within normal limits.
(5) Hemoglobin and hematocrit decreased.
(6) Mean corpuscular volume (MCV) increased or within normal limits.
(7) Mean corpuscular hemoglobin concentration (MCHC) decreased. The changes in the blood indices—hemoglobin, hematocrit, MCV, and MCHC—are due to the swelling of the red blood cells together with all other body cells.

b. With a drop in the plasma sodium level to 125 mEq/L or lower, observe the patient for signs and symptoms of water excess: behavioral changes of inattention, confusion, drowsiness, delirium; weight gain; increased rate and depth of respiration; neuromuscular changes of muscle cramping after use; isolated muscle twitching, weakness, headache, incoordination, signs of increased intracranial pressure (increased blood pressure, slowed pulse rate, slowed respirations, projectile vomiting, papilledema). Symptoms of water excess are not usually significant until the 125 mEq/L level has been reached. This complication is frequently called water intoxication.

Observation for these symptoms is especially important in the person with SIADH because the onset is very rapid, often bypassing the earlier symptoms of changes in sensorium, drowsiness, and presenting with far advanced symptoms (i.e., delirium, psychotic behavior, or convulsions). Treatment must be rapid to prevent coma or even death from occurring; therefore, changes should be reported as soon as identified and with adequate emphasis and follow-up to elicit immediate response on the part of the physician.

c. With falls in serum sodium levels, an error frequently seen is an attempt to replace the sodium by giving broth or some other high-sodium food. Since the concentration of total body sodium is not known, all that the nurse can be sure of is the presence of excess water, and treating excess water with sodium chloride is inappropriate.

6. *Nursing implications related to decreased plasma sodium due to sodium loss:*

   a. Assure that any patient having nasogastric or intestinal suction is receiving not only ounce-for-ounce water replacement, but also mEq-for-mEq electrolyte replacement.
   b. Irrigate any nasogastric or intestinal tubes with normal saline solution. This precaution is not always observed in the clinical setting. The individual at risk for water imbalance can be pushed into excess by irrigation with water.

7. *Teaching needs for persons at risk* for, or diagnosed as having, fluid imbalance are dependent on the diagnosis, current status, previous knowledge, and the ability to learn. Some content areas concerning prevention are:

   a. Instruct those persons who will be involved in active sports, or who will begin work in a hotter environment, or who will be moving to a hotter climate, to replace salt lost in perspiration by judicious use of salt together with fluid replacement. (*Caution:* Hypernatremia can occur with the use of salt tablets.) Fluids containing sodium, or taking salty foods such as potato chips, should be recommended and warning given against drinking only water to slake thirst.
   b. Teach individuals who will be taking diuretics at home the signs and symptoms of sodium deficit and excess, as well as water excess and deficit. Stress the need to take medication only as prescribed, without variation. Teach those signs/symptoms that should be reported to the physician as well as what steps the individual can take independently to prevent imbalance (as given above). A family member or responsible home caretaker should be included in all teaching.
   c. Teach patient/family/home caretaker to read labels on all foods and medications for sodium content.
   d. Instruct patients on a low-sodium diet which foods to avoid, those to be used in moderation, and those low enough in sodium to be used freely. (The American Heart Association has free booklets available that describe mild, moderate, and strict sodium-restricted diets. They are usually distributed through physicians, dieticians, or nurses. The nurse doing teaching related to diet should acquire copies of the booklet for distribution.) The following is a list of some frequently used foods that are high in sodium.

(1) Meat: bacon, luncheon meats, frankfurters, ham, kosher meats, sausages, salt pork.
(2) Vegetables: sauerkraut and other vegetables prepared in brine, or with salt added during or after cooking.
(3) Fish: sardines.
(4) Miscellaneous: processed cheese, meat tenderizers, relish, horseradish, bouillon cubes, peanut butter, catsup, mustard, olives, pickles, Worcestershire sauce, potato chips, pretzels.

e. Instruct the person about high sodium content of ingestates other than diet: for example, toothpastes, powders, certain drugs (laxatives, pain relievers, sedatives, cough syrups, even some antibiotics), and chewing tobacco or snuff.

1.2 SERUM CHLORIDE

Synonym: plasma chloride

Normal Ranges

Adult	97–108 mEq/L
Senior adult	not available; could be assumed to mirror sodium concentration changes
Pediatric	
Cord	96–104 mEq/L
Newborn	93–112 mEq/L
Infant	95–110 mEq/L
Child	101–105 mEq/L

This chemical may be one of the least important electrolytes to measure, particularly in a screening procedure. Often, an emergency study will omit the chloride measurement. Its frequent use may be more a factor of historical interest, as well as its inclusion in the automated electrolyte series. Serum chloride was the first electrolyte that could be easily measured, and clinical laboratories established and used chloride tests long before sodium, potassium, or pH measurements were available. Emphasis on the "chloride shift" as a discrete, physiological, compensatory measure, rather than use of the shift of other ions (i.e., hydrogen, sodium, potassium) is based on that fact. It must, however, be included in electrolyte studies if the purpose is to detect the presence of unmeasured anions (the "anion gap"; see Appendix A). Even though measurement of serum chloride may not be essential, it is not unimportant, particularly when assessing acid-base balance (Davidsohn and Henry, 1969).

Chloride is the most plentiful of the extracellular anions. Eighty percent of the total body chloride is in the ECF and chloride constitutes two-thirds of the anions in the plasma. However, its actual concentration is greater in the lymph and interstitial fluid than in the plasma. Although its intracellular amount is very low, it is believed to be significant, since it is found in highly specialized cells (e.g., nerve cells) (Stroot et al., 1977). The body does not produce any chloride. It is fully derived from exogenous sources, yet increased amounts ingested will affect the serum levels only slightly (Howard and Herbold, 1978). Dietary sources of chloride include dairy products, meat, and some vegetables and fruit. The food content of chloride is roughly proportional to the sodium content. Foods high in sodium are also high in chloride. Exact daily minimum requirements of chloride have not been established, but the normal adult usually takes in from 60 to 100 mEq daily.

Chloride and sodium usually vary proportionally in the plasma of a healthy person. Serum concentrations of chloride do not vary markedly during development from infant to adult, the highest concentrations being found in the first few months of life, nor is there a difference between the sexes.

Physiology. Once ingested, absorption of chloride appears to occur in the ileum and, in even greater amounts, in the colon in exchange for bicarbonate. Net absorption of chloride from the colon exceeds that of sodium. Absorption is not an active process. Chloride seems to be absorbed as a paired ion with sodium. Absorption of ingested chloride is almost total (Tietz, 1970). If there is inadequate chloride available, bicarbonate will be absorbed with sodium. Chloride's functions in the body include a principal role, with sodium, in the regulation of osmotic pressure and water distribution. One of its major solo functions is as an integral part of the production of hydrochloric acid for digestion. The serum level will actually decrease about 2 mEq/L at the height of gastric secretion. Almost twice the amount of chloride found in the serum is actually secreted for this purpose only, and then reabsorbed. Chloride plays a role in acid-base balance since it combines with sodium in competition with bicarbonate. It also acts as a coenzyme for digestive amylases (Howard and Herbold, 1978).

Chloride is regulated secondarily to the sodium concentration. Usually, about 90% is excreted in urine, the rest in feces and sweat. The rate at which it is excreted depends on the amount ingested and the presence of adequate fluid. It is reabsorbed in the renal tubules under the indirect control of aldosterone and in response to the pH of the ECF—chloride being excreted and bicarbonate reabsorbed when pH is low, and vice versa.

Pathophysiology. Changes in chloride concentration, when proportionate to changes in Na+ concentrations, indicate variations in fluid balance. (The pathophysiology is discussed with plasma sodium.) When chloride concentrations change independently of serum sodium, the situation is usually one of an acid-base imbalance. Loss of chloride requires an increase in serum bicarbonate to maintain the total concentration of anions in the ECF and to combine with sodium. (The total anions of the ECF must always equal the total cations.) This state is called hypochloremic metabolic alkalosis. Increased retention or ingestion (as with chloride-based drugs) of chloride ions leads to a commensurate excretion of bicarbonate in the urine, leading to a decrease in the base bicarbonate and a state of hyperchloremic metabolic acidosis.

In hypochloremia, greater amounts of sodium are reabsorbed secondary to increased aldosterone concentrations in the tubules (decreased chloride assumes decreased sodium, as they are usually paired). Bicarbonate is reabsorbed with the sodium, in the absence of chloride, increasing the base content of the body—metabolic alkalosis. Sodium will be reabsorbed in preference to potassium, or even hydrogen, despite the increasing alkalosis (Frolich, 1976). If serum potassium is low, the hydrogen ion is the major cation excreted, potassium being given priority for reabsorption. This leads to an acidic urine with hypokalemic, hypochloremic alkalosis. The renal compensatory mechanism does not function. Excretion of chloride decreases when serum levels are decreased unless aldosterone secretion has not been stimulated, as in adrenal cortical insufficiency. Respiratory compensation for metabolic alkalosis attempts to increase hydrogen concentration by retaining carbonic acid through decreasing the rate and depth of respirations.

SERUM CHLORIDE DECREASED IN:

1. *Conditions causing respiratory acidosis,* such as pulmonary emphysema, pneumonia, pneumothorax, pulmonary edema and hypoventilation secondary to poliomyelitis, anesthesia, or other restrictive conditions. The decrease is due to increased excretion of chloride to compensate for increased anions in the serum (bicarbonate).

2. *Conditions causing decreased intake of chloride,* such as starvation or severely restricted intake of sodium chloride in treatment of heart, kidney, or liver disease.

3. *Conditions leading to increased loss of chloride,* such as:
   a. Vomiting, especially in pyloric obstruction.
   b. Nasogastric suctioning. As in item a, gastric secretions are lost which contain much greater concentrations of chloride than of sodium, because of the loss of hydrochloric acid.
   c. Diarrhea secondary to bacterial infections, which decreases the transit time in the colon of nutrients and thus decreases the absorption of the major part of ingested chloride.
   d. Diarrhea secondary to either congenital (rare) or acquired chloridorrhea. It is thought that the accompanying potassium deficit in chloridorrhea may affect the permeability of the intestinal mucosa, interrupting the chloride bicarbonate exchange. The acquired form of chloridorrhea is characterized by an inability to absorb chloride adequately. The increased concentration of chloride in the feces further increases the diarrhea, since it acts as an osmotic cathartic (Sodeman and Sodeman, 1974).
   e. Excessive use of diuretics (mercurial or chlorothiazide), which act to reduce sodium reabsorption and, indirectly, chloride reabsorption (Collins, 1975).
   f. Addison's disease, with a marked decrease during Addisonian crisis, due to the loss of aldosterone stimulation of sodium reabsorption and with it the indirect stimulation of chloride reabsorption.
   g. Primary aldosteronism, due to an increase in serum bicarbonate, secondary to the increase in sodium retention and the resultant metabolic alkalosis.
   h. Chronic pyelonephritis, due to a lack of tubular reabsorption despite a serum deficit of chloride. (All conditions listed so far can lead to metabolic alkalosis.)
   i. Diabetic ketoacidosis, even in the face of hemoconcentration, due to chloride loss in osmotic diuresis, vomiting, gastric dilatation, paralytic ileus, and the return of sodium to the blood as sodium bicarbonate rather than as sodium chloride, in an attempt to maintain acid-base balance.

      In other metabolic acidotic states the chloride level may be lower than would be expected because other negative ions, acetate, phosphate, or lactic acid are present.

4. *Hypokalemic metabolic alkalosis.* A severe decrease in the serum chloride itself can lead to, or maintain, a hypokalemic alkalosis

as well as follow it. A decrease in the availability of chloride ions as anions to pair with sodium leads to a decrease in sodium reabsorption. The compensatory mechanism causes an increase in the excretion of potassium in the urine in exchange for sodium with bicarbonate reabsorption (Jones et al., 1978).

5. *Conditions leading to retention of fluid in the vascular space,* causing a dilutional, rather than an actual decrease (see "Plasma Sodium Decreased in" in Section 1.1). Conditions such as acute renal failure with suppression and congestive heart failure are examples.

SERUM CHLORIDE INCREASED IN:

1. *Conditions leading to intravascular fluid decrease* with a relative, rather than an actual, increase in chlorides in the serum (see "Plasma Sodium Increased in" in Section 1.1).
2. *Some forms of metabolic acidosis,* such as that secondary to drug poisoning (salicylate), or renal tubular acidosis, due to a primary deficiency of base bicarbonate.
3. *Excessive treatment with chloride medication,* such as ammonium chloride.

IMPLICATIONS FOR NURSING

1. Prevention of metabolic alkalosis is frequently possible, and therefore *identification of individuals at risk* for hypokalemia or hypochloremia is an important first step (see "Implications for Nursing" in Section 1.3).
2. *Any patient who has* a nasogastric tube in place and functioning, has been vomiting, has a dietary restriction in sodium and thereby is restricted in chloride intake, has diarrhea, is on diuretics that do not replace potassium, or has an adrenal dysfunction should be considered at risk for hypochloremia and thus, at risk for metabolic alkalosis.
3. *Closely monitor plasma potassium and CO_2 content* (or combining power, or venuous CO_2 direct measurement), indicating bicarbonate or base concentrations, for possible decrease and compare to serum chloride levels in the populations at risk. Tests for blood

gases are not routinely ordered and are usually not necessary to monitor these individuals adequately.

4. *Check for signs and symptoms of metabolic alkalosis.*
   a. Complaints of circumoral numbness and tingling.
   b. Hypertonicity of musculature.
   c. Decreased rate and depth of respirations.
   d. Alkaline urine (other causes for alkalinity must be taken into account, such as immobility or the tendency toward sodium conservation and thus extracellular alkalosis after surgery).
   e. Complaints of nervousness or other signs of central nervous system stimulation.
   f. Indications of tetany, due to the binding of calcium to protein in metabolic alkalotic states.
      (1) Trouseau's and Chvoestek's signs: carpopedal spasm with constriction of the upper arm musculature as with a tourniquet; twitching of the facial muscles in response to a tapping of the VII cranial–the facial–nerve at the angle of the jaw in front of the ear.
      (2) Complaints of numbness or tingling of the extremities.

5. *Assure replacement of chloride as well as potassium* in preventative electrolyte therapy for risk populations, or when metabolic alkalosis is present. Potassium chloride can be given. Small amounts are effective; 100 mEq/L is enough to correct severe metabolic alkalosis (Davidsohn and Henry, 1969).
   a. Call attention to the need for chloride if it is not being given.
   b. If the individual is allowed oral intake and sodium chloride is not contraindicated, provide salty foods to replace chloride by diet. Recall that most of the chloride ingested is absorbed.

6. After treatment for metabolic alkalosis the nurse should *assess for laboratory outcomes indicating success:* for example, serum chloride and potassium increase to within normal limits; venous CO_2 decreases to within normal limits; urine pH becomes acid (i.e., 6).

   Recall, however, that urine pH is not a good indicator of response in hypokalemic metabolic alkalosis. It may be acid even at the height of alkalemia. Response to therapy would be indicated by an initial increase in pH as the bicarbonate begins to be excreted.

7. *Any person at risk for, or diagnosed as in, fluid inbalance* is equally at risk for chloride imbalance. The nursing implications are identical (see "Implications for Nursing" in Section 1.1).

8. *In children a positive serum chloride balance* is particularly important in order to expand the ECF compartment. Therefore, all children should be considered risk populations for chloride imbalance.

9. *Mature adults and the aged* should be considered risk populations because:
   a. Renal response to pH changes is less precise and imbalances occur more rapidly.
   b. Anemia is a frequent accompaniment of age (for many reasons) and thus a major buffering system would be depleted (i.e., the chloride shift of hemoglobin).
   c. Pulmonary function is frequently compromised in the elderly and this will interfere with both carbon dioxide elimination and the ability to maintain adequate oxygen blood levels, which would seriously interfere with respiratory compensation for metabolic alkalosis.

10. *Patient teaching about specific preventative measures* in risk populations is an important and often neglected nursing responsibility. Content, including appropriate electrolyte replacement in conditions causing chloride loss, and assessments the individual can make to check the effectiveness of electrolyte replacement should be covered.

1.3 PLASMA POTASSIUM

Normal Ranges	
Adult	3.5– 5.5 mEq/L
Senior adult	
Male	3.5– 5.6 mEq/L
Female	3.5– 5.2 mEq/L
Pediatric	
Premature (cord)	5.0–10.2 mEq/L
Premature (48 hr)	3.0– 6.0 mEq/L
Newborn (cord)	5.6–12.0 mEq/L
Newborn	5.0– 7.7 mEq/L
Infant	4.1– 5.3 mEq/L
Child	3.5– 4.7 mEq/L
Thereafter	3.4– 5.6 mEq/L

This test measures the concentration of potassium in the plasma. Sampling of plasma rather than serum is recommended by many laboratories because there is a release of potassium during blood clotting and the serum potassium will be falsely elevated. Plasma potassium is more stable and should be used for potassium determinations. Potassium is the major cation of the intracellular fluid (ICF); close to 90% of total body potassium is in the ICF. Potassium plays an essential role in maintenance of excitability of both nerve and muscle tissue. A proper balance among potassium, sodium, and calcium is highly important for all muscular function, but imperative to cardiac muscle function.

Potassium exerts effects on almost all cellular metabolism. In carbohydrate metabolism, decreased potassium causes a decrease in glucose uptake in the liver. In protein metabolism, growth retardation occurs secondary to decreased potassium because there is a potassium-dependent step in protein synthesis. Enzyme reactions of adenosine triphoshate (ATP), coenzyme A, and adenosine diphosphate (ADP) all depend on potassium for part of their activation (Welt and Blythe, 1973).

Potassium must be ingested daily since the body does not store it in any large amounts. Either an increase or a decrease in potassium levels may precipitate physiologic problems.

1.3.1 Hyperkalemia

Hyperkalemia is defined as a plasma level of greater than 5.5 mEq/L. With adequate renal function it is virtually impossible to maintain a state of hyperkalemia because it is so readily excreted by the kidney (Stroot et al., 1977). Significant potassium increase is found primarily in severe renal failure with azotemia (excessive amounts of nitrogenous waste). Increased plasma levels of potassium occur much less frequently than do decreased levels (Sodeman and Sodeman, 1974).

Physiology. There is a constant exchange between extracellular sodium and intracellular potassium. With an increase in extracellular potassium, the membrane potential is decreased and the cell becomes highly excitable. As a result there is increased irritability of all nerve and muscle cells. This is not a steady state and in a short time the cell activity is exhausted, resulting in muscle weakness and flaccid paralysis.

The compensatory mechanism to increased extracellular potassium is increased renal excretion and decreased reabsorption of potassium in the colon, both in response to aldosterone. An increase of extracellular potassium promptly stimulates aldosterone release so that more sodium and less potassium will be reabsorbed by the kidney. The ratio of reabsorption of sodium and potassium is usually 2:1 in favor of sodium (SHMC, 1978).

PLASMA POTASSIUM INCREASED IN:

1. *Any condition causing severe oliguria or anuria,* for example, states of renal failure with azotemia. A not uncommon cause of death in renal failure is potassium intoxication leading to cardiac arrest (Sodeman and Sodeman, 1974). Even with no potassium intake, it is probable that potassium levels will increase secondary to tissue catabolism in renal failure. Congesitve heart failure with decreased cardiac output is a frequent cause of prerenal kidney failure, resulting in oliguria and increased plasma potassium.
2. *Chronic adrenal insufficiency* (Addison's disease) with diminished aldosterone output can lead to increased plasma potassium levels. Untreated adrenal insufficiency is a contra-indication for giving potassium.
3. *In the first 24 hours after severe burns,* hyperkalemia is marked due to the release of large amounts of potassium into the circulation from burned tissue. This situation is reversed in the next stage of the burn injury course, that of diuresis as edema fluid is remobilized into circulation. Crushing injuries increase plasma potassium in much the same way.
4. *Excess administration of potassium,* especially with inadequate urinary output, can lead to hyperkalemia. Excess ingestion may be due to a lack of knowledge on the part of the person taking potassium-containing medications. Too rapid, or excess, intravenous administration of potassium is a fairly frequent cause of increased levels.
5. *A transitory state of hyperkalemia* occurs after strenuous exercise. Potassium leaves the cell with muscle use due to the sodium potassium exchange in cellular contraction. This, plus lactic acidosis, is believed to be the cause of muscular fatigue and pain (Kee, 1978). A similar process may account for the transitory increase of potassium found after convulsions.
6. *Defective potassium secretion due to tubular defects* has been found to occur at times with pyelonephritis (Levinsky, 1973).
7. *Overuse of aldosterone antagonist diuretics* (e.g., spironolactone) can lead to a hyperkalemic state due to increased reabsorption of potassium by the kidney.
8. *False increases in plasma potassium levels* can occur and are related to states of venous stasis due to a combination of tourniquet compression and muscular activity prior to venipuncture (repeated fist clenching to "bring up the veins"). False increases

are also found in patients with thrombocytosis or leukemia. This increase is thought to be due to release of potassium from platelets or white blood cells in the clotting process after the blood is removed from the body.

1.3.2 Hypokalemia

Defined as a plasma level of less than 3.5 mEq/L. Syndromes of potassium deficit are relatively common. If potassium deficiency is sufficiently severe, both functional and actual structural changes occur in the kidney (Sodeman and Sodeman, 1974), perpetuating fluid, electrolyte, and acid-base imbalances.

Physiology. When plasma potassium is depleted, for whatever cause, the resting cell membrane potential is increased. During excitation, potassium should move out of the cell to replace the deficit and sodium inward, to maintain electrolyte balance, depolarizing the membrane. But because of the decrease in extracellular potassium, the resting membrane potential (the ratio between intracellular and extracellular potassium) is increased and the cell is less excitable. Muscular weakness and atony are hallmarks of potassium deficit.

However, even with plasma potassium depletion, the ratio between intracellular and extracellular potassium is not always out of balance, and the classic signs and symptoms may not occur. Slowly developing potassium depletion may allow time for both compartments to experience commensurate drops and the resting potential of the cell membrane would be close to normal (Welt and Blythe, 1973).

Mechanisms to compensate for potassium depletion are not fully known, but suppression of renal tubular cell secretion is thought to occur. This mechanism is less prompt, and certainly less effective than the mechanism for sodium control. In part, this decrease in effectiveness is due to the fact that conditions leading to potassium deficit often stimulate aldosterone secretion, which causes potassium loss (Sodeman and Sodeman, 1974). Even when potassium intake is reduced to nothing, the urine excretion will still be at least 5 to 20 mEq over 24 hours. Therefore, potassium depletion will occur if intake is less than 5 to 20 mEq/day, or when potassium losses occur from extrarenal sources (e.g., excessive loss in feces). Potassium excretion varies with diet, but usually ranges between 26 and 123 mEq/24 hours. The amount would be higher in infants because of the immaturity of the kidney, resulting in decreased reabsorption.

Alkalotic states tend to perpetuate potassium deficits since potassium is excreted in exchange for hydrogen in the kidney and potassium shifts into the cell in exchange for hydrogen.

Periods of stress favor excretion of potassium secondary to the increased secretion of steroids, notably aldosterone and cortisone.

PLASMA POTASSIUM DECREASED IN:

1. *Diarrhea states.* Potassium is normally secreted into the colon in large quantities. The amount of this unbound potassium that will be reabsorbed depends on (a) the rapidity with which it transits the colon, and (b) the amount of aldosterone activity, since the colon is sensitive to steroid hormones in a manner similar to the kidney. A frequent cause of diarrhea in older adults has been laxative abuse. In children the more frequent cause is infection, viral or bacterial.
2. *Large losses of gastrointestinal fluids.* This may be due to prolonged vomiting, gastrointestinal suctioning (primarily intestinal), fistula, or ileostomy drainage.
3. *Massive diuresis or continuous, prolonged diuresis.* Potassium is lost in proportion to the diuresis. Diuresis occurs for a number of reasons:
   a. Administration of diuretics over a prolonged period without adequate follow-up to determine electrolyte levels and/or without adequate electrolyte replacement. This can occur due to lack of knowledge on the part of the patient about the need for potassium replacement in the diet, or lack of follow-through on the part of the health care team.
   b. Glycosuria with concomitant, obligatory loss of water and electrolytes.
   c. The diuretic stage of burns (usually 24 to 48 hr post injury).
   d. The diuretic phase of acute renal failure.
4. *Postoperative patients with multiple losses of potassium.* Potassium deficits can occur secondary to cellular trauma with loss of intracellular potassium (surgical trauma); increased catabolism of cells for nutritional needs due, in part at least, to the NPO state of most surgical patients; gastrointestinal surgery in which patients frequently encounter stress postoperatively; and nasogastric suction, causing alkalosis, which favors potassium loss.
5. *Patients after treatment for diabetic ketoacidosis.* Administration of insulin drives glucose and potassium into the cell. Usually, this has been preceded by a loss of potassium in osmotic diuresis secondary to an increase in EC potassium in exchange for hydrogen at that time.
6. *Stress response.* An increased secretion of steroid hormones is a major part of the stress response. Steroids favor sodium retention

and potassium loss, as discussed previously. Vomiting and diarrhea and/or anorexia can also occur secondary to stress (see Appendix B).

7. *Lack of adequate intake of potassium* (anorexia, lack of potassium-rich foods in the diet, starvation). This can occur as a response to illness or as an effect of inadequate finances. Patients at risk include the unconscious patient.
8. *Endocrine disease,* such as Cushing's syndrome and primary aldosteronism. The increase in corticosteroid production favors potassium loss.
9. *Malabsorption syndromes,* where the gut is not able to absorb nutrients. Malabsorption occurs in cystic fibrosis and adult-onset sprue, as well as many other conditions.
10. *Inappropriate use of enemas.* This is not a frequent cause of potassium loss in recent years, but cannot be overlooked. The use of multiple enemas prior to diagnostic procedures (enemas until clear), particularly in a patient at risk for electrolyte imbalance, could induce rather rapid hypokalemia. Enema fluid, if not returned out of the body, can be absorbed through the bowel wall, thereby diluting the potassium in the interstitial space and ultimately all extracellular fluid. Hypertonic enemas can damage bowel mucosa, leading to an increased potassium loss in feces.

IMPLICATIONS FOR NURSING

1. The nurse can make a most useful contribution to community health by helping to *prevent the occurrence of potassium imbalances,* as many, if not most, are preventable.
2. *Prevent hyperkalemia* by:
   a. Identifying persons at risk (see "Plasma Potassium Increased in").
   b. Preventing false increases by discouraging the "hand pump" method of vein distention for venipuncture. Use warm arm or hand packs instead.
   c. Assuring that patients receiving glucocorticoid therapy (e.g., those with Addison's disease) do not abruptly discontinue the use of drugs.

d. Assuring that persons receiving potassium supplements have plasma levels checked appropriately, perhaps once a month if otherwise stable.
e. Monitoring both potassium and sodium levels in the patient at risk for potassium imbalance.
f. Teaching high-risk patients self-care by:
   (1) Identifying and correcting their lack of knowledge about potassium-rich foods.
   (2) Providing information about the approximate potassium content of such foods.
   (3) Helping the patient and home caretaker to plan the diet, calculating the proper potassium intake so as not to exceed their personal intake limit.
g. Protecting any patient receiving potassium IV from hyperkalemia. Administer slowly, never in undiluted or concentrated form, at no more than 20 mEq/hr, unless by direct, written physician order and, even then, not unless the patient is on a cardiac monitor. Usually, only peripheral lines are used for potassium infusion. If a central line is used, monitoring of administration is particularly important, since there is less opportunity for dilution of the potassium. Plasma potassium levels exceeding 8 mEq/L may cause fatal arrhythmias as they reach the heart (Levinsky, 1973). Slow, or discontinue potassium infusion if redness, swelling, or complaint of burning occurs at the infusion site. Never "speed up" a potassium infusion except by direct written order. Urine output must be at a minimum of 30 ml/hour during 24 hr for potassium administration.
h. Placing any patient at risk for potassium imbalance on strict intake and output.
i. Observing for and preventing metabolic acidosis.

3. *Protect patients with hyperkalemia* by:

   a. Providing monitoring (cardiac) if possible.
   b. Observing for pulse irregularity, slowing (bradycardia).
   c. Observing for ECG changes. The following depicts the progression of changes that may be found in untreated hyperkalemia.
      (1) The amplitude (vertical) of T waves increases with narrowed base and peaking. (Commonly occurs in humans when the plasma K^+ reaches about 7 mEq/L.)
      (2) The amplitude of R and S waves increases.
      (3) Atrioventricular and intraventricular block occurs.

(4) Loss of P waves—atrial arrest at a plasma K+ of about 9 mEq/L.

(5) Depression of the ST segment (obliteration of the segment with the T wave originating from the S).

(6) Spread of QRS and T waves into a smooth biphasic curve (sine wave) [plasma K+ level about 10 mEq/L or above (Sodeman and Sodeman, 1974)].

d. Assessing for ascending muscular weakness which can progress to flaccid quadriplegia.

e. Being alert for complaints of dyspnea (air hunger), signifying respiratory paralysis.

f. Providing fresh blood, if possible, for transfusions. The breakdown of older blood cells releases potassium.

g. Assuring that patients in acute renal failure are adequately and promptly dialyzed. Sudden death occurs frequently in patients with anuria of 1 week's duration, due to potassium intoxication and cardiac arrest (Sodeman and Sodeman, 1974).

h. Teaching the patient/family/home caretaker the purpose of medical treatment to decrease anxiety and increase cooperation and compliance.

(1) The physician may opt to use calcium infusions as rapidly effective therapy in emergency situations where the sine wave has appeared and there is not time to decrease the potassium level. Increased calcium levels antagonize the effects of hyperkalemia on the cardiac membrane. Hypocalcemia intensifies the problem.

(a) This therapy should not be used in patients taking digitalis, since digitalis intoxication can be precipitated with even moderate reduction in serum potassium.

(b) Once begun, the treatment with calcium must be continued until the potassium imbalance has been corrected (Finch, 1972).

(2) IV glucose with insulin is often given as a treatment in moderately severe hyperkalemia that does not warrant calcium. Potassium will shift into the cells with the glucose and insulin, and plasma potassium levels will decrease by as much as 1 to 2 mEq/L. This decrease will persist for several hours. Nondiabetic patients may not require insulin.

(3) Hypertonic sodium, such as in the form of sodium bicarbonate with isotonic saline, is given IV in patients with hyperkalemia to increase renal excretion of potassium and to cause alkalosis, which drives potassium into the cells. Potassium levels will be decreased because of di-

lution as well as the increased renal excretion of potassium. Lactate or bicarbonate may be given if the hyperkalemia exists concurrently with acidosis.

(4) Polystiperne sulfonate (hypertonic kayexalate) can be given by mouth or as a retention enema in the patient unable to take oral fluids. Kayexalate is an exchange resin which removes excess potassium from the blood via the colon in exchange for sodium and hydrogen. The patient will need to be encouraged to retain the enema fluid. Many kits come equipped with a flanged tube, which, when blocked after administration of the enema, helps to retain the solution in the patient who is unable to do so.

(5) Debridement of necrotic tissue, such as after a burn or crushing injury, may be necessary to decrease the amount of potassium being released into the system from the injured and dead cells. Measures to prevent decubiti should be undertaken to prevent necrosis and increased potassium release.

4. *Prevent hypokalemia* by:
   a. Identifying persons at risk (see "Plasma Potassium Decreased in").
   b. Assessing for signs and symptoms of deficit with particular attention to the sequence of occurrence in an attempt to help differentiate from long-term hyperkalemia. Hypokalemia causes the following problems not seen in prolonged hyperkalemia: presence of complaints of muscle pain; hyporeflexia; fairly early nausea and vomiting; paralytic ileus and orthostatic hypotension.
   c. Monitoring intake and output.
   d. Checking plasma potassium levels frequently. If the patient has several risk factors (e.g., on diuretics, has intestinal drainage, is NPO, and without replacement of electrolytes), at least weekly levels should be available. If not, collaborate with physician.
   e. Being aware of potassium available in foods. Teaching of the patient/family/home caretaker in menu planning to include foods high in potassium (see item 2f above).
   f. Checking if salt substitute is made with potassium for a patient who is also on a low-salt diet. If not, check with the physician as to the advisability of change.
   g. Being aware of the availability of potassium-sparing diuretics [spironolactone (Aldactone), triamterene (Dyrenium)] which

can be used in place of, or in conjunction with, thiazide diuretics.

h. Monitoring other electrolyte levels important in the maintenance or assessment of potassium levels: for example, chloride because a decrease in chloride perpetuates potassium deficit; serum sodium because decreased levels foster potassium loss; and urinary potassium to evaluate effectiveness of interventions. Return to normal concentrations of potassium in a 24-hr urine specimen indicates successful treatment.

i. Requesting ounce-for-ounce and mEq-for-mEq replacement for any losses via gastric/intestinal suction.

j. Collaborating with physician and/or x-ray department to find alternatives to multiple enemas prior to diagnostic testing in the patient at risk for hypokalemia, or making sure that serum levels are monitored.

k. Being alert for signs and symptoms of metabolic alkalosis which could cause, or be due to, decreased potassium.

5. *Protect the patient with hypokalemia* by:

a. Observing closely for signs of digitalis intoxication in the hypokalemic patient taking the drug. Even a moderate decrease in potassium levels can enhance the effect of digitalis and precipitate a toxic state.

b. Checking serum digitalis levels if available and assessing for signs and symptoms of digitalis intoxication. These are not unlike symptoms of hypokalemia, so it is necessary to be alert for complaints of vision changes—colored vision—which are symptoms more specific to digitalis intoxication. Pure glycosides are thought to produce fewer of the early gastrointestinal symptoms and thus give less warning of intoxication.

c. Instructing the patient on oral potassium supplements concerning side effects and measures to be taken to alleviate or prevent the side effects. The major side effect is gastric irritation.

(1) Prevention:

(a) With the exception of "controlled-release" preparations, such as slow-K, which should not be dissolved, dilute with cold water or orange juice any potassium, whether liquid, powder, or effervescent tablet. Dissolve completely.

(b) Instruct the patient to sip slowly, and to take the medication either with meals or immediately after meals.

(2) Symptoms to be reported to physician:
  (a) Abdominal pain.
  (b) Nausea, vomiting.
  (c) Distention.
  (d) Evidence of gastrointestinal bleeding (tarry stools, hematemesis).

1.4 SERUM GLUCOSE

Synonyms: blood glucose or sugar; plasma glucose or sugar

*Normal Ranges**

Adult	
Younger than 50	60–110 mg/dL
Older than 50	60–125 mg/dL
Senior adult (fasting)	
Male	52–135 mg/dL
Female	58–135 mg/dL
Pediatric (fasting)	
Premature	20– 60 mg/dL
Newborn	30– 80 mg/dL
Child	60–100 mg/dL

*Normals for tests done on whole blood, as opposed to serum or plasma, will vary, usually being somewhat lower.

Glucose is the principal body fuel, obtained primarily from the diet but can be produced by the body's own metabolism. Sugars other than glucose are usually converted to glucose within the body, as are most carbohydrates that are ingested. Simple sugars such as glucose are used quickly, but other nutrients, such as proteins, when ingested in greater quantity than needed, are gradually converted to glycogen and stored to be used to maintain normal serum glucose level between meals. The maintenance of normal fasting serum levels depends on the interaction of a number of body structures, among them the liver, peripheral tissues, and hormones, all of which act to raise or lower serum glucose levels. Since serum glucose levels generally become abnormal only when there is serious disruption of this interaction, checking the serum glucose level helps evaluate the function and integrity of this system. Two measurements of serum glucose have been found to be most useful as screening tests and will be discussed here. A third, *random glucose measurement,* which is done without any preparation of the individual being tested, has been found to be of little value clinically since the results may vary so widely, depending on the intake or lack of intake of food prior to obtaining the blood sample. The two tests used most frequently, which provide the most information in their results, are the *fasting glucose test* and the *2-hr postprandial* (after meals) [or postcibum (after eating)], usually written as *serum glucose 2-hr p.p. or p.c.*

The *fasting glucose test* roughly evaluates the body's ability to regulate glucose and provides information about the kind of abnormality, if one occurs. No food or drink, other than water, is given for 8 hr prior to taking the blood sample.

The *2-hr p.c. test* is a simple screening test to demonstrate the ability of the body to adjust to, and dispose of, a glucose load. A fasting blood sample is usually drawn first. The person is then given approximately 100 g of glucose by diet, or in a solution, and a second blood sample is drawn exactly 2 hr later. If both values are within the normal limits, the mechanism is considered normal. If the blood value has not returned to the upper limit of normal in the 2-h p.c. sample, the mechanism is considered abnormal and further testing may be necessary to identify the precise nature of the problem. Some authorities feel that the use of an intravenous glucose load is more accurate than oral administration and that indications for the oral test are few (Scipien et al., 1975).

1.4.1 Hyperglycemia

Hyperglycemia is defined simply as an excess of glucose in the blood above the upper range of normal for a given age. Although increases in fasting serum glucose are most frequently related to the presence of diabetes mellitus, the number of diseases and physiological conditions that can result in major increases is vast and the nurse should be alert to the need to assess for cause. Also it is well for the nurse to be aware that whereas a normal fasting blood glucose level rules out an active and acute diabetic problem, it does not rule out the diagnosis of diabetes mellitus. Only 30 to 40% of diabetics can be diagnosed by a fasting serum glucose. The 2-hour p.c. test is an excellent screening test for diabetes, however, with levels above 160 mg/dL usually being considered diagnostic. (A new test, the glycosylated hemoglobin level, may ultimately replace the 2-hr p.c. glucose as the most useful screening test. See Section 8.3.)

Physiology. Serum glucose is maintained by several different processes in the body. Absorption of all sugars from the small intestine is rapid, with glucose being immediately available in the bloodstream. The liver is extremely important in the control of blood sugar levels. It synthesizes glucose to glycogen and fat when uptake is excessive (glycogenesis), or, when the supply is low, the liver can convert the glycogen to glucose (glycogenolysis) as well as synthesizing glucose from some of the amino acids or from the glycerol of fat breakdown (gluconeogenesis).

It also converts other forms of sugar to glucose, as does the intestine. Glucose is preferred to fat or protein for energy supply, but when insulin is insufficient, fat is mobilized. The action of liver regulation is influenced by several hormones, including, and primarily, insulin. These are thyroid, adrenocortical hormones (glucocorticoids in particular), epinephrine, and glucagon. Glucagon's role is not clearly understood, but is vital. To be properly utilized, glucose must enter the cell, and for this, insulin is required. Normally, very little glucose is excreted in the urine, usually a maximum of 0.5 to 0.75 g over 24 hr. If serum glucose exceeds 170 mg/dL, the level of the renal threshold for glucose, excretion increases. Table 1.2 gives a brief overview of the roles played by hormones in glucose regulation. All of these roles can be triggered by physiologic activities such as exercise or nervous excitement.

TABLE 1.2 *Roles of hormones in glucose regulation*

Hormone	Action	Result
Insulin	Facilitates transfer of glucose across cell membrane for all cells except brain cells	Decreases blood glucose
Thyroid[a]	Stimulates intestinal and renal absorption of glucose	Increases blood glucose
	Increases metabolic rate, thus increasing utilization of glucose in the periphery	Decreases blood glucose
Glucocorticoids	Mobilize protein and fat stores and influence hepatic gluconeogenesis;	Increase blood glucose
	thought to decrease the cell's ability to utilize glucose	Increase blood glucose
Epinephrine	Influences conversion of glycogen to glucose in both liver and muscle (glycogenolysis); blocks insulin release	Increases blood glucose
	Increases glucose uptake in tissue cells	Decreases blood glucose
Glucagon	Promotes conversion of glycogen to glucose in the liver	Increases blood glucose
Growth hormone	Believed to reduce the rate of glucose utilization in the cells	Increases blood glucose
	May also increase insulin resistance of cells and lead to destruction of beta cells of the pancreas (this mechanism is not well understood)	Increases blood glucose

[a]The two responses given are dependent on the concentration of hormone in the serum.
Source: Data from Carnevali and Patrick, 1979; Collins, 1975; and Sabiston, 1977.

SERUM GLUCOSE INCREASED IN:

1. *Stress response* due to acute trauma, anoxia, hypoglycemia, severe exercise, hemorrhage, severe pain, emotional excitement, or exposure to extreme heat or cold. In the first few hours of stress response liver glycogen is broken down to glucose, which is released to the blood and raises serum glucose concentration. The rate of glucose production is usually increased and hyperglycemia results. With continued stress, and in the absence of adequate intake of glucose to meet metabolic needs, fat is mobilized from depot stores by hydrolysis to free fatty acids (FFAs) and glycerol. Finally protein is oxidized when glycogen stores are depleted. The rise in serum glucose is unaccompanied by an appropriate rise in insulin, probably related to the concomitant rise in epinephrine production in response to stress (Sabiston, 1977), which maintains the hyperglycemia. Increased serum glucose secondary to stress can be seen in myocardial infarct, cerebral infarct, some malignancies, gestational diabetics (carbohydrate metabolism would be normal between pregnancies; the increase in glucose during pregnancies may be totally stress related), following acute injury and fright as in automobile accidents, and with surgery. Levels as high as 400 mg/dL have been found in some individuals during anesthesia despite normal carbohydrate metabolism (SHMC, 1978); see Appendix B.
2. *Cushing's disease,* or any condition that will increase glucocorticoid secretion, due to increased gluconeogenesis and decreased peripheral utilization of glucose. All the 11-oxygenated adrenocortical hormones act in a manner directly opposite to that of insulin.
3. *Diabetes mellitus,* usually due to lack of insulin, but can be due to a lack of effective insulin (insulin resistance). Fasting blood sugars over 150 mg/dL are highly suggestive of diabetes mellitus. Levels found in diabetic ketoacidosis/coma are usually between 400 and 800 mg/dL. If the values are higher than 800 mg/dL, it is suggestive of concomitant renal failure (SHMC, 1978).
4. *Acromegaly,* due to insulin resistance and decreased cellular utilization of glucose. Usually, both the fasting and the 2-hr p.c. values are increased.
5. *Hyperthyroidism,* due to increased absorption of glucose and other carbohydrates from the gut. Peripheral utilization of glucose is increased, leading in a normal serum glucose in some individuals, but the 2-hr p.c. test will be increased (see Table 1.2).

6. *Pheochromocytoma,* due to the increased secretion of epinephrine in which insulin release may be blocked and glucogenolysis increased. Again the fasting value of glucose may be normal, but the 2-hr p.c. test will be elevated.
7. *Chronic pancreatitis,* an unusual finding, however, due to a reduction in insulin production secondary to destruction of the islet cells of the pancreas. There may also be a slight decrease in glucose uptake in the liver and decreased cellular utilization.
8. *Administration of some drugs* (e.g., the chlorothiazide diuretics), due to suppression of insulin release—mechanism unknown—and dilantin, due to a membrane-stabilizing effect on the pancreas, inhibiting effective insulin release (Govoni and Hayes, 1978).
9. *Postsurgical patients,* temporarily, due in part to the hyperglycemic properties of the stress response (see item 1 above), but frequently due more directly to the intravenous infusion of dextrose, which is often run rapidly in an attempt to replace lost fluid volume and depleted stores of glucose, causing a slight, temporary increase in serum concentrations.
10. *Nonketotic, hyperosmolar coma,* which usually occurs in the insulin-dependent diabetic due to inadequate insulin secretion for peripheral utilization of glucose, but with adequate secretion to prevent fat breakdown. Serum glucose can reach levels as high as 1000 mg/dL with minimal or negative ketones. This condition is usually triggered by body water loss. Marked hypernatremia is a helpful diagnostic sign (Blevins, 1979).

1.4.2 Hypoglycemia

Hypoglycemia is a disorder characterized by a serum glucose below the lower range of normal for the age group—less than 46 mg/dL (previously 60 mg/dL) in the adult. Symptomatic hypoglycemia usually does not occur until the serum glucose level is 50 mg/dL or lower, or when the serum glucose level drops rapidly. Documented, significant hypoglycemia is distinctly uncommon except in certain select patient populations. In many instances there seems to be no demonstrable cause for the deficit. The serum sugar falls after eating (reactive hypoglycemia), and may do so several hours after a meal or following exercise. Hypoglycemia may also be symptomatic of a variety of disorders. Newborns frequently show a low serum glucose, which may be asymptomatic unless extremely low. Infants are especially susceptible to hypoglycemia because of their extremely high metabolic rate. Newborns who are not fed by mouth during the first few hours of life are at particular risk. Hypoglycemia also occurs in more than half of the newborns of diabetic mothers and is a frequent cause of seizures in the infant, as are elevated temperature and hypocalcemia. The frequency of its occurrence increases with premature infants or below-birthweight infants. The stressed infant is also at risk (sepsis, respiratory distress syndrome) (Scipien, et al., 1975). However, the largest population of persons with hypoglycemia are those with no demonstrable cause, so-called "functional" hypoglycemia (Burke, 1979).

As can be seen by reviewing the physiology of regulation of serum glucose concentrations, the mechanisms tend to foster increases of serum glucose.

Physiology. Symptoms of acute hypoglycemia reflect the widespread response in the body as the sympathetic nervous system is activated. Glycogenolysis is stimulated by low serum glucose concentration as a compensatory mechanism, influenced by epinephrine. When the hypoglycemia is corrected and serum glucose levels rise to the upper range of normal, secretin is released, which, in turn, stimulates the islet cells of the pancreas to increased insulin production and the liver output of glucose is inhibited. Again, the carefully integrated mechanism, discussed previously, for control of serum glucose concentration is totally involved. If there is pathology of any of the mechanism's areas, imbalance will occur.

Whereas glucose is added to the blood from only three sources (intestinal absorption, glycogenolysis, and gluconeogenesis), it is removed from the blood in innumerable ways, all the reductions being essential to the function of the part and the body as a whole. Only when glucose is stored as adipose tissue or lost in the urine is its removal not essential to body function. Levels of urine glucose are usually not indicative of hypoglycemia. The amount found in urine does not correspond in any ratio to the serum level of glucose.

In summary, hypoglycemia occurs in response to both the lack of food and to the ingestion of it, particularly ingestion of high-carbohydrate meals (Sodeman and Sodeman, 1974).

SERUM GLUCOSE DECREASED IN:

1. *Liver disease,* due to impaired gluconeogenesis and depleted glycogen stores in advanced liver disease. "Hypoglycemia occurs so frequently it should be the first problem suspected when a

patient with liver disease becomes confused" (Sodeman and Sodeman, 1968).

2. *Islet cell adenoma,* due to excessive and unregulated insulin release. Islet cell hyperplasia, carcinoma, and retroperitonal sarcoma can also be the source of increased production of insulin.
3. *Addison's disease,* due to impaired gluconeogenesis, or panhypopituitarism due to decreased glucocorticoid production and decreased intestinal absorption. In panhypopituitarism (anterior pituitary insufficiency) hypothyroidism probably adds to the problem, as may the decrease or absence of growth hormone.
4. *Malnutrition,* due to decreased intake, leading to depletion of the liver stores of glycogen.
5. *Postgastrectomy,* due to rapid passage of glucose to the intestine, sharply increasing insulin production and rapid depletion of the serum glucose (tachyalimentation of glucose).
6. *Subclinical diabetes mellitus* (prediabetes), due to a delayed but excessive insulin secretory response to carbohydrate intake. Hypoglycemia occurs 3 to 5 hr after eating.
7. *Excessive administration of insulin in a diabetic patient,* due to improper insulin regimen, dietary omission, or excessive physical activity (insulin reaction).
8. *Functional, or spontaneous hypoglycemia,* with the cause or mechanism unknown.
9. *Alcohol intake in fasting state:*
   a. In prediabetic individuals due to impairment of gluconeogenesis-depleted glycogen.
   b. In individuals with inadequate liver function (e.g., cirrhosis).
10. Rare instances by the *intake of certain commonly prescribed drugs,* other than known hypoglycemic drugs taken for that purpose, [e.g., salicylates, haloperidol (Haldol), propoxyphene (Darvon)] (Jones, 1978).
11. *Infants born to diabetic mothers,* probably due to maternal hyperinsulism and/or maternal hyperglycemia. As mentioned before, the incidence of hypoglycemia is increased in premature, or low-birthweight infants, and is not an uncommon finding in any stressed infant due to rapid depletion of glucose stores.

12. *Sudden removal of intravenous glucose in an infant,* due to increased levels of insulin secreted in response to the available glucose.
13. *Leucine sensitivity,* which is more common in infants than adults. It produces signs and symptoms of hypoglycemia shortly after a high-protein feeding. The hypoglycemic response also occurs on fasting. The cause of the fasting hypoglycemia is not known, but is possibly due to an accumulation of endogenous leucine. The initial hypoglycemia due to this sensitivity occurs early in the first year of life (Faulkner et al., 1968).
14. *Lowered renal threshold maximums* (TMs) for glucose.

IMPLICATIONS FOR NURSING

1. *Patient preparation* for the test:
   a. NPO except for water for 8 hr prior to the test.
   b. Insulin should be withheld for any diabetic having blood drawn for glucose determinations. Give insulin promptly after blood is taken and assure that food is given within 2 hr thereafter.
2. *Identify individuals at risk* for glucose imbalance. The extremes of age, the very young and the very old, are always a high-risk group if only because of a lack of an intact system for integrating blood glucose regulation.
3. *Protect the patient at risk* by:
   a. Knowing and assessing for early signs and symptoms of glucose imbalance in persons at risk. Recall that onset is more rapid in infants and children and profound changes can occur with great speed; therefore, *frequent* observations are necessary.
      (1) Hypoglycemia–signs and symptoms. The sequence given is typical, but the pattern varies.
         (a) Mild/early: hunger, tremor, perspiration, weakness, blurred vision, impaired mentation, headaches, feelings of anxiety.
         (b) Moderate: mental confusion, neuromuscular function impairment–staggering gait, irrational, hostile behavior (often misinterpreted as drunkenness).

(c) Profound: coma, epileptoid seizures. Permanent brain damage or death will occur if untreated.

(d) Mental retardation in the infant or young child. In the infant signs and symptoms are similar to that of seizure activity (e.g., jittery, listless, yet hyperirritable and restless).

(2) Hyperglycemia—signs and symptoms

(a) Mild: increased thirst, increased intake of fluids, increased appetite, polyuria, loss of weight due to catabolism of muscle cells and loss of body fluid, decrease in muscle mass, fatigue.

(b) Precoma: drowsiness, dryness of skin, increased rate of respiration, nausea, vomiting, abdominal pain, acetone breath (may occur now or later).

(c) Coma: Kussmaul breathing, weak thready pulse, decreased temperature (unless increased due to dehydration) and blood pressure, loss of consciousness.

b. Awareness of factors that vary the need for glucose and the need for or utilization of insulin in those persons at risk for glucose imbalances (e.g., changes in diet, amount of exercise, presence of infection, other stressors) (see Appendix B).

c. Placing all persons at risk for blood glucose imbalance on strict intake and output recording.

d. With sudden onset of coma, especially in the known adult diabetic, assessing for signs, symptoms, and history of both hyper- and hypoglycemia, but also bearing in mind the possibility of nonketotic hyperosmolar coma. Risk group for this pathology is usually the diabetic with insulin-dependent diabetes, in the upper age group, with some cardiovascular or renal complications, and a recent history of acute infection or other acute stress. Obtain as detailed a record of the individual's intake and output of fluids as possible. It is well to be aware that ketoacidosis, hyperosmolar coma, and lactic acidosis *can* occur together. Most frequently, one of these conditions progresses to another if untreated (MacBryde and Blacklow, 1970).

e. Acquiring accurate knowledge of the possible and planned medical treatment to provide anticipatory teaching for the patient and family; to help reinforce any teaching done by the physician; and to assure decreased anxiety as well as knowledgeable compliance with the medical plan of care by the family and patient.

4. *Prevent hyperglycemia* by:
   a. Adequate and knowledgeable urine testing and recording to provide baseline data about glycosuria and ketonuria. Significant hyperglycemia must be present to produce glycosuria in most cases (see "Physiology" in Section 1.4.1). Urinary threshold maximums (TMs) vary with people and glucosuria is not a true indicator of serum levels. Therefore, compare urine findings with serum glucose level.
      (1) Research types of testing materials available and those being used. It is important to know what a given method actually tests for and what false positives or negatives are possible.
      (2) Follow directions exactly as provided with the test being used. Always use the color scale that is provided with the test being used.
      (3) Some controversy surrounds the need to use only second voidings (double-voided specimen) for urine testing, but such a procedure is followed in many places in expectation of more accurate results. The presence of acetone with sugar may indicate impending diabetic ketoacidosis; check for adequate food intake and acetone odor of urine. If present, inform physician of the appearance of ketones.
   b. Giving insulin or oral hypoglycemic medication as prescribed, carefully noting and reporting response.
   c. Storing medication properly between use to help maintain its effectiveness.
   d. Applying a sound knowledge base concerning dietary needs in helping the patient select a diet he or she can live with, thereby increasing the probability of compliance to the dietary plan.
   e. Using testing agents other than Clinitest for pregnant women, nursing mothers, or patients taking large doses of ascorbic acid. Clinitest reacts to lactose as well as glucose and these populations tend to spill lactose. Use of the cephalosporin antibiotics (Keflin, Keflex) will also produce false positives for urine glucose when tested by Clinitest. Ingestion of large doses of aspirin has the same effect.
   f. Teaching the patient and home caretaker all of the foregoing precautions, providing a rationale, and also including necessary information about weight reduction, when indicated. The signs and symptoms of imbalance must also be taught and the steps that should be taken immediately upon the occurrence of an imbalance. The diabetic also needs to be made aware of the possibility of sugar content in items other than food,

such as medications. Teaching must be tailored to the level of the learner and his or her ability to learn. Techniques can be adapted for many physical and mental deficits so that self-care is possible and error-free. Special materials are available for people with vision problems, for instance. The reader is referred to the many excellent resources available for preparation in teaching diabetics.

5. *Assess hyperglycemia and prevent complications* by:
   a. Notifying the physician at first indication of hyperglycemia so that adequate insulin and glucose coverage can be instituted and an adequate number of serum glucose determinations made.
   b. Observing for any changes in level of consciousness.
   c. With increases in insulin dosage, observing for signs and symptoms of hypoglycemia.
   d. Checking plasma potassium levels in any patient with hyperglycemia, or after administering large doses of insulin. Since the cells cannot utilize glucose without insulin, cellular catabolism occurs and potassium is released from the cell to be excreted in the urine. Excessive amounts may be excreted because, in the presence of increased serum glucose, there is an accompanying increase in serum osmolality and an osmotic diuresis and hypokalemia result. It is important to recall that total body potassium is not always reflected in the plasma levels, however, so it is necessary to assess for signs and symptoms of potassium deficit as well. Hypokalemia can also occur following administration of large doses of insulin, due to K^+ entering the cells.
   e. Checking the urine for glucose and acetone at least four times during the day. The presence of acetone without glycosuria is usually indicative of inadequate food intake, primarily of carbohydrates.
   f. With an increase in blood glucose, or with a repeated pattern of glucosuria in the first urine check of the day prior to administration of insulin, in the face of previous increases in dosage to rectify the problem, checking the serum CO_2 content if available (or any *venous* CO_2 measurement; decrease in venous CO_2 usually indicates a metabolic, acidotic state, as it is a measure of the bicarbonate reserves of the body). If the venous CO_2 remains within normal limits, the cause of the glycosuria may be an actual overdosage of insulin rather than a lack of insulin. The condition is called the *Somogyi reaction.* This reaction is a fairly common occurrence in teenagers (Price and Wilson, 1977) and, unfortunately, not

that uncommon in adults. A nurse aware of this possibility will apply a high index of suspicion in assessing the "hard to control" or "brittle" diabetic. Taking a thorough history will help identify the presence of the reaction. Provide an adequate care plan that will document data necessary for identification. (See also Appendix G.)

6. *Prevent hypoglycemia* by:
   a. Being especially alert for signs and symptoms of the condition in all infants, especially newborn, premature, and low-birth-weight children.
   b. Acquainting yourself with the expected time of peak effect of the type of insulin in use for diabetic patients and observe carefully at that time for any signs or symptoms of hypoglycemia.
   c. Providing distribution of food throughout the day.
      (1) Provide to coincide with the peak effect of the hypoglycemia agents; frequently the third hour after meals is a critical time.
      (2) Provide frequent, low-carbohydrate, small, high-protein meals, regularly spaced throughout the waking hours.
      (3) Plan with physician, dietician, and patient to have simple sugar food immediately on hand for use with early signs and symptoms of hypoglycemia. Hard candies, orange juice, lump sugar, or a candy bar are all good possibilities. A candy bar with nuts is preferable, as this will not only supply the quick glucose needed, but will also provide some protein to help maintain increased glucose levels.
      (4) Be alert for hypoglycemia in the risk population in the early morning hours, as it typically occurs after an 8- or 9-hr fast.
   d. Noting early evidence of confusion which might be due to hypoglycemia in patients with liver disease. To differentiate from other possible causes of confusion, it is helpful to keep records of dietary intake on these patients.
   e. Observing the patient at risk for hypoglycemia during sleep, checking for restlessness and diaphoresis, which can indicate serum glucose deficit.
   f. Teaching patient and family the purpose for and administration of glucagon for emergency use in case of hypoglycemia if it has been ordered for the patient.
   g. Seeking alternatives to prolonged periods NPO for individuals at risk for hypoglycemia. Discuss with physician and/or laboratory personnel.

7. *Treat hypoglycemia reactions* by:
   a. Taking seizure precautions for individuals with confirmed hypoglycemia, or with fragile compensatory responses to changes in serum glucose levels. This is especially pertinent in the care of infants.
   b. Keeping a record of the time of day the hypoglycemia reaction occurs. This can help provide clues to the underlying cause if unknown.
   c. Getting a history of nutritional intake prior to attack to help identify precipitants.
   d. Providing high-carbohydrate foods with or without a direct order from the physician as soon as hypoglycemia has been validated. Follow through after the attack, collaborating with other members of the health team to prevent yet another reactive hypoglycemic episode secondary to the high-carbohydrate intake given to treat the original episode. Glucose is rapidly assimilated and, in individuals capable of producing their own insulin, insulin production will increase. In the person not able to produce insulin, the glucose may well not use up all the available insulin, causing a second drop in serum glucose concentration when the glucose is assimilated. Providing high protein with adequate carbohydrate foods will accomplish some control.
   e. If the individual is unconscious, administering glucagon subcutaneously or intramuscularly if available. If not available immediately, contact a physician and request a stat order for the drug. It is possible to provide some immediate glucose to the unconscious person if a high-carbohydrate substance, such as a sugar cube, is placed in the buccal cavity. Absorption is fairly rapid in this area. However, this should only be done if there is no possibility of the individual aspirating. Usually, the glucagon dose can be repeated once or twice if the original dose was not adequate. The person should awaken in 10 to 20 min after receiving the glucagon. If not, repeat the dose.
   f. Starting an IV at the TKO (to keep open) rate if the patient is unconscious or at risk of unconsciousness. Also, prepare and have ready for administration 1 L of intravenous glucose, 5% in water, or saline, depending on the problems other than glucose concentration that the patient is facing.
   g. Providing oral carbohydrate intake as soon as the patient awakens.
   h. If residual signs and symptoms persist, reassuring the patient and family that it is not unusual to continue to feel weak,

have a headache, or be nauseated. At the same time, take what measures are available to diminish such discomforts. Since the patient will be weak and may be confused, it is imperative to provide for his safety.

8. *Protect patients in any imbalance by providing a safe environment.* Some decrease in mentation or alertness accompanies both hypo- and hyperglycemia, and visual disturbances are a frequent accompaniment. Persons with hyperglycemia are also poor risks in dealing with infections. Hypoglycemia states foster accidents due to weakness or dizziness.

1.5 SERUM CREATININE

Synonyms: blood creatinine; plasma creatinine

Normal Ranges

Adult	0.7-1.5 mg/dL
Senior adult	0.6-1.2 mg/dL Within lower range of adult normals
Children	Less than 1 mg/dL 0.3-1.1 mg/dL

Creatinine is the least variable of the nonprotein nitrogen substances in the serum. It is an end product of muscle metabolism which is liberated from the muscle and excreted in the urine at a virtually constant rate. Therefore, the serum level is also constant in the healthy person. Of all the nonprotein nitrogenous substances, only creatine—which is the precursor of creatinine—is used by the body. It is stored for energy in muscle metabolism.

Creatinine is correlated with changes in the serum urea nitrogen (BUN) for diagnostic purposes but is more accurate as an index of the glomerular filtration rate (GFR) because it is produced in amounts related to muscle mass, which changes very little while the BUN rises in response to many factors (see Section 1.6). It is, therefore, used as an indicator with known renal disease or in those instances where the cause of an elevated BUN is uncertain.

Creatinine is a relatively unstable compound, especially in urine, and prevention of some destruction is accomplished in the laboratory by freezing separated serum, or urine. Clinical use of serum creatinine measurement has increased with the introduction of automated, and therefore rapid, methods.

Physiology. Creatine, an amino acid of nonprotein base, is an ingredient of muscle tissue formed through the action of creatine phosphokinase (CPK) when energy is needed for metabolic processes. When used for energy, it forms the inactive metabolic creatinine. This is liberated from the muscles into the blood at a constant rate. Higher levels are produced in males than in females because of their greater muscle mass. The glomerulus of the kidney filters the creatinine, and it is not reabsorbed by the tubules. Thus the rate of excretion in the urine is also constant. Blood levels appear to fluctuate even less than do urinary levels, perhaps due to the ability of the tubules to secrete creatinine in the presence of increased serum levels (Price and Wilson, 1978). Creatinine is excreted unchanged in the urine, as it is little modified in its passage through the nephron. It is more readily excreted by the kidneys than is urea or uric acid.

SERUM CREATININE DECREASED IN:

1. *Any severe muscle wasting process,* such as muscular dystrophy, due to a reduction in the total body muscle mass and, hence, the amount of creatine converted to creatinine each day. Decreases may be found in myasthenia gravis as well, for much the same reasons.
2. *Thyrotoxic states,* at times, apparently due to the effect of excess thyroxin on creatine phosphokinase (CPK) activity. There is a concomitant increase in serum and urinary creatine levels, which is not metabolized, thus decreasing serum creatinine. Not all authorities agree wtih this effect, however, feeling that thyroxin levels have no effect on serum creatinine (Silver et al., 1969).
3. *Some methods of testing,* with false decreases in levels, related to an elevated bilirubin which interferes with the test (ACA).

SERUM CREATININE INCREASED IN:

1. *Chronic renal insufficiency* (uremia) secondary to chronic glomerulonephritis, diabetic nephrosis, polycystic kidney, nephrosclerosis, chronic pyelonephritis, and gout, to name a few, due to the inability of the kidneys to excrete creatinine. Serum creatinine may be normal in some cases of *acute* uremia or *mild* chronic renal disease. An elevated serum creatinine indicates severe, long-standing renal impairment. An increase of over 4 to 5 mg/dL is evidence of marked impairment. Chronic nephritis with uremia can produce levels as high as 20 to 30 mg/dL (SHMC, 1978).
2. *Obstructive uropathy of long standing,* which can occur in prostatic hypertrophy, bilateral ureteral stricture, and renal calculi-

bilateral, due to the compromise of free urine flow and the GFR. Renal clearance is depressed.

3. *Chronic decreases in glomerular filtration rate,* due to prerenal causes, as seen in chronic congestive heart failure.
4. *False values reported in some methods of testing* (ACA), which produce secondary interference from hemoglobin and lipemia (SHMC, 1978).
5. *Some people with remarkably enlarged muscle mass,* which produces increased amounts of creatinine. The elevation is usually slight.
6. *Some instances of acromegaly,* due to an increased muscle mass. Again, the serum value will show only slightly increased levels.
7. *Diabetic ketoacidosis,* due to a false elevated reading caused by the increase of ketones in the serum (Ring, 1969).
8. *Rejection of kidney transplant,* due to decreasing filtration of waste products by the failing kidney. In such cases serial determination of the serum creatinine may be the more sensitive indicator of renal function (Harrington and Brener, 1973).

IMPLICATIONS FOR NURSING

1. There is usually *no patient preparation necessary* for testing serum creatinine. It is preferable, however, but not required, that the person be without food and drink, other than water, for 8 hr prior to having the blood sample drawn.
2. The nurse can be instrumental in *the prevention of some types of damage to the renal system* and thereby help prevent renal insufficiency characterized by increased creatinine levels in the serum. Identifying the population at particular risk (prolonged bed rest coupled with decreased self movement, individuals with diabetes mellitus, individuals with lupus erythematosus and other collagen disorders, or those with a history of urinary tract infections to list a few only) is important. Providing adequate fluid intake (minimum of 30 to 50 mL/hr for 24 hr) and maintaining an acid urine help prevent stone formation in the urine with the probable superimposed infection. Meticulous technique in dealing with urinary catheterization is imperative.
3. *Prevention of renal impairment* is part of the nurse's responsibilities *when giving nephrotoxic drugs.* Thorough knowledge of the side

effects of drugs to be administered is the minimal acceptable base for patient care. Observe for increases in the serum creatinine level and in the BUN when these drugs are being given. Any person with a history of renal impairment, regardless of present level of renal function, should be safeguarded particularly diligently and alternate nonnephrotoxic medication substituted when at all possible. Collaborate with the physician. (A few drugs found to be highly nephrotoxic yet quite frequently used include Gentamycin, the cephelothins as a group, Colchicine, and Kanamycin.)

4. *The patient in early renal failure* with only slight, if any, increases in creatinine levels has a decreased ability to concentrate urine. Note changes in urine concentration by doing daily specific gravity determinations on patients at risk for, or in, early renal failure. As it advances, the specific gravity tends toward 1.010—isothenuria. Observe these individuals for nocturia, polyuria, and polydipsia. Note changes in urine color.

5. *With increased serum creatinine levels,* bearing in mind that this measurement is considered the most specific test of renal function, all other parameters of renal function should be assessed. All parameters should be looked at for interrelationships so as to validate the finding of the elevated creatinine and to begin the task of preventing complications. Other parameters include:
   a. Strict intake and output recording.
   b. Daily weights, same time, same clothing.
   c. Observations of blood pressure—sitting and lying—pulse, and neck vein distention for potential fluid overload or deficit.
   d. Serial assessments for fluid retention in edema—periorbital and pulmonary.

6. *Monitor BUN levels and compare with creatinine levels.* The BUN rises and falls more rapidly than does the creatinine level. One could expect the BUN increase to precede serum creatinine rise in early failure. If there is no increase in the creatinine levels, other possibilities should be explored to explain the elevated BUN (see Section 1.6).

7. *Check red blood cell count and the other blood indices.* Almost all persons with chronic renal failure (indicated by an increased serum creatinine) become anemic.

8. *Observe for easy bruising or oozing from mucous membrane.* This is more likely to occur in the individual who has advanced renal insufficiency such as uremia. Provide for protection from injury. Shoes while up and about to prevent slipping; oral medi-

cations whenever possible and the use of the smallest possible gauge needle for injections when they cannot be avoided. (See Section 3.12 or "Implications for Nursing" in Section 2.3.2 for more precise suggestions.)

9. *Prevent infection by all means available* that are consistent with the person's individual needs when serum creatinine levels are increased. The person with uremia is particularly susceptible to infection, and infection is difficult to treat because of the altered antibiotic metabolism (Hekelman and Ostendarp, 1979). Infection also tends to increase the severity of the azotemia (presence of urea or other nitrogenous substances in the blood) because of the increase in cellular catabolism. Observe the person with elevated serum creatinine levels for signs and symptoms of infection to include observations other than increased temperature and white blood count. The individual in end-stage renal failure may have a low body temperature in face of an infection or may have an increased white blood count without an infection being present (Harvey et al., 1976).

10. *Observation of the serum creatinine level is imperative for the person who has had a kidney transplant.* If all data suggest a rejection, the nurse should of course report the information immediately and prepare to take whatever isolation precautions are used in the facility housing the patient. Observations that indicate rejection include decreased urine output, increased specific gravity of urine, increased blood levels for BUN and serum creatinine, and the appearance of protein in the urine.

11. *Patients on chronic dialysis* are often dialyzed based on changes in creatinine levels. BUN, because of its more rapid change, is preferable in determining the effectiveness of dialysis. Serum creatinine levels of 8 to 15 mg/dL have been given as an indicator for dialysis in end-stage renal disease. However, such criteria vary depending on the physician and the institution involved.

12. Since elevation of serum creatinine is usually accompanied by an elevation of the BUN, *nursing implications for azotemia apply* (see "Implications for Nursing" in Section 1.6).

13. *Any drug that remains in the plasma in solution* will be filtered at the glomerulus, as is creatinine. Dosage of such drugs is usually modified by the physician in cases of impaired renal function. The nurse should know how drugs given are excreted and should observe the individual for evidence of overdosage and/or prolonged effect if the medication is excreted through the kidney (e.g., penicillin). Extreme caution in administration of drugs is

imperative. If the person will be administering any drug himself or herself, adequate understanding of the possible side effects and what actions to be taken in the face of their occurrence is needed by that person and a responsible family member. Instruction by the nurse must be thorough and well evaluated for adequate learning on the part of the person or family.

14. *Persons with renal insufficiency and increased serum creatinine* require more than usual attention paid to getting adequate rest, balanced with enough exercise to maintain muscle tone and circulation. Increase in physical exercise does not usually increase serum creatinine in the healthy individual, although it may increase BUN due to increased cellular catabolism. However, exercise should be done with caution because of the related problems of elevated BUN causing changes in awareness and judgment and because of the weakness that is associated with anemia.

15. *Since creatinine is produced only within the body,* there are no dietary restrictions related to it. However, the person with renal insufficiency is likely to have some fluid and/or dietary restriction with which the nurse should be conversant in order to provide teaching and to oversee intake.

1.6 SERUM UREA NITROGEN

Synonyms: BUN; blood urea nitrogen

Normal Ranges

Adult	4–22 mg/dL
Senior adult	8–18 mg/dL
Pediatric	Less than 20 mg/dL
Newborn/infant	5–15 mg/dL
Thereafter	10–20 mg/dL

Urea is one of the more abundant nonprotein nitrogen (NPN) constituents in the body. Besides urea, these constituents include creatinine, uric acid, ammonium, and amino acids. At one time all constituents were measured together (NPN), but because testing for individual compounds is fairly simple and yields more precise data, the NPN test has been almost completely replaced by the individual tests.

Urea is the major nitrogenous waste product of protein catabolism and is produced solely in the liver. In the United States urea is commonly measured as urea nitrogen, whereas in Europe the measurement is expressed as urea only. Urea is found in equal concentrations in all body fluids, with the exception of whole blood due to a difference in the percent concentration of serum and erythrocytes. Therefore, serum or plasma is preferred to whole blood for urea nitrogen analysis.

Serum urea nitrogen and serum creatinine are the two most commonly ordered tests of the kidney's ability to excrete metabolic waste. Increases in these values are used, among others, as indicators for the need for dialysis in chronic kidney failure patients. Interpretation of urea nitrogen values requires a knowledge of exogenous protein intake, fluid intake, and conditions which can increase endogenous production (e.g., muscular activity, trauma, infection, strict dieting/fasting/starvation). Any of these variables can cause increased concentrations in blood or urine that are not a true reflection of renal clearance of urea per se.

The two tests can be used, with the foregoing precautions in interpretation, as crude indicators of improvement or deterioration of the individual's kidney function.

Although the urea nitrogen determination is much less specific than is the serum creatinine, it is widely used—particularly in pediatrics, as a screening test for kidney function and as one that tells something of the individual's state of hydration. Lesser degrees of renal impairment require more sophisticated testing, such as clearance tests (Scipien et al., 1975).

Physiology. Urea is produced through a process of protein degradation being transformed from amino acids to ammonia (oxidated deamination), thence to urea (ornithine cycle) within the liver. Since the body does not use urea, it is carried in the blood from the liver until excreted in the urine. Levels vary physiologically depending directly on protein intake in diet (exogeneous), the state of hydration (the ratio of solute to solvent in the body), or indirectly on the rate of tissue catabolism (rapid cellular breakdown causing increased nitrogenous waste), or the rate of tissue anabolism (decrease in levels due to the increased rate of tissue building such as occurs in pregnancy, growth spurts, or convalescence) (Collins, 1975). Urea is excreted in the glomerular filtrate and reabsorbed (probably through diffusion) in the nephron tubule. Only a fraction of all waste material contained in the glomerular filtrate is excreted, but as urea is poorly reabsorbed by the tubules, little urea is reabsorbed, a beneficial effect.

SERUM UREA NITROGEN DECREASED IN:

1. *Little clinical significance* is attached to decreased levels of urea nitrogen, as it is not a necessary substance for body function. Decreased values are seen less frequently than increased values. It

has been suggested that a low urea nitrogen may well be a good prognostic sign, as it indicates good renal function with adequate output (Danovitch et al., 1971).

2. *Any condition with increased secretion of androgen hormones or growth hormones,* probably due to the anabolic effect of these hormones.
3. *Normal pregnancy,* also probably due to the anabolic state of the body.
4. *Severe hepatic insufficiency,* particularly that associated with obstruction of portal vein flow, due to the inability of the liver to convert ammonia to urea. A concomitant rise in blood ammonia would be expected.
5. *Rapid changes in hydration,* such as in:
   a. Rapid rehydration when no nitrogenous compounds have been added to the intravenous solution.
   b. The individual who has been overhydrated and then rapidly diuresed. The decreases in urea nitrogen levels associated with rapid changes in hydration are in themselves temporary and are usually of academic interest only.

Azotemia. Before examining the conditions in which serum urea nitrogen is increased, we need to discuss azotemia—that is, the consistent and marked elevation of nitrogenous products in the blood. Consistent elevations of urea nitrogen levels occur only when the renal function, specifically the glomerular filtration rate, is reduced by 40 to 60%. The GFR can be altered not only by renal disease, but also by prerenal deviation of water (loss of circulating volume for whatever cause), which leads to an increase in urea nitrogen retained. Azotemia occurs generally due to loss of circulating volume, excessive protein catabolism, or impairment of renal function. Interpretation of increases in urea nitrogen depends on knowledge of both renal and extrarenal factors and their relative importance.

SERUM UREA NITROGEN INCREASED IN:

1. *Renal failure,* second stage (renal insufficiency) and third stage (end stage or uremia), due to the inability of the diseased kidneys to excrete urea. Temporary increases of urea nitrogen levels can occur in the first stage of renal failure (decreased renal reserve) if the renal mechanism is stressed. Therefore, increases could be expected in chronic glomerulonephritis, diabetic nephrosis, polycystic kidney, nephroschlerosis, and chronic pyelonephritis, all of which exhibit parenchymal kidney damage of some type.

2. *Dehydration,* due to decreased circulating plasma volume.
3. *Water or saline losses in children,* particularly infants. The urea nitrogen rise is often spectacular due to the infant's proportional increased amount of body water compared to adults.
4. *Starvation,* due to increased protein catabolism and hypoproteinemia. This situation is also seen temporarily in long-term, high fevers.
5. *Bleeding gastric ulcer,* due to increased production of urea from breakdown of blood (protein) dumped into the gastrointestinal tract. There is also an accompanying decrease in circulating volume which may be of more importance than the increase in protein catabolism.
6. *Congestive heart failure,* due to the decreased cardiac output, causing a decrease in renal blood flow and decreased GFR. A serum urea nitrogen is usually determined in general cardiac assessment to learn whether kidney function has been disturbed.
7. *Shock* (hypovolemic, cardiogenic, vasomotor collapse, septic), due to the accompanying decrease in GFR. Adequate kidney perfusion is mandatory for excretion of urea.
8. *Obstructive uropathy,* which usually must be severe and bilateral because of the remarkable reserves available for kidney function. Increased urea nitrogen is due to a decrease in the renal clearance of urea. This occurs in conditions such as prostatic hypertrophy, bilateral ureteral strictures, renal calculi, and arteriosclerosis or thrombosis of the renal vasculature.
9. *Ingestion or inhalation of nephrotoxic drugs,* such as carbon tetrachloride, or heavy metals such as mercury, due to damage of the kidney parenchyma. Since damage to the liver often occurs first, signs and symptoms of liver damage (jaundice) would precede the elevation of the urea nitrogen (MacBryde and Blacklow, 1970).
10. *Thyrotoxicosis,* due to excessive protein catabolism. Increased protein catabolism may also lead to an increase in urea nitrogen in states of uncontrolled diabetes mellitus, adrenocortical hyperfunction, and some neoplastic diseases.
11. *Rejection of kidney transplant,* due to decreasing urine output.
12. *Athletes after extraordinary activity,* due to excessive muscle breakdown.
13. *Intestinal obstruction,* due to loss of plasma volume by "third spacing" of fluids into the gut.

IMPLICATIONS FOR NURSING WITH INCREASED SERUM UREA NITROGEN LEVELS

1. *Patient preparation* for having a blood sample taken for urea nitrogen determination is usually minimal. However, in the person to whom it is particularly important that the test reflect the actual urea nitrogen levels as closely as possible, intake should be restricted to water only for 8 hr prior to taking the blood sample. Most laboratories do not require this restriction, although it is the preferable procedure [see also item 2d(2) below].
2. *The amount of the rise in the BUN* can provide clues as to probable cause, which in turn will assist the nurse in planning care.
   a. In true hypernatremia (increased ratio of salt to water in the ECF) the BUN can be three to four times the normal level.
   b. Hospitalized persons' normal levels are slightly higher than those seen in active "normal" adults, possibly due to an increased catabolic state.
   c. While BUN values can go as high as 400 mg/dL, they usually do not exceed 200 mg/dL, which is the level one would expect in the person with severe kidney disease and with coma or stupor. In any case, levels in excess of 100 mg/dL are usual in severe kidney disease.
   d. With values above 40 mg/dL in the adult, in absence of dehydration, the nurse should initiate the following observations.
      (1) Individuals with increased urea nitrogen levels should have careful records kept of fluid intake and output. This is particularly important in the care of infants and children or those adults with a history of renal dysfunction.
      (2) History of food intake should be taken for the 24 hr prior to the blood test.
      (3) Validate the presence of dehydration as a probable cause of increased serum urea nitrogen by checking the hematocrit level and the urine specific gravity. They will be increased if dehydration due to saline deficit is present. Urine output will also be decreased unless severe diuresis is occurring due to renal disease or the second stage of response to a burn.
3. *Increases in serum urea nitrogen levels* frequently cause lethargy and confusion. Adequate nursing care would include maintaining

safety for the individual (creating a safe environment and preventing injury) by providing supervision over self-care, restriction of activity, and by providing psychological security through reality orientation, realistic reassurance as to the reason for the changes and the possibility of improvement, and by assessing for change in intellectual function. This last can be done by instituting a daily repetition of some intellectual task for which the individual's normal mental ability can be determined (e.g., mathematical problems or riddles that require clarity of thought).

4. *Prevent further increases in urea nitrogen levels* by prevention of avoidable stress, such as infection, great increases in muscular activity, or psychological stresses, whatever they may be, as identified for the individual.

5. *An increase in serum urea nitrogen not due to dehydration* may be treated by a decrease in dietary protein by the physician and, in the absence of the physician, the nurse can do no harm by restricting protein intake until such time as the physician may be consulted.

6. *Persons with high levels of serum urea nitrogen who are undergoing hemodialysis,* particularly for the first time, should be monitored closely for the occurrence of a syndrome known as dialysis disequilibrium. This is demonstrated by the occurrence of nausea, vomiting, mental confusion, hallucination, and/or convulsions about 2 hr after start of dialysis. The responsibility of the nurse is to identify the syndrome correctly and report the fact immediately. Dialysis may be discontinued depending on the standing procedure of the unit involved. (See Appendix C for more information on this syndrome.)

7. *In any person who has had a serum urea nitrogen taken when not in the fasting state* described above, the nurse should obtain and record a history of food and drink intake for the 8-hr period prior to testing.

8. *Check for an increase in serum ammonia levels* in the person with liver disease and increased BUN. This is particularly important when there have been changes in the level of consciousness or mentation. Treatment for hepatic encephalopathy should not be omitted because the mental confusion or decreased level of awareness is thought to be due only to the increased BUN.

9. *Plasma potassium levels should be noted* in the person with known renal dysfunction and an increased BUN. The nurse should also

monitor the individual for signs and symptoms of hyperkalemia (see Section 1.3.1).

10. *Compare BUN with serum creatinine levels* for a more accurate interpretation. A person with a low protein intake may well have a normal BUN even in the face of severe renal impairment. An elevated BUN wiht a normal serum creatinine would indicate probable intestinal bleeding or other increased intake of protein.
11. *Note the RBC for the appearance of anemia.* Increased serum urea nitrogen over 200 mg/dL reduces the life span of red blood cells to about half of normal, and in some patients anemia is also secondary to decreased erythropoietin production.
12. *Observe for signs and symptoms of pericarditis* if serum urea nitrogen remains elevated above 100 mg/dL (Harrington and Brener, 1973).

1.7 SERUM URIC ACID

Synonym: serum urate

Normal Ranges

Adult	
Male	3.9–9.0 mg/dL
Female	2.2–7.7 mg/dL
Senior Adult	
Male	2.9–8.8 mg/dL
Female	2.4–7.2 mg/dL
Pediatric	2.0–5.5 mg/dL
Male: 5 months to 11 years	1.5–7.5 mg/dL
Female: 5 months to 11 years	1.8–7.2 mg/dL
Both: 11½ to 16 years	Elevates sharply to adult levels

Uric acid is another of the nitrogenous waste products found in the blood. It is derived from the breakdown of purines from the nucleic acids of cells and from xanthines. (Xanthines are purine compounds found in most body tissues.) To date, it is the one means of quantifying the nuclear metabolic process. The test is a fairly simple determination that can be used for identification of certain diseases, gout being the primary example, and is helpful in differentiating among several diseases. There are numerous foods that add an exogenous source of purine, and thus uric acid production. Ingestion of those foods tends to influence the amounts of uric acid excreted daily more than the serum levels, given normal kidney function. Normal serum levels tend to increase with age, and normal values are consistently higher in males than in females after the age of 4.

Although it had been thought that the only sources of urate production were those given above, it has been determined that simple compounds in the body, such as carbon dioxide, glycerine, and ammonia, can be synthesized into uric acid and this knowledge has made the dietary treatment of hyperuricemia of less importance (Howard and Herbold, 1978).

Pathologic conditions related to increases or decreases in serum uric acid levels are confined to adults for the most part. Response to myleoproliferative disease, and/or its treatment, and genetic abnormalities are the major causes of increases in children.

Physiology. The normal metabolism of uric acid is not as yet fully determined. The hypothesis which is generally accepted concludes that it is produced from purines through amino metabolism in organs having a high metabolic rate, such as the liver, bone marrow, and possibly muscle (Davidsohn and Henry, 1969). The production from synthesis of simple compounds mentioned previously is even less well understood. Purines that are ingested as complex proteins are degraded in the intestine and absorbed into the blood, where they are carried to the liver and catabolized into the waste product, uric acid. Once formed, uric acid is not catabolized further but joins the "uric acid pool" of the body. Approximately 50 to 75% of this pool is excreted from the body daily. Uric acid is totally filtered and excreted at the glomerulus, then totally reabsorbed in the proximal tubule. The filtrate is then actively secreted in the distal tubule, which is responsible for the total urinary urate. Blood and urine levels vary with purine ingestions as well as protein and caloric intake. A second avenue of excretion is by way of the intestinal lumen. As much as one-third of the total amount of uric acid lost daily is thought to be lost by this route (Harvey et al., 1976).

Pathophysiology of Hyperuricemia (Gout). Excessive accumulation of uric acid occurs in the blood by mechanisms not truly understood. One well-defined pathway is overproduction and destruction of cells causing excessive purine for catabolism to uric acid. A second mechanism, less well defined, is that of a defect in the purine biosynthetic enzyme. A third possibility is a defect in excretion.

Decreased renal excretion has been hypothesized as secondary to a defect in the renal secretion mechanism given above (Groer and Shekleton, 1979), or, when associated with nitrogen retention as well, probably results from decreased renal clearance and tubular secretion, at times secondary to obstructive or suppressive urinary flow problems (Davidsohn and Henry, 1969).

Uric acid crystals do not precipitate until serum levels exceed 6.5 mg/100 mL. The crystals collect largely in the synovial fluid of the joints. A rapid inflammatory process occurs in a matter of hours, with leucocytic phagocytosis of the crystals, followed by a release of lysosomal enzymes which cause injury and inflammation, as well as great pain. Because of this metabolic activity, the synovial fluid can become more acidic, which fosters further urate crystal formation and an extension of the inflammatory process. Urate crystals are deposited in relatively avascular tissues such as tendon and cartilage, as well as the synovial fluid, and in the interstitial tissues of the renal pyramid. With recurrent attacks, additional areas of the body will be included and damaged. Accumulations in tissue, such as cartilage, are called *tophi,* which are hard, translucent swellings that can be noted frequently in the helix of the ear. The presence of increased levels of urate in the urine has a high potential for development of uric stones, particularly in acid urine, which ultimately cause renal damage. Some 10 to 20% of individuals with hyperuricemia develop urate stones–renal calculi (Harvey et al., 1976).

SERUM URIC ACID DECREASED IN:

1. *Conditions that have been treated with specific drugs,* for example:
   a. Large doses (4 to 6 g/24 hr) of salicylates. Salicylates have a paradoxical, dose-related effect on uric acid retention and excretion. Low dosage blocks the distal tubule secretion of uric acid, while high doses block reabsorption from the proximal tubule. Salicylate is one of a number of *urocosuric drugs* with this dose-related response.
   b. Butazolidin (phenylbutazine) and Tandearil (oxyphenibutazone).
   c. Benemid (probenecid).
   d. Zyloprim (allopurinol).
   e. Corticosteroids.
   f. Coumarin compounds.
   g. Anturane (sulfinpyrazone).
2. *Massive hepatic necrosis,* due to the diminished ability of the liver to catabolize purine. Serum levels are greatly depressed.

3. *Fanconi's syndrome* ["a familial, slowly progressive kidney disease with progressive degeneration of the renal parenchyma and metabolic disorders" (Miller and Keane, 1972)], due to the lack of tubular reabsorption of uric acid.
4. *Wilson's disease* (Hepatolenticular degeneration), due to the lack of tubular reabsorption of uric acid.

SERUM URIC ACID INCREASED IN:

1. *Gout,* due to varying causes not fully understood. The primary form is thought to be due to a metabolic defect in purine metabolism, causing increased production of uric acid or a defect in uric acid excretion. Secondary gout occurs in a variety of diseases associated with overproduction and destruction of cells (see "Pathophysiology" above). The total urate pool may be increased from 3 to 25 times normal.
2. *Starvation,* due to the increase in cell turnover (catabolism), coupled with decreased excretion, probably related to the accompanying metabolic acidosis, which favors urate stone formation.
3. *Lesch-Nyhan syndrome,* a congenital form of gout, associated with mental retardation, compulsive self-mutilation, and neurological problems similar to cerebral palsy. First identified in childhood (Frolich, 1976).
4. *High-fat diet and nondiabetic ketosis,* due to depletion of hepatic glucogen, causing gluconeogenesis, which in turn increases the formation of purine breakdown products (Davidsohn and Henry, 1969).
5. *Some instances of renal disease,* such as chronic glomerulonephritis, due to a decreased renal clearance and tubular secretion. A similar picture occurs in other obstructive or suppressive urinary flow problems.
6. *Eclampsia* (toxemia of pregnancy), due to a decreased renal clearance of uric acid, the mechanism of which is not understood. With eclampsia the BUN is within normal limits, which helps in the differential diagnosis among other toxic or inflammatory conditions (Collins, 1975).
7. *Leukemia,* due to increased production and destruction of white blood cells, resulting in an increased rate of turnover of the nucleic acid of those cells, leading to increased purine catabolism.

Increased uric acid levels are also found in polycythemia vera, multiple myeloma, lymphoblastoma, lobar pneumonias, and remission stages of pernicious anemia due to this same augmentation of nuclear catabolism.

8. *Diabetic glomerulosclerosis and some collagen disorders* when renal function has been compromised, leading to a decrease in renal clearance and tubular secretion of uric acid.
9. *Renal hypertension*—when the BUN rises above 25 mg/dL, there is a sharp rise in uric acid.
10. *Psoriasis and sarcoidosis,* as well as other diseases that may cause joint pain and swelling. Uric acid increases in these situations are due to renal retention of uric acid.
11. *Individuals who are on long-term diuretic therapy,* believed to be due to inhibition of tubular secretion of uric acid.
12. *Conditions that have been treated with specific drugs,* for example:
    a. Small doses of salicylate (less than 2 g/24 hr) (see "Serum Uric Acid Decreased in" item 1a).
    b. Thiazide diuretics (see item 11 above).
    c. Diamox (Acetazolamide). Can actually cause an increase or decrease in uric acid secretion. Increase is due in part to its ability to increase the alkalinity of the urine.
    d. Spironolactone (Aldactone).
    e. Methyldopa.

IMPLICATIONS FOR NURSING

1. *Patient preparation* for serum uric acid test includes no food or drink other than water for 8 hr prior to the test. There is no special preparation necessary for testing urine uric acid levels.
2. *With any increase in serum uric acid levels,* gout is suspected and must be ruled out before proceeding with other diagnoses. The nurse should collect significant data to facilitate this process.
    a. A detailed family history for incidence of gout is important because of the strong familial factor in its incidence.
    b. Age. Occurrence is almost nonexistent prior to puberty. Increased incidence is seen in early middle age and on into the fifth decade. Tophi formation can occur earlier, however.

c. Sex. Rare in females, especially before menopause. Tophi formation is also rare in females.

d. Laboratory data. Check indicators of *acute* gout other than increased serum uric acid, which is essential for the diagnosis of gout.

(1) White blood count for leukocytosis.

(2) Erythrocyte sedimentation rate for increase.

(3) Increase in urinary uric acid levels in a 24-hr specimen.

In *chronic* gout the laboratory changes listed above would be present in a variable degree. Not all persons with increased serum uric acid will overexcrete. Indicators to be checked include:

(1) BUN for evidence of increased nitrogenous waste retention, which could indicate inadequate blood flow to the kidney rather than increased uric acid due to gout.

(2) Plasma creatinine for evidence of kidney damage, possibly related to gouty nephropathy, or other cause of renal destruction.

e. Question for a history of "arthritis" symptoms, particularly involving the lower extremities. Check history of/or presence of exquisite pain, usually in a joint, redness, and swelling, all of which are characteristic of gouty arthritis.

f. Check the helix of the ears for the presence of tophaceous deposit.

g. Report increased uric acid levels found in infants and children not having known malignancy or treatment for malignancy. Assess for signs of Lesch-Nyhan syndrome, which includes failure to thrive at about 6 months, and orange urate crystals on the diaper. Although no treatment has been found for the neurological disorders, the extent of renal damage can be reduced by giving allopurinol, which reduces the formation of uric acid (Finch, 1972). This drug is useful in all patients with increased uric acid levels and renal disease. It does not produce its effect in the kidney, as do the uricosuric drugs (Probenecid, Anturane). Rather, it blocks the metabolic pathway of uric acid production (Harvey et al., 1976).

3. *Prevent increased uric acid levels,* and possible occurrence of acute gout, in susceptible individuals by:

a. Preventing the occurrence of precipitants of acute gout or hyperuricemia when logical or feasible. Precipitants include trauma; certain drugs (see "Serum Uric Acid Increased in," item 12); possibly overeating, especially of foods with a high purine content (organ meats, such as liver, heart, kidney; wild game; goose; anchovies; herring; sardines; mackerel; scallops; meat extracts, broth, and gravy), minor or major surgical procedures, ingestion of beer, wine, or ale, sudden weight loss, and high-fat diet (Howard and Herbold, 1978).

b. If not preventable, being sure that the physician is aware of the possibility of hyperuricemia so that Colchicine can be administered prophylactically.

   Usually, a serum uric acid level greater than 9 mg/dL is one of the major indications for beginning a preventative program.

c. Assisting the individual to select an optimum diet. Exclusion of all purine foods is rarely done and rarely satisfactory when done, but elimination of the high-purine-content foods listed above is feasible. A high-carbohydrate diet tends to increase uric acid excretion.

d. Observing for evidence of early prodromal symptoms and signs of an acute attack: diuresis probably due to increased urinary solutes, mood changes possibly due to increased retention of nitrogenous waste, and increased pain or discomfort in affected joints.

e. Teaching affected individual and home caretaker the precautions given above, as well as the necessity of taking maintenance medication exactly when, in amounts, and for as long as directed by the physician. The action of uricosuric drugs is dose dependent (see "Serum Uric Acid Decreased in," item 1a). Colchicine and Allopurinal produce cumulative dosage effect, and Probenecid may be given on a life-long schedule.

4. *Prevent development of complications* due to increased serum uric acid levels, or modify the severity of the complications by:

   a. Observing the response of the individual in an acute gouty attack to the administration of Colchicine, or other gout medications.

      (1) Colchicine relieves the pain due to gout only. It has no effect on pain due to other joint inflammations. The specific pain relief is helpful in establishing a diagnosis, or supporting one.

      (2) Report the lack of pain relief. The drug is usually administered every hour, or 2 hr until pain is relieved or gastrointestinal side effects occur. Pain and swelling should subside within 8 to 12 hr, disappearing in 24 to 72 hr (Govoni and Hayes, 1978).

      (3) By itself Colchicine does not reduce serum urate. It can be given in combination with probenecid (Colbenemid) which has a uricosuric effect (excretion of uric acid in the urine). Given alone Probenecid aggravates acute gout, increasing serum uric acid levels.

(4) Monitor serum uric acid levels. Goal of treatment is 6 mg/dL, preferably less.

b. Keeping accurate intake and output records. Daily output should be from 2000 to 3000 mL/day at a minimum. A high fluid intake helps minimize uric acid precipitation, thereby preventing the formation of urate stones and kidney damage. Excellent hydration is imperative when uricosuric therapy is used. Since gout is a fairly chronic condition with remissions and exacerbations, the affected individual should be taught this process and its rationale. Monitor serum creatinine levels as well as BUN for evidence of renal damage.

c. Testing urine pH with nitrazine paper and teaching the procedure to the affected person and home caretaker. Urate stones form best in acid media, so urine pH of 7.0 (alkaline) is optimal. Urine acidity will increase with onset of an acute attack. The physician may order sodium bicarbonate, sodium citrate, or other medications such as Diamox to help alkalinize the urine. Any indication of heart disease, hypertension, or renal insufficiency should be reported prior to beginning this therapy, as they could be contraindications to the increased sodium intake.

d. Providing alkaline ash foods when not otherwise contraindicated, to assist in urine alkalinization. Although not vital if medication is being given, such intervention can be of use. Alkaline ash foods include most fruits and vegetables, with the *exceptions* of corn, lentils, plums, prunes, and cranberries, which are acid ash.

e. Assuring that acetaminophen (Tylenol) is given in the place of aspirin, particularly when uricosuric medications are in use (Benemid, Anturane), because salicylates nullify the action of these drugs.

   Check urinary uric acid levels, if available, for increase when uricosuric drugs are being given. Twenty-four-hour specimens give the most reliable data. Increase indicates effective drug action.

f. Monitoring serum glucose levels of individuals on oral hypoglycemic agents and on Anturane or Benemid at the same time. These drugs have hypoglycemic qualities which potentiate the antidiabetic medicaton. False-positive Clinitest reactions occur with Benemid as well.

g. Monitoring the complete blood count, hemoglobin, and platelets of individuals on Colchicine and Allopurinol because of the potential for bone marrow depression. If possible, periodic checks during therapy should be evaluated against a baseline determination done prior to initiation of the medication.

h. Monitoring the prothrombin time of persons on oral anticoagulants and Allopurinal for increased levels because of an increase in the half-life of the anticoagulant in the face of Allopurinal administration (Govoni and Hayes, 1978).

1.8 SERUM TOTAL PROTEIN

Synonyms: total protein, T.P.

Normal Ranges

Adult	6.0–8.2 g/dL
Senior adult	6.0–7.8 g/dL
Pediatric	
Premature	4.3–7.6 g/dL
Newborn	4.6–7.6 g/dL
Child	6.2–8.1 g/dL

The term plasma protein may be found to be used interchangeably with serum, or total protein, but there is a difference. Plasma protein contains the coagulation factor fibrinogen and serum protein does not. Reliable measurements can be made on either plasma or serum, but serum protein is the measurement most used. Plasma proteins as a group include fibrinogen, hormones, serum enzymes, and conjugated proteins (lipoproteins, glycoproteins, and metal binding proteins). They comprise the major part of the solids in plasms. Interstitial fluid is very similar to plasma. It is the presence of albumin, globulin, fibrinogen, and prothrombin that differentiate the two. These proteins in plasma exert the colloid osmotic pressure that maintains equilibrium in the capillaries, one of the major functions of plasma protein. Besides maintaining normal distribution of water between blood and tissues, another major function of plasma protein is as a transport agent to cells; many vital metabolites, metal ions, hormones, and lipids are bound to, and carried by, specific proteins (Tietz, 1970). Plasma proteins are also concerned with nutrition, acid-base balance (serum proteins are amphoteric and can combine with acids or bases—given a normal range of blood pH, protein acts as an acid and will combine with cations) (Harper, 1971), immunity, and enzyme action. Serum protein, or total protein, is a measurement of albumin and the many different globulin fractions only. Serum and plasma proteins are the most conveniently available body protein for examination and measurement.

Because total protein determination represents several different proteins, it is not a good indicator of change in any one individual fraction. Changes in total protein concentration occur in many disease states, and information about these changes are of clinical value in evaluation of the course of disease or response to treatment, although rarely of assistance in diagnosis. Changes in total protein may occur in one, several, or all fractions. Changes can occur in different directions in different fractions without changing the total protein concentration itself. In the past, for more definitive information, the physician would order testing of total protein, serum albumin, globulin, and an albumin/globulin ratio (A/G ratio). Although these tests are still in use, a more valuable and accurate examination of the protein fractions is that of protein electrophoresis (see Chapter 10).

Physiology. Proteins are taken into the body in the diet. Many research experiments have shown a direct relationship between the formation of plasma protein, to include antibody formation, and the amount and quality of dietary protein ingested (Harper, 1971). Almost all of the protein taken in food is fully digested to amino acids in the small intestine. According to Howard and Herbold (1978), "If the dietary protein lacks even one of the essential amino acids, the body reacts as if all essential amino acids are deficient," and unless all are available at much the same time, complete protein utilization does not occur. Amino acids are transported to the liver by the bloodstream, where albumin, the alpha and beta globulins, prothrombin, and fibrinogen are synthesized exclusively. Gamma globulins are produced by B lymphocytes and carried out primarily in plasma cells and lymphoid tissue. The plasma cell is the end-stage production and storage cell. Once synthesized, plasma proteins are released into the bloodstream. All body proteins form a large pool which can be drawn on by any tissue that needs protein. The protein pool is in dynamic equilibrium. For instance, a single molecule, synthesized in the liver and released into the plasma pool may make up a part of an enzyme of some cell, yet eventually be incorporated into the hemoglobin in an erythrocyte. All body cells contain protein that can be used to meet caloric requirements when dietary protein is unavailable. Amino acids are utilized for energy, or to form substances such as the enzyme mentioned above, hormones, or any other of the many protein substances essential to the body. Approximately 15 to 20 g of plasma proteins, about one-tenth of the circulating plasma proteins, are formed daily from this protein pool, and an equal amount are broken down by complete degradation daily. Marked elevation of total protein occurs rarely.

Slight elevations are not uncommon. When there is an increase in the level of a protein, particularly one of low molecular weight, large amounts are excreted. Evidently, having passed through the glomerular sieve of the kidney, the protein saturates the reabsorptive capacity of the tubule (Frolich, 1976).

The ultimate fate of protein is not clear. Any albumin that seeps into the ECF is returned to the blood via the lymph. The body protein reserve is well assimilated and only a very small portion is excreted. The protein that is filtered through the glomerulus is almost totally reabsorbed—it is assumed by the proximal tubules. Only about 1/100 of albumin filtered is excreted in urine. Plasma proteins are destroyed by way of the digestive tract as well as the kidney, and by catabolism in tissue cells, particularly in the liver. Amino acids liberated by catabolism and leaked into the gastrointestinal tract are presumed to be reabsorbed into portal circulation and reutilized in protein synthesis.

Regulation of protein synthesis is also unclear. It seems obvious that an equilibrium exists among protein synthesis, catabolism, and dietary intake, with the body constituents being replaced rapidly at a constant rate (Sodeman and Sodeman, 1974). As noted above, the quality and quantity of amino acids available in the diet influence the rate of synthesis. Also affecting protein synthesis is the metabolic rate of the body and the action of certain hormones. Growth hormone, androgens, and insulin increase protein synthesis. Protein catabolism increases in response to glucocorticoids and high concentrations of thyroid. However, if these hormones are present at physiologic levels, there is an anabolic affect on protein metabolism.

When there is a limited intake, or supply, of carbohydrates, adipose tissue—followed by the nonnitrogen fraction of protein—is used for energy. An ample supply of carbohydrate allows conservation of body stores of protein for tissue maintenance and growth. Thus carbohydrate has a protein-sparing action.

Pathophysiology. Total protein concentration will decrease in several conditions, which is almost always a reflection of decrease in the albumin fraction. Globulins, most frequently the alpha globulin fraction, usually increase at the same time and the result may be a total protein concentration that is within normal limits. Edema almost invariably occurs when the total protein concentration falls below 5.3 gm/dL, which is considered the critical level. Hypoproteinemia occurs slowly and insidiously in many unrelated disease states. It can occur secondary to inadequate intake of protein—to include the lack of one or all essential amino acids—and impaired absorption; secondary to inadequate protein synthesis within the body (as in liver disease or genetic disorders); or secondary to an increased loss of protein which occurs with renal dysfunction, or pathologic states that increase the amount of low-molecular-weight proteins in circulation that can be filtered and lost (intravascular hemolysis). Loss also occurs due to increased protein catabolism (cachetic wasting in malignancies), increased levels of catabolic hormones, or in gastrointestinal enteropathies.

Hyperproteinemia usually occurs secondary to pathologic loss of fluid, or marked decrease in water intake. The absolute amount of serum proteins is unchanged, but there is an increase in concentration due to the loss of solvent water. Absolute increase in serum protein is seen in multiple myeloma, discussed later.

SERUM TOTAL PROTEIN INCREASED IN:

*1. *States of severe fluid loss,* such as in severe vomiting diarrhea, Addison's disease, diabetic acidosis, or early stages of burns. In burns of highly vascular tissue a great fluid shift occurs by extravasation into deeper tissues and dehydration of the non-damaged tissue occurs. More fluids and sodium are lost initially than is protein. Later hypoproteinemia can occur as protein is lost into the burned area.

*2. *States of prolonged, inadequate fluid intake.* Without adequate water intake dietary protein cannot be properly metabolized and water is drawn from the interstitial and intercellular spaces to supply the necessary volume to excrete the increased solute load (Metheny and Snively, 1979). Eventually, without replacement, total body water stores will be depleted and serum total protein concentration will rise.

*3. *Post albumin infusion in therapy* has shown transient increases in total protein concentration.

*4. *The condition known as multiple myeloma.* This is considered an immunoproliferative disease—a plasma cell tumor that produces excessive amounts of abnormal immunoglobins (gamma globulin). Serum albumin is often decreased. Abnormal proteins which sometimes appear in the urine are called Bence-Jones protein, which are light chains from immunoglobulin molecules. Serum hyperviscosity can occur. Bence-Jones proteins are almost entirely secreted in the urine 12 hr after synthesis, which can cause an excretion of as much as one-half of the daily nitrogen

---

*In this list and the one that follows (pp. 66-69), asterisks indicate states in which changes of albumin concentration parallel serum protein changes.

intake (Harper, 1970). Quantities of serum protein other than gamma globulin are unaltered except for a decrease in serum albumin which is not characteristic of the disease. More likely it reflects malnutrition related to the increased protein demand of malignant process, or renal loss when the kidney is affected by the myeloma.

SERUM TOTAL PROTEIN DECREASED IN:

1. *Conditions causing impaired utilization or synthesis,* such as:
   a. Potassium deficit. Potassium is an essential element in protein synthesis. Any person with a prolonged disturbance in body fluids can be at risk for protein deficit since the causes of abnormalities of body fluid are often causes of protein deficit as well.
   *b. Chronic liver disease. Lack of adequate functioning hepatocytes causes a decreased production of albumin, primarily in conditions such as portal cirrhosis. There is often a simultaneous increase in globulin which may cause a total protein concentration that is within normal range; or in less frequent occurrence, the total protein is increased. Changes in serum proteins are important in the diagnosis and evaluation of liver disease since so many are formed there.
   c. Pancreatic insufficiency, as with chronic pancreatitis, because of the impaired digestion or absorption consequent to the inadequate amounts, or total absence, of proteolytic enzymes produced in the pancreas.
   d. Idiopathic steatorrhea. There is impaired absorption from the intestine of not only protein, but also carbohydrate and fat, which causes use of plasma protein for energy, which further diminishes the serum total protein. There is a decrease in albumin and all globulin fractions. Other malabsorption syndromes may cause similar problems (e.g., cystic fibrosis, adult-onset sprue*).
2. *Conditions causing increased protein loss,* such as:
   *a. Inflammatory gastrointestinal disease as with ulcers or colitis. The rate and amount of protein leakage into the gastrointestinal tract is increased, which significantly increased the amount of protein lost in the feces. Ordinarily, amino acids are reabsorbed and reused.
   *b. Nephrotic syndrome. The glomerulus becomes increasingly permeable, allowing greater amounts of protein, usually albumin, to be filtered out and excreted in the urine. The

syndrome can occur secondary to glomerulonephritis, amyloidosis, lupus erythematosus or Kimmelstiel-Wilson disease. Both albumin and gamma globulin fractions are decreased. There is protein loss from the body of more than 50 to 70 mg/kg/day. The total protein pool is greatly decreased with the loss of albumin, and its rate of synthesis, as well as catabolism, increases. A *reduction* in synthesis rate sometimes occurs and may be due in part to the usually poor nutritional state of the individual (Frolich, 1976).

c. Hemorrhage. Loss of large portions of intravascular components, both water and solute, stimulate release of ADH and water conservation. Replacement of the circulating volume is primarily water and the total protein concentration is decreased.

*d. Acute and chronic infections, primarily bacterial. Infections, particularly those accompanied by fever, tend to reduce appetite, especially for protein foods, and to decrease the absorption rate from the gastrointestinal tract. The increased metabolic rate due to fever increases caloric need and protein catabolism can occur in the absence of adequate carbohydrate intake or fat stores. Negative nitrogen balance ensues (Howard and Herbold, 1978). The major decrease is in albumin. A concomitant rise in both alpha and gamma globulin may produce a total protein that is within normal range.

e. Burns. (See "Serum Total Protein Increased in," item 1.)

*3. *Conditions related to inadequate intake* lead to varying degrees of malnutrition, so-called protein-calorie malnutrition. There is decreased synthesis of all plasma proteins, even alpha globulin, which is usually raised in hypoproteinemias, and increased use of plasma protein for energy. Fasting alone results in a decrease of albumin synthesis of 30 to 40% (Frolich, 1976). Concentrations of nitrogenous waste products in the plasma (BUN, urea, creatinine) usually decrease as well. Protein deficits occur slowly, so any decrease in total plasma proteins indicates prolonged protein deprivation. The causes of malnutrition are extensive. Some causes include the inability to eat due to decreased level of consciousness or anorexia nervosa; decreased ability to chew secondary to myotonia or loss of molars; incomplete protein intake, lack of one or more of the essential amino acids secondary to fad diets, or cultural or economic strictures; increased metabolic requirements secondary to malignancy or hyperthyroidism; or inadequate intake of carbohydrates to spare protein for growth and metabolism.

4. *Conditions causing dilution and relative decrease in serum protein concentrations,* such as:
   a. Excessive administration of water and sodium after acute trauma (e.g., surgery). The basic drive of the body after acute trauma is to retain water. Aldosterone is stimulated to conserve sodium, which in turn helps conserve water, and there is loss of potassium in order to conserve sodium. The body can then be easily overwhelmed by fluid (Sabiston, 1977), and total protein levels appear depressed due to increased solvent in the extracellular space.
   *b. Transudation of plasma protein, particularly albumin, into ascitic fluid.
   *c. Early phase of pregnancy in which hydration changes occur (Davidsohn and Henry, 1969).

IMPLICATIONS FOR NURSING

Prevention of malnutrition and protein deficiency is a major need that can be accomplished by the nurse, both in the hospital and in the community. Oddly enough, deficiency states are more frequently encountered in the hospital in the United States. Nursing actions to meet this need may include any or all of the following.

1. *Patient preparation.* No food or drink other than water for 8 hr prior to the test is preferred, although not essential.
2. *Education of all clients,* regardless of diagnosis, educational level, occupation, or setting in which they are met, in the elements of basic nutrition. Such education may be sorely needed not only by the health care consumer, but also by many health care providers.
3. *Acquisition of knowledge of the essential amino acid content of foods* so that diet planning will include adequate combinations of foods to provide all essential amino acids, despite dietary restrictions. Vegetarian diets can include all essential protein, but not without great care in planning.
4. *Identification of risk populations* in which nutritional assessment should be carried out.
   a. Nutritional screening and assessment should be done for all pregnant women on the initial visit if possible. Risk factors

to look for relate to age, socioeconomic status, and past history of medical or obstetrical problems (Holloway, 1979).

b. Persons with renal disease, especially if on protein restriction.
c. Persons with chronic liver disease.
d. Persons presenting with anemia, cause unknown.
e. Persons with pathology that causes increased metabolic demands (e.g., acute infections, malignancy, hyperthyroidism).
f. Persons with decreased intestinal absorptive function (e.g., chronic diarrhea, acute diarrhea in children, colitis, adult-onset sprue, cystic fibrosis, and new ileostomates).
g. Persons not receiving food by mouth (e.g., NPO, postsurgical, unconscious, on tube feedings).

5. *Assessment of the nutritional status of risk populations:*
   a. Check height and weight. Compare height for age and weight for height. This will give more useful information about nutritional status than does weight for age. A height deficit could be present due to chronic malnutrition. The height for age and weight for height approach is especially useful in children, as they may be both wasted and stunted. In the adult, determining height of parents and siblings is helpful. Also useful in the adult is determining weight at age 25 as a baseline for comparison (Phipps et al., 1979). Assess for recent change.
   b. Check for presence of edema, skin lesions, dullness, dryness, and/or loss of hair.
   c. Check for history of change in affect (increasing apathy?), frequent infections (there is an increased susceptibility to infection with malnutrition because of depression of the immune defense system), or history of delayed wound healing.
   d. Check pertinent laboratory data when available. If not available and other assessment data indicate malnutrition, request that tests be performed.
      (1) Total protein. Will be normal or decreased, with decreased albumin, which is the protein primarily responsible for colloid osmotic pressure and probably is the primary nutritional source of body tissues.
      (2) Red cell count. May be decreased because of lack of available protein for production; because of lack of iron absorption, which will cause a hypochromic, microcytic anemia; because of lack of vitamin B_{12} aborption, which will cause a macrocytic, normochronic anemia.
      (3) Blood indices:
         (a) Hemoglobin may decrease due to iron or protein deficiency.

(b) MCV: decreased with hypochromic microcytic anemia; increased with hyperchromic, macrocytic anemia.
(c) MCHC: decreased with hypochromic, microcytic anemia; increased with hyperchromic, macrocytic anemia (rarely seen).

(4) White blood count. Polymorphonuclear neutrophils will increase in the presence of acute infection; check the lymphocyte count in children with a history, or presence, of infection. If less than 6300 per mm^3 (the average for a 2-year-old), it could indicate an impaired defense against infection. This can lead to further difficulties in assessment (e.g., false negative on a tuberculin skin test) (Howard and Herbold, 1978).

(5) Plasma potassium. Potassium is essential for protein synthesis. Decreased in malnutrition states.

(6) BUN, urea, creatinine. Will be decreased in long-term malnutrition. (Other laboratory values may be decreased secondary to the decrease in protein. Chemicals such as calcium are transported in the blood by being bound to protein. Therefore, a decrease in available protein will cause a decrease in circulating calcium).

e. Note the presence or absence of teeth and any prosthesis. Determine if prostheses are usually worn. Persons with partial lower molar dentures frequently leave them out, thereby decreasing their ability to chew, and increasing the probability of selecting soft, easily masticated foods. This can eliminate many good sources of protein.

6. *For the individuals identified at risk for protein deficiency,* or so diagnosed, the nurse can help assure adequate intake and utilization of all essential amino acids.

a. The greater the amount of protein intake, the greater the water requirement. This need is especially important in the person on tube feedings, the person with a fever, the person with a high catabolic rate, or the person who has a decreased ability to concentrate urine. Aged persons may require increased water intake even without an increase in protein intake because of the frequent occurrence of impaired renal function in the elderly.

With ingestion of a high-protein diet, urine volumes will be increased, even if not extra fluids are given. This can lead to excessive saline loss and dehydration. Fluids are therefore imperative with a high-protein diet.

b. Individuals who are nutritionally depleted and have non-elective surgery which necessitates prolonged periods NPO should be closely monitored when returned to a diet to assure adequate and complete protein intake. Anorexia is one of the symptoms of malnutrition, making the process of encouraging protein intake particularly challenging for the nurse. Malnutrition is more common in the elderly than in young adults in the United States, requiring special awareness with this population.

c. It is well to remember that there is a starvation effect in the first few days postsurgery for almost all ill persons. Weight loss of ½ lb/day in the adult is not unusual. Weight loss may be thought of as a benefit for the obese individual but the obese person can be, and usually is, malnourished despite an excessive intake of food. Check for dilutional hypoproteinemia before instituting measures to replace protein (see "Serum Total Protein Decreased in," item 4).

d. Measurement of muscle mass is helpful in determining protein loss, but without exercise such measurement is of no value in checking the effectiveness of protein replacement. Without exercise, body protein may continue to be lost despite adequate intake. Provision of active and passive bed exercises (described in Section 3.10) and early ambulation may assist the nutritional status, as well as improve appetite. Teach the patient and family members the rationale for exercise to increase their compliance with the action and independent effort on their part.

e. Obtain a diet history to determine what types of protein would be most acceptable to the individual and his or her frequency of eating. Provide these choices if possible.

f. Provide foods with adequate potassium to assure protein synthesis.

g. Provide adequate carbohydrate in the diet, especially in the presence of fever, to spare protein from being used for energy. Minimum daily requirements of carbohydrates have not been established. The general rule is 100 g/day; 150 g/day if fasting to prevent muscle breakdown (Howard and Herbold, 1978).

h. Protect the individual who is malnourished from exposure to infection.

i. When protein intake is restricted, as in some types of renal disease, about 70 to 75% of the allowed protein in the diet should be from foods with high biological value—that is, containing complete amino acids and able to assimilate readily.

The following foods are given in order of their effectiveness: fresh and dried beef serum and lactoalbumin (milk protein) are most effective; next are egg white, beef muscle, liver casein, and gelatin (Harper, 1971).

7. *The person with hypoproteinemia due to the nephrotic syndrome* may lose large amounts of clotting factor IX and must be monitored for bleeding tendencies. Conversely, the plasma levels of fibrinogen and other coagulation factors may be increased so that some authors feel there is an increased frequency of thrombosis in these individuals (Frolich, 1976). Observation of peripheral circulation, use of TED hose, and early ambulation can be helpful.

8. *The average daily protein requirements of infants* can be more than three times that of adults (2 to 3.5 g/kg of infant weight; 1.0 g/kg of adult weight) and increases markedly during illness. Absorption is less than in adults since food is propelled very rapidly through the digestive tract because of that system's immaturity (Whaley and Wong, 1979). Therefore, malnourishment in the infant tends to be even more serious and have more permanent outcomes than in the adult. Frequent nutritional assessment should be carried out in the infant and growing child and parents should be taught the process as well as its importance.

1.9 SERUM PROTEIN FRACTIONS

1.9.1 Serum Albumin

Synonym: plasma albumin

Normal Ranges

Adult	3.5–5 g/dL
Senior adult	3.2–4.5 g/dL (salt fractionation)
Pediatric	
Newborn infant	2.9–5.5 g/dL
Child to age 3	3.8–5.4 g/dL

Albumin is the major constituent of the serum protein. It can be directly measured and alterations in its serum concentration parallel many alterations of the serum total protein (see abnormalities indicated by an asterisk under "Serum Total Protein Increased in" in Section 1.8). Albumin has a half-life of approximately 30 days and is considered a reliable index of the severity and prognosis in patients with chronic hepatic disease (Davidsohn and Henry, 1969). Those patients showing a rise in serum albumin have a more favorable prognosis than those who do not. Albumin measurement is not as useful as measurement of fibrinogen or prothrombin, in dating the onset of liver cell failure because its half-life is much longer (Sodeman and Sodeman, 1974).

Physiology. Albumin is the most important serum protein in maintaining intravascular oncontic pressure. Should it decrease, edema results. Albumin is considered the primary nutritional source for body tissue. Serum albumin is important in transport, being the major vehicle for calcium, magnesium, bibirubin, and fatty acids transport, as well as the transport of many drugs. Effective blood levels of such drugs are altered by a decrease in serum albumin concentration. There is some evidence that the production of albumin may be regulated by osmotic effects, rather than—or as well as—the change in serum albumin concentration itself, but the rate of snythesis usually increases when serum levels are decreased. Synthesis occurs in the liver. With a failure in dietary intake of protein, such as in fasting, there is a marked decrease in synthesis. The liver is believed to be responsible for about 10% of normal albumin catabolism (Frolich, 1976).

Pathophysiology. In disease states affecting protein concentrations, serum albumin tends to decrease or remain the same and does not rise above normal except with hemoconcentration or dehydration. Decrease in albumin frequently is associated with an increase in globulin (see "Pathophysiology" in Section 1.9.2). Albumin is lost in pathology by extravasation (burns, ascites), in urine with tubular dysfunction (nephrosis), or by increased leakage into the gut (colitis). Synthesis of albumin is decreased in conditions causing a lack of protein intake or absorption (liver disease). Decreases in serum albumin levels usually lead to edema, due to the loss of intravascular oncotic pressure.

For conditions in which albumin concentration increases or decreases, see serum total protein increases and decreases in Section 1.8.

IMPLICATIONS FOR NURSING

See "Implications for Nursing" in Section 1.8.

1.9.2 Serum Globulin

Synonym: plasma globin

Normal Ranges

Adult	2.1–3 g/dL
Senior adult	
Male	3.1–3.4 g/dL
Female	2.8–3.2 g/dL*
Infant	No specific variation from adult

*Computed from total protein and albumin ranges as given in Carnevali and Patrick (1979).

Serum globulin is the major constituent, after albumin, of the total protein, or serum protein. The total protein measurement can be used to estimate globulin concentration. The globulin concentration is the remainder when albumin—corrected for nonprotein nitrogen—is measured directly and subtracted from the total protein concentration. The globulin fraction of the serum protein is a very complex mixture with functions that are also multiple, complex, and not fully understood. The serum globulin is a relatively imprecise measure and gives little or no specific information for diagnosis. The rapid increase in knowledge of the molecular structure of proteins has outdated much terminology used in protein classification—even terms such as albumin and globulin (Harper, 1971). Generalizations about serum globulins are of even less value than those about albumin because of the complexity of the group of proteins given this name, both in function and molecular structure. The one feature they all share is their insolubility in water and concentrated salt solutions and their solubility in weak, neutral salt solutions (Davidsohn and Henry, 1969). Globulin fractions are usually classified as alpha, beta, and gamma, and subclasses have been defined for each fraction.

Physiology. Serum globulins are produced at several sites in the reticuloendothelial system of the body. Most of the alpha and beta globulins originate in the liver, but gamma globulins are produced from plasma cells and lymphoid tissue and are made up of amino acids only (Harvey et al., 1976). The antibody activity of the plasma, interstitial fluid, and body secretions is associated with the gamma globulin fraction, called immunoglobulins, the symbol for which is Ig. The collective group of immunoglobulins have been defined and are known as G, M, A, D, and E (e.g., IgG, IgM). They provide protection against bacterial and viral infection, parasites, allergens, and malignancy. Distinct function specialization has been described for some of the Ig subclasses. The alpha and beta globulins are made up principally of mucoproteins and glycoproteins. Beta globulin is also made up of lipoproteins. Transport is a major function of these globulin fractions and beta provides a vehicle for transport of fat in plasma. Transferrin, a beta globulin, is one of the many metal binding globulins which provides transport for copper and iron. Both alpha and beta globulins transport fat-soluble vitamins and certain hormones: for example, corticosteroid binding globulin (CBG), thyroid binding globulin (TBG), and antihemophillic globulin (AHG) or factor VIII, a protein involved in the clotting process (Harper, 1971). Cryoglobulins are cold-precipitable gamma globulins (Davidsohn and Henry, 1964).

The human fetus is capable of forming antibodies, but the greatest amount of immunity of an infant is that obtained through the placenta from the mother. This is usually IgG, which makes up 75 to 85% of the Ig function (Frolich, 1976). By the end of his or her first year, the infant is able to produce adult concentrations of immunoglobulin.

The protein from which both albumin and globulin are made is found in the "protein pool," described with serum proteins, and the same general processes of formation and degradation apply. Little is known, however, about regulation of globulin production other than its response to antigen stimulation. Although the area is currently under intensive study, much is still theoretical or totally unknown.

Pathophysiology. Very few generalizations can be made about globulin response in disease. In acute infections a slight increase, particularly of gamma globulins, reflects synthesis of antibodies to the infecting agent. A greater rise occurs in chronic infections (Tietz, 1970). When there is a state of hypoproteinemia in the body, the level of alpha globulin concentration increases, which is thought to reflect an increase in glycoproteins and lipoproteins (plus C reactive protein). This is seen frequently in advanced metastatic cancer, but no diagnostic pattern has been noted (Davidsohn and Henry, 1969). Acute cellular necrosis is also frequently accompanied by an increase in alpha globulin, $alpha_2$. However, this globulin has been seen to decrease in acute hepatocellular necrosis, so the generalization is not always true. Beta globulins have not been associated with specific disease processes with any regularity. Changes in transferrin concentrations are reflected by changes in beta globulin and increases in accumulation of lipids are reflected by increases in beta globulin. The possible relationship as a cause of atheroclerosis is being studied (Harper, 1971).

In many diseases there is a constant association between a decreased albumin concentration and an increased level of alpha globulins (nephrosis, cirrhosis, acute infections), but little is known of the process.

Decreases in the immunoglobulins produce, not surprisingly, an increased susceptibility to infections, since humoral immunity, as opposed to cellular immunity, is immunity due to circulating antibodies in the gamma globulin fraction of the plasma protein.

SERUM GLOBULIN INCREASED IN:

1. *Familial idiopathic dysproteinemia,* due to a genetic defect causing an increased production of globulin in relation to albumin.
2. *Diseases associated with continuing cell necrosis* or tissue destruction:
   a. Viral hepatitis, due to the immunologic response to the virus and to the necrotic process in the liver cells, as well as to proliferation of reticuloendothelial cells in the liver. All globulin fractions increase. The increase begins before the onset of jaundice, peaks in 8 to 10 days, and does not return to normal for an extended time, 3 to 4 months. Increases are also seen in diffuse hepatocellular diseases, such as cirrhosis and chronic active hepatitis. The liver is often infiltrated with plasma cells and lymphocytes.
   b. Acute febrile disease, due to increased tissue breakdown.
   c. Cancer, due to tissue wasting.
   d. Advanced tuberculosis, also probably due to tissue wasting.
3. *Multiple myeloma,* due to gamma globulin increase secondary to production of the abnormal immunoglobulin (monoclonal or M protein, e.g., Bence-Jones' protein). The alpha and beta fractions occasionally increase. Ultimately, in some cases, a secondary decrease in gamma globulin production can occur, causing hypogammaglobulinemia or agammaglobulinemia.
4. *Nephrotic syndrome,* due to loss of gamma globulin in the urine. Alpha and beta globulins increase.

SERUM GLOBULIN DECREASED IN:

1. *Hypogammaglobulinemia,* due to decreased production of gamma globulin, cause unknown.
2. *Agammaglobulinemia,* whether congenital, physiological, idiopathic, or acquired secondary to conditions such as multiple myeloma, leukemia, or Hodgkin's disease, due to a marked decrease or total absence of gamma globulin production.

IMPLICATIONS FOR NURSING

1. *Any individual with either a decrease, or an increase, in globulin* can be expected to exhibit some degree of immunological deficiency specific to the person. Therefore, a nursing history should be taken when changes in globulin concentrations occur to determine:
   a. Frequency of occurrence of infections.
   b. Evidence of chronic infection.
   c. Failure to recover from infections.
   d. Frequent reinfection.
   e. Infection with unusual agents (history may reveal no logical source of infection).
   f. Familial history of deficiency.

2. *Observation of infants* with a familiar history of immunoglobulin deficiency for evidence of the disease process may not be fruitful until around 3 months of age because of the maternal transfer of immunoglobulins. Observe for:
   a. Validating laboratory findings: decreased serum lymphocyte count and a lack of increase in lymphocytes in response to antigens; bone marrow showing a lack of plasma cells.
   b. Evidence of graft vs. host response (fever, skin rash, alopecia, hepatosplenomegaly, diarrhea and ulceration of mucous membrane of gastrointestinal tract, mouth, and anus) 7 to 20 days after administration of any blood supplements or other foreign tissues.

   Immunodeficient infants have a poor prognosis. Histocompatible bone marrow transplant is the only effective treatment, although injections of gamma globulin provide a passive immunity that is transitory. A very few infants have been kept alive by provision of a totally sterile environment, but to be effective, this environment must be provided before the infant has *any* infection.

3. *Nursing care of immunodeficient infants* consists of:
   a. Assisting in preventing infection and teaching family members the process (isolation, skin and mouth care).
   b. Providing support to the family in the care of a fatally ill child.
   c. Providing family support against feelings of guilt and impotency in the very likely occurrence of chronic fungal infections of mouth and nails despite the family's vigorous efforts to prevent or treat such infections.

d. Providing access to genetic counseling for the family (Whaley and Wong, 1979).
e. The infant may exhibit symptoms similar to rheumatoid arthritis as one form of allergic manifestation. The reader is referred to Scipien et al (1975, pp. 808-810) for nursing care.

4. *Acquired forms of hypogammaglobulinemia, or agammaglobulinemia,* should be suspected in persons with malabsorption syndromes because of the possibility of defective synthesis of globulin. A high index of suspicion should be held also for any adult with a malignancy, particularly those involving the lymphatic or reticuloendothelial systems. Any individual with such a diagnosis should be carefully guarded against infection and a thorough history taken of types of infections to which the person has been particularly susceptible.
5. *The most common secondary immunodeficient state* includes not only exaggerated susceptibility to infection, but also thrombocytopenia. This implies the need for observation of unusual bleeding tendencies and nursing measures to protect the person from bleeding (see "Implications for Nursing" in Section 2.3.2; Section 3.12; and "Implications for Nursing," item 6, in Section 1.8).

1.9.3 A/G Ratio

Synonyms: Albumin/globulin ratio; plasma A/G ratio

Normal Range

Adult	1.0–2.0

The A/G ratio is an expression of the ratio of albumin to globulin in the blood and can also be determined from the urine. It is used to express protein changes in disease. It is computed by dividing the albumin concentration by the globulin concentration. Prior to the advent of electrophoresis and immunophoresis techniques, the A/G ratio was the best indicator available for looking at the component parts of serum total proteins, for in any one individual the A/G ratio is quite constant.

In several disease states there is a fairly constant relationship between the increase in globulin and the decrease in albumin (e.g., cirrhosis, nephrosis, acute infections, pneumonia, rheumatic fever, typhus), and following the A/G ratio was one of the best tools available for watching the response to treatment. Generally, albumin tends to decrease in abnormal conditions and globulin exhibits a simultaneous increase. Both the albumin and the globulin can be measured reliably in either plasma or serum.

The A/G ratio is felt to be less important than the actual changes in albumin and globulin (Ring, 1969), to be needlessly awkward and imprecise, and to no longer have clinical application because of incomplete separation of albumin from globulin (Davidsohn and Henry, 1969). Tietz (1970) believes that the analysis of disease states would be enhanced were the A/G ratio to be abandoned.

Physiology. See "Physiology" in Section 1.8.

A/G RATIO DECREASED IN:

Any condition that decreases the albumin fraction of total protein (see Sections 1.8 and 1.9.1).

A/G RATIO INCREASED IN:

Any condition that increases globulin over albumin (see Sections 1.8 and 1.9.2).

1.10 TOTAL SERUM BILIRUBIN

Synonyms: total bilirubin; total plasma bilirubin

Normal Ranges

Adult	0.1–1.2 mg/dL	
Senior adult	0.2–1.2 mg/dL	
Pediatric		
	Premature	*Full term*
Cord	<2	<2 mg/dL
0-1 day	<8	<6 mg/dL
1-2 days	<12	<8 mg/dL
3-5 days	<16	<12 mg/dL
Thereafter	<2	<1 mg/dL

Bilirubin is one of two substances making up the bile pigments, biliverdin being the other. Approximately 85% of bilirubin formed is derived from the conversion of the heme from hemoglobin (Frolich, 1976). The total bilirubin test can be done equally well on either serum or plasma and is one of the tests included in a "liver profile," being a test based on the secretory and excretory functions of the liver, and therefore of major importance in the profile. In itself it is not specific for any one disease, but is extremely helpful in sorting out liver or biliary dysfunction when correlated with a thorough history and physical examination. Total serum bilirubin is useful in measuring the depth and progress of jaundice and is of considerable value in detection of "latent" jaundice (serum levels greater than 2 mg/dL) (see "Pathophysiology," below). Serum bilirubin, of all the tests included in a liver profile, is probably the most informative. Knowledge of bilirubin metabolism has increased knowledge and understanding of liver physiology. Its estimation has immense importance in the newborn, where it serves as a prime index of exchange transfusion necessity and effectiveness in prevention of kernicterus.

Total bilirubin and the direct-reacting (conjugated, water-soluble) fraction can be accurately measured, but the indirect-reacting (unconjugated, water-insoluble) fraction is inferred by subtracting the direct from the total. Total bilirubin value represents the sum of both conjugated and unconjugated bilirubin. Bilirubin is destroyed by exposure to white light, artificial light, or sunlight. Although a breakdown of bilirubin into its fractions is helpful in differential diagnosis of jaundice, the total bilirubin is an excellent screening test to indicate hyperbilirubinemia, whatever the cause.

Physiology. The mechanism of bilirubin metabolism is complex and not completely understood (see Fig. 1.1). Approximately 6 to 8 g of hemoglobin is released each day, and some 263 mg of bilirubin is produced daily in the normal adult—with 5 L of blood and a hemoglobin concentration within normal limits. Many molecules share the same binding site on the albumin molecule with bilirubin, and when present in large numbers will compete for binding. With even a slight decrease in available albumin, the binding sites may become inadequate and bilirubin or other molecules will appear in increased concentrations in the serum. The compensatory mechanism for increased concentrations of bilirubin is an increased rate of excretion of the conjugated fraction, or an increased rate of binding or conjugation, when possible, of the unconjugated fraction. When hepatic reserve is exceeded, the indirect (unconjugated, water-insoluble) bilirubin rises and a pathologic state exists. This provides a rationale for the pale jaundice seen in advanced malnutrition.

Conjugation enzymes mature late in fetal development and are not fully developed until the tenth month after conception. All premature infants, and a variable number of full term, but underweight newborns, will have impaired conjugation in differing degrees of severity (Sodeman and Sodeman, 1974). This, coupled with excessive RBC breakdown due to change from the hypoxic uterus to the air at birth, causes what is termed "physiologic hyperbilirubinemia." The liver "learns" to conjugate bilirubin within 3 to 5 days and serum bilirubin levels return to normal in most instances (Beck, 1971).

Bilirubin metabolism provides the only source of endogenous carbon monoxide, and measurements of its production rate are used in some testing methods to determine the rate of heme product catabolism, and thereby infer the rate of hemolysis (Sodeman and Sodeman, 1974).

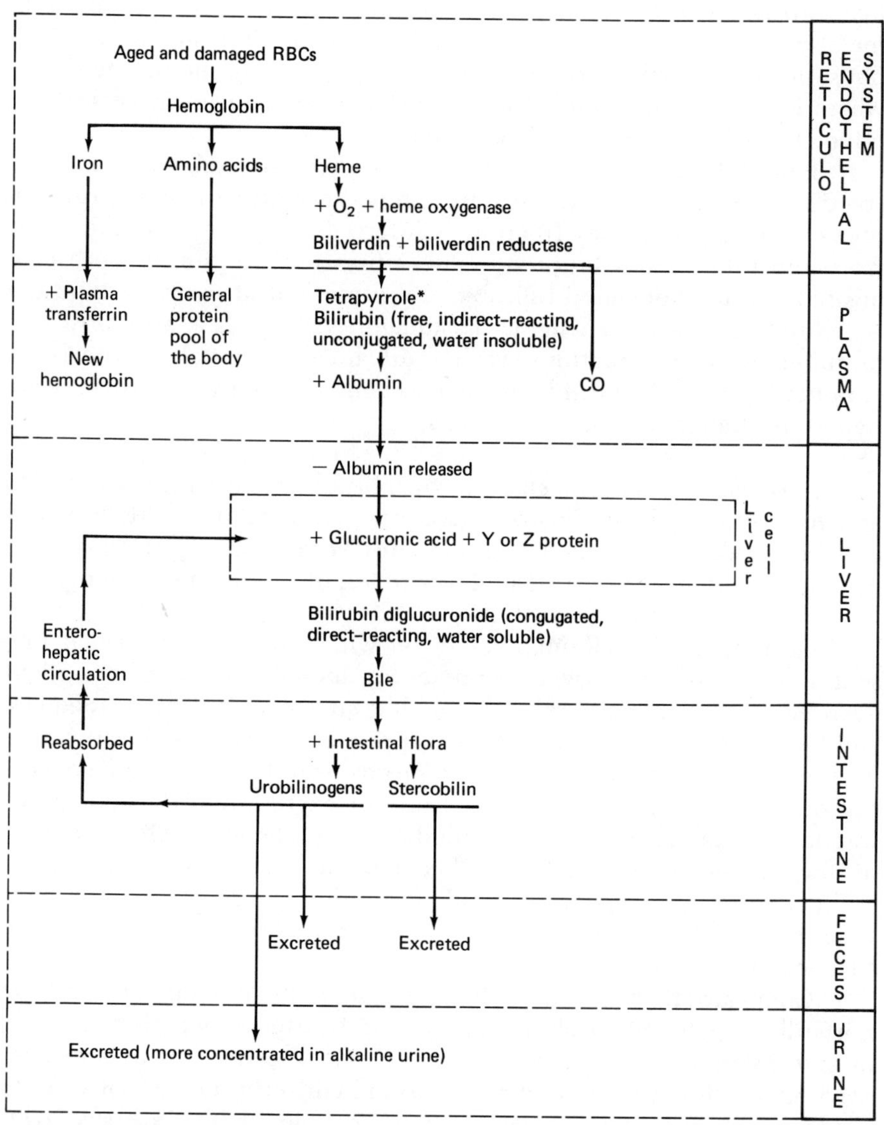

*Defined as a complex cyclic compound and an important component of myoglobin, cytochrome, catalase as well as hemoglobin (Levinsky, 1973).

FIGURE 1.1 Bilirubin metabolism. (Source: data taken from Beck, 1971; Carnevali and Patrick, 1979; Sabiston, 1977; and Steffes, 1979.)

Pathophysiology. Jaundice is the major, overt indicator of a pathologic state in bilirubin metabolism. It occurs when bilirubin is not removed or excreted, or is formed in excessive amounts. At any point in the bilirubin metabolism mechanism a congenital abnormality (an inborn error in metabolism), or an acquired abnormality can occur. Congenital abnormalities are often called constitutional hyperbilirubinemia. An example of such an abnormality would be Gilbert's syndrome. Decreased levels of bilirubin occur rarely and are of little clinical significance.

Increases in total bilirubin are categorized into three mechanisms of jaundice production:

1. *Prehepatic* (retention, hemolytic) jaundice, due to overproduction of bilirubin or ineffective red cell formation.
2. *Hepatic* (also included in the retention class), due to liver cell damage or inadequate albumin availability.
3. *Posthepatic* (regurgitation, obstructive), due to mechanical obstruction of extrahepatic bile passages, causing decreased excretion.

Hepatic and posthepatic jaundice often occur together, since a degree of obstruction usually occurs with liver cell damage, blocking the bile canaliculi. When there is liver cell damage the cells lose their ability to conjugate bilirubin, a function normally found only in those cells. The cell damage allows the bilirubin, which has been conjugated by healthy cells, to pass freely into all liquids of the body when under normal conditions it is confined to the liver cell, the liver canaliculi, and the bile. Its distribution is determined by the protein (particularly albumin) content of the fluid. The invaded tissue is stained, and jaundice becomes apparent when serum bilirubin concentration exceeds 2 mg/dL in the adult or child (Harvey et al., 1976) or 5 mg/dL in the premature infant (Whaley and Wong, 1979).

Unconjugated (free, indirect-reacting, water-insoluble) bilirubin accumulates in adipose tissue and can be best seen in subcutaneous fat of the abdomen and extremities, and will be excreted in the feces in increasing amounts in the adult. Also in the adult, severe hemolysis will cause serum bilirubin elevations rarely exceeding 5 mg/dL. The jaundice will be a mild pale yellow, and urine will be free of bilirubin (recall, the elevation is of the water-insoluble, unconjugated fraction). If urine becomes darker, it will be due to an increased conjugation and excretion of direct-reacting bilirubin by the liver because of the increased loads of unconjugated bilirubin presented to it (Price and Wilson, 1978).

For the adult, chronic overproduction of bilirubin with mild serum increases, although it may lead to the production of gallstones—which are made up primarily of bilirubin—causes little harm. But in the full-term infant, levels of unconjugated bilirubin over 20 mg/dL may lead to kernicterus, a condition in which the unconjugated, unbound, and lipid-soluble bilirubin is able to cross the blood-brain barrier and is deposited in the basal ganglia of the brain, capable of causing severe damage or death. The exact mechanism is not known, but the pathogenesis is seen to be almost identical with that observed in hypoxia (Whaley and Wong, 1978). Several factors affect the occurrence of kernicterus besides the initial elevation of the serum bilirubin. They are:

1. Conditions that decrease binding capacity of the serum: for example, metabolic acidosis, decreased albumin levels in the serum, drugs that compete for albumin binding sites (e.g., salicylates, sulfonamides, vitamin K), or other chemicals with similar competitive binding properties (e.g., increased free fatty acids).
2. Any condition that increases oxygen demand (e.g., fetal distress).
3. Any condition that increases glucose demand (hypoxia). All of these factors serve to increase the amount of unbound, unconjugated bilirubin, thus increasing the risk of kernicterus occurring.

Physiologic jaundice, due to immaturity of hepatic functions or increased RBC destruction, is more severe and prolonged in the premature infant. The infant is also more susceptible to the disorders listed above that contribute to increased, unconjugated serum bilirubin levels. Because of this, the premature infant is at greater risk for the occurrence of kernicterus.

TOTAL SERUM BILIRUBIN INCREASED IN:

1. *Conditions causing overproduction of bilirubin,* as in:
   a. Hemolytic disease causing saturation of available albumin binding sites due to the massive amounts of bilirubin presented to the liver: for example, erythroblastosis fetalis, abnormal hemoglobins (e.g., hemoglobin S in sickle cell anemia), and abnormal red blood cells (e.g., hereditary spherocytosis).
   b. Ineffective red cell formation (sometimes called shunt hyperbilirubinemia): for example, thalassemia (Cooley's anemia), pernicious anemia, porphyria.

c. Physiological jaundice of the newborn, particularly in the premature infant, due in part to the reduced life span of RBCs in the newborn, lack of intestinal flora for conversion of conjugated bilirubin to urobilinogen, inability of the liver to conjugate bilirubin, and possibly adaptation of the infant's liver to the postnatal hypoxic state after the closing of ductus venosus at birth (Whaley and Wong, 1979).
d. Infants of Oriental or Asian descent, which in this instance includes American Indian, who tend to have bilirubin levels almost twice that seen in the black or white races (the cause is unknown). Hyperbilirubinemia is also seen in newborns of eastern Mediterranean heritage (e.g., Greek). Whether these increases are due to overproduction or excretion defects is also unknown, but the condition has been placed in this category for convenience.
e. Gilbert's syndrome, a retention type of constitutional (inborn error of metabolism) dysfunction with the true cause unknown. A high serum indirect (unconjugated, water-insoluble) bilirubin may be produced. This condition is occasionally associated with a hemolytic anemia as well (Davidsohn and Henry, 1969).
f. Escape of blood from circulation into tissues, causing large hematomas or infarcts.

2. *Conditions causing hepatic intracellular conjugation defects,* as in:

a. The specific marked decrease of glucuronyl transferase activity which occurs in all newborns, or Crigler-Najjer syndrome.
b. Inhibition of glucuronyl transferase in some breast-fed infants due to chemicals excreted by their mothers into their milk. This dysfunction can occur prior to birth in some infants when the chemical reaches a high level in the mothers and disappears after the birth, producing a transient, familial, neonatal hyperbilirubinemia—Lucey-Driscoll syndrome.
c. Administration of certain drugs to the near-term, pregnant mother, or to the newborn (e.g., sulfonamides, vitamin K).
d. Decreased production and stores of albumin due to the immaturity of the liver.
e. Administration of drugs that inhibit glucuronyl transferase [e.g., novobiocin (Albamycin)] (Frohlich, 1976).
f. Viral hepatitis, which affects not only the cellular activity of the liver in bilirubin metabolism, but will quickly lead to intrahepatic cholestasis so that both the direct and indirect fraction increase in serum concentration.

g. Laennec's cirrhosis (portal cirrhosis) in advanced stages, due to degeneration and fibrosis of the liver structure.

3. *Conditions causing obstruction of intrahepatic or extrahepatic biliary passages,* as in:
   a. Choledocholithiasis (gallstones in the common bile duct), causing increases in direct bilirubin in both blood and urine, producing the characteristic dark, "Coca-Cola" color. Clay-colored stools also occur because of the decrease in fecal urobilinogen and stercobilin.
   b. Cancer of the head of the pancreas, causing an increase in direct bilirubin levels in much the same manner as given for choledocholithiasis above.
   c. Certain women evidencing a jaundice in the third trimester of pregnancy. These same women often develop jaundice with the use of contraceptive agents. The mechanism of jaundice is not clear.
   d. The Dubin-Johnson syndrome, in which the reduced capacity to excrete bilirubin is due to an inborn error of metabolism.
   e. The presence of renal failure, the mechanism of which is unclear.

IMPLICATIONS FOR NURSING

1. *Preparation* for the test includes abstention from any intake other than water for 8 to 12 hr prior to drawing blood to prevent lipemia, which interferes with the test. Hemolysis of the sample should be avoided to prevent falsely low results in some testing methods (diazo) (Tietz, 1970).

2. *Implications related to the apperance of jaundice:*
   a. Relieve pruritis, if present, as this symptom can be physically exhausting and emotionally demoralizing. It also tends to lead to tissue breakdown, especially when damage is done by scratching.
      (1) Prevention of scratching is impossible; the person will scratch, at least in their sleep, unless totally restrained, and the outcomes of such restraint are usually more difficult to deal with than the outcomes of scratching.
      (2) Suggest alternatives to scratching:
         (a) Use a soft cloth instead of fingernails.

(b) Use of counterstimulation by tickling with a feather or long-napped material such as fake fur, or by small, sharp slaps. (The last should be used sparingly. Not only can the slaps become painful in themselves, but pruritis will be aggravated by the resultant capillary dilitation.)

(3) Keep the environment cool and clothing and bedding light and nonrestrictive. Woolen blankets or clothing should not be used, because wool fibers often cause itching and many people react strongly to wool.

(4) Do not allow perspiration to remain on the skin or in the clothing. Salt crystals can aggravate itching.

(5) Provide tub soaks with *tepid* water (to prevent capillary dilitation secondary to temperature extremes or secondary to physical stimulation of shower spray).

(6) Addition of soothing substances such as cornstarch or oatmeal to the tub soak or application of calamine lotion to affected areas should be considered independent nursing, but may require a physician's order.

(7) Provide diversion in whatever form is acceptable to the individual and not contraindicated by his or her status. However, assure that the activity does not unduly increase the body's metabolic rate, as this would increase the body temperature and aggravate the pruritis.

(8) Administer medications ordered for pruritis (tranquilizers, sedatives, antihistamines) after first assuring they are not principally metabolized by the liver, or if so metabolized, that the dosage has been adjusted accordingly. Careful observation for signs and symptoms of overdosage must be maintained as well as measures for safety of the individual [decreased level of consciousness (LOC) is a common side effect] and observation for effectiveness.

b. Prevent skin breakdown by:

(1) Keeping fingernails clean and clipped short.

(2) Suggesting use of clean, white, cotton gloves, especially during sleep.

(3) Keeping bedding smooth and well secured. (Wrinkles lead to excess localized venous stasis, which also aggravates itching.)

(4) Frequent changes of position and instructing individual in the need for this to prevent venous stasis, increased body heat in localized areas, and capillary dilitation.

c. Assess for extent and change in jaundice, or existence of latent jaundice if serum bilirubin is above 2 mg/dL (adult/child), or 5 mg/dL (premature infant).

(1) Inspect skin in daylight rather than in artificial light. Normally olive skin, or a fading suntan, may appear to be jaundiced in artificial light.
(2) Note color distribution. If sclera, mucous membrane, palms of hands, or soles of feet are not involved, the color change is probably normal. Color change only in areas usually tanned is probably not jaundice.
(3) Note quality of color. A somewhat bronze color, rather than golden or bright yellow, indicates hepatic or posthepatic jaundice. A light lemon-yellow tone is more indicative of pre-hepatic jaundice.
(4) Jaundice is not seen well in edematous areas because of the increased fluid and decreased protein—especially albumin—in such areas.
(5) Latent jaundice may be validated by:
 (a) Looking for scratch marks.
 (b) Applying pressure over bony prominences (sternum, tip of the nose) to blanch skin, which makes the jaundice more apparent.
(6) Monitor urine and feces for color change.
 (a) In early hemolytic jaundice, the urine color should be normal.
 (b) Tea-colored urine that will stain clothing indicates the presence of increased urobilinogen—found in posthepatic jaundice.
 (c) In hepatitis, bilirubin may appear in the urine before jaundice is evident. Urine will be dark brown and frothy ("Coca-Cola") when the concentration is high.

d. Compare serum total bilirubin with related laboratory tests to measure the effectiveness of treatment and/or progress of the disease process.
(1) The reader is referred to Wallach's *Interpretation of Diagnostic Tests* (1970) for rapid retrieval of information on specific tests in given diagnoses. Any thorough medical-surgical nursing test should also provide such information.
(2) In all cases of jaundice the fractions of serum total bilirubin can be particularly useful in following the course of the disease or response to treatment.
(3) In prehepatic, or hemolytic, jaundice, tests frequently used include: red cell fragility, reticulocyte count, peripheral blood smear, red cell survival test, Coombs' test, hemoglobin, hematocrit, serum haptoglobins, WBC, and Sickledex.
(4) In hepatic, or posthepatic, jaundice, tests frequently used include: serum transaminases [particularly gamma

glutamyl transpeptidase (GGT) or serum glutamic pyruvic transaminase (SGPT or ALT)], hepatitis B surface antigen (HB_sAg), serum total protein, serum albumin, protein electrophoresis or immunophoresis, plasma prothrombin, urobilinogen, and urine bilirubin.

e. Monitor the adult with chronic elevated serum bilirubin for the occurrence of gallstones and when appropriate, provide dietary instruction related to fat intake.

f. There is no indication in the literature of the use of phototherapy to reduce jaundice in the adult, probably because the disease effects in the adult are so much less severe than in the neonate. If, however, pruritis is a major problem and the possibility exists that reduction of the jaundice may also relieve the pruritis, further investigation of this modality could be undertaken by the nurse in collaboration with the physician.

3. *Implications related to care of the neonate with hyperbilirubinemia.* [This is only a brief synopsis of the material so well covered by Whaley and Wong (1979) with some expansion of laboratory data. The reader is referred to that text for in-depth nursing care.]

a. Prevent neonatal hyperbilirubinemia.
   (1) Early introduction of feeding, even if only water, will help prevent neonatal jaundice by increasing peristalsis to remove sterile meconium and by introducing normal intestinal flora to convert conjugated bilirubin to urobilinogen and stercobilin.
   (2) Encourage prenatal medical supervision and prenatal identification of blood group Rh type.
   (3) Follow Rh-negative women during pregnancy for increased serum bilirubin and the presence of antibodies in the mother, amniocentesis, and indirect Coombs' test.
   (4) Administer RhoGAM as ordered to Rh-negative women at delivery or at time of abortion. If there is no order for RhoGAM, follow up vigorously to attain the order. Many hospitals require mothers to sign a release if they refuse the medication.

b. Identify risk population of infants.
   (1) Amniotic fluid may be dark, due to the infant's increased urobilinogen or bilirubin.
   (2) Assess infant for jaundice at birth.
   (3) Check infant's hemoglobin and hematocrit for possible anemia due to an excessive RBC lysis.
   (4) Check for variations from normal CNS activity: irritability—tremors, twitching, high-pitched cry, convulsions,

opisthotnos—and depression—absent Moro and/or sucking reflexes, diminished deep tendon reflex, hypotonia, lethargy—as indicators of the onset of kernicterus.

c. Prevent onset, or minimize effect, of kernicterus.
   (1) Assess for, and prevent if possible, metabolic acidosis (decreased venous CO_2, blood gases).
   (2) Check serum protein electrophoresis (or serum albumin) for decreased albumin concentration. Report if low so that albumin may be given if indicated.
   (3) Discourage use of drugs that compete with bilirubin for binding sites on albumin molecule (e.g., salicylates, vitamin K, sulfonamides).
   (4) Decrease metabolic demands for oxygen or glucose by:
      (a) Placing infant in position for optimal respiratory exchange. Check that oxygen is delivered at concentration ordered. If not on oxygen, request order for oxygen if indications suggest need. Suction as indicated.
      (b) Preventing hypothermia by appropriate measures.
   (5) Check serum bilirubin response if phenobarbital given. Purpose of phenobarb administration is to increase protein synthesis/albumin production. Desired outcome: decreased concentrations of bilirubin.

d. Assist with care of complications.
   (1) Phototherapy (see Whaley and Wong, 1979, pp. 300-302). Usually instituted when bilirubin levels reach 10 mg/dL. Provide 25% additional fluid to make up for increased insensible losses. Outcome criterion: decrease in serum bilirubin levels by 3 to 4 mg/dL after 8 to 12 hr of therapy.
   (2) Exchange transfusion (see Section 14.5).

e. Provide parental support to alleviate feelings of responsibility for infant's illness, to allow mother-child bonding to occur, and to provide a realistic, positive awareness of the progress of the infant. The mortality rate in kernicterus is almost 50% during the first month.

f. Do follow-up care and teaching for the family of any full-term infant whose serum bilirubin levels approached 20 mg/dL at birth.
   (1) Parents need to keep other members of the health team informed of the child's history of hyperbilirubinemia at birth.
   (2) An early developmental and hearing assessment should be planned to determine any possible deficits due to central nervous system damage.
   (3) The infant's blood should be checked during the first 2 months for possible anemia and need for supplemental

iron. Hemolysis may continue in mild erythroblastosis fetalis, even though bilirubin levels are controlled.

1.11 SERUM CHOLESTEROL

Synonym: plasma cholesterol

Normal Ranges

Adult	
40-70 years	140–270 mg/dL
Less than 40 years	150–330 mg/dL
Senior adult	150–250 mg/dL
Pediatric	
Cord	45–100 mg/dL
Newborn	45–170 mg/dL
Infant	70–175 mg/dL
Child	120–240 mg/dL
Thereafter	150–250 mg/dL

Cholesterol is a fat-related chemical, a complex alcohol that can be synthesized by all body cells except the brain, and which can be ingested in the diet through animal protein. As an alcohol it can form esters ["a compound formed from an alcohol and an acid by removal of water" (Miller and Keane, 1972)] with fatty acid, which are the storage form of cholesterol. Cholesterol esters make up about two-thirds of the cholesterol in plasma. Free cholesterol is also found in the plasma as a lipoprotein. Cholesterol itself is insoluble in plasma, but when bound as a lipoprotein it becomes soluble and can be transported. Although these two forms of cholesterol are different, for the purpose of this discussion they can be considered together because of their closely allied role in the body.

Cholesterol is a primary constituent of the low-density lipoproteins (LDL), but can be found in the high-density lipoproteins (HDL) as well as in the very low density lipoproteins (VLDL). "Cholesterol is the most important sterol ['a solid alcohol of animal or vegetable origin with properties like fat' (Miller and Keane, 1972)] in animal metabolism" (Sodeman and Sodeman, 1974). It is found only in foods of animal origin.

Although cholesterol is considered a body lipid, it does not, as do other lipids, serve as a source of energy for metabolism. The body is unable to disintegrate the sterol ring. It is the only lipid that is excreted in appreciable amounts. The others are metabolized, stored, or utilized in body anabolism. Cholesterol probably acts as a framework in the body cells for the essential metabolic changes of the other constituents of the protoplasm. It is important in maintaining the permeability of cell membranes and is important in the synthesis of steroid hormones as a precursor of steroids of the adrenal cortex and ovary (Davidsohn and Henry, 1969). It is a major constituent of bile and bile acids.

Serum cholesterol determinations alone are of limited value. It is when they are considered together with other clinical data and bio-chemical tests, such as triglyceride levels, that they provide useful information for the diagnosis or evaluation of management of a number of diseases. Because of its medical prominence and importance, there are more methods for its measurement than for any of the other lipid fractions. Serum cholesterol measurement is essential in checking both the cardiovascular system and liver function (Kasanof, 1972).

Physiology. The serum level of cholesterol remains remarkably constant from day to day in a healthy person, but does tend to increase with age and change with populations, and there is wide variation among individuals.

The greater part of body cholesterol is produced by synthesis, about 1 g/day. Only about one-third of that amount is provided by the diet. Although an inverse ratio of synthesis to oral intake does occur, endogenous production is not completely suppressed by dietary intake, as only the hepatic synthesis is depressed. No specific serum cholesterol level has been determined as being the critical abnormal level. However, for individuals over 30 years of age, an elevated cholesterol remains one of the better indicators of risk populations for the development of ischemic heart disease (Harvey et al., 1976).

Cholesterol is synthesized by the body from small molecules in a long and complex series of condensations, transformations, and ring closures. Of these one vastly important reaction is that with acetyl CoA and acetoacetyl CoA, because this pathway is shared with both carbohydrate and fatty metabolism. Carbohydrates, amino acids, and other fats can be converted to cholesterol by this route, making the reduction of serum cholesterol by dietary means a complex and frustrating effort. The major sites of cholesterol synthesis are the liver and the intestines in humans. Not only is synthesis depressed with dietary intake of cholesterol but also with increases in insulin or thyroid hormone, and increased estrogen levels shorten the half-life of cholesterol, thereby lowering its plasma level (Sodeman and Sodeman, 1974).

Cholesterol is readily absorbable from the diet. Plants do not contain cholesterol but have other sterols, poorly absorbed by the body, which inhibit cholesterol absorption when given in large quantities —one basis for increased nonsaturated fat dietary regimes in the treatment of elevated serum cholesterol (Howard and Herbold, 1978).

Cholesterol and all lipids are digested in the duodenum. After bile emulsification, cholesterol diffuses into the blood or lymph.

Cholesterol is removed from the circulation only by the liver. It is directly secreted into bile and has a slight secretion to bile acids. Most of the cholesterol in bile is reabsorbed from the intestine, but a small amount is excreted with feces. This small amount is approximately half of all cholesterol excreted from the body. Neutral sterols, also excreted in the feces, make up most of the rest of the total cholesterol excreted. Waste products from steroid hormone synthesis are eliminated in the urine, making it a minor cholesterol excretory pathway (Davidsohn and Henry, 1969).

Cholesterol is discharged from the liver into both blood and bile, including bile acids, and the first step in the formation of steroid synthesis from cholesterol takes place within the liver. Approximately three-fourths of the cholesterol esterified by the liver is transported to the body tissues, where it is ingested and utilized. In the adrenal cortex cholesterol acts as a precursor for pregnenolone, which itself is a precursor for progesterone, testosterone, estrogen, aldosterone, and cortisol. In the skin, cholesterol is a precursor of vitamin D, activated with the application of ultraviolet light (Howard and Herbold, 1978). It also helps to provide the skin with its water-resistant quality (Harvey et al., 1976).

SERUM CHOLESTEROL DECREASED IN:

1. *Malnutrition,* due to insufficient intake of dietary protein to provide liver synthesis of lipoproteins, but when caloric intake is adequate to prevent mobilization of lipid stores.
2. *Idiopathic steatorrhea,* due to lack of intestinal absorption of amino acids, causing decreased hepatic synthesis of lipoprotein. Blocks in carbohydrate and lipid absorption contribute, but are not the major problem.
3. *Hepatocellular liver disease,* such as hepatitis. There can be marked depression with severe heptatitis or in portal cirrhosis, due to the inability of the damaged liver cell to convert protein and carbohydrate to fat. Determination of serum cholesterol levels is a frequently used tool in the diagnosis of hepatic disease. With liver disease there is a relatively larger decrease in esterified cholesterol than in free cholesterol.
4. *Hyperthyroidism,* although the depression is variable and is therefore of little use in patient evaluation. Serum cholesterol is the oldest *in vitro* measurement of thyroid function. Although it is known that thyroid stimulates removal of cholesterol by direct secretion into bile and bile acids, some authorities believe that

thyroid also stimulates cholesterol synthesis (Krueger and Ray, 1976), which may account for the variability of the serum level changes in both hyper- and hypothyroidism.

5. Decreases have been seen in *acute infection and anemia,* possibly due to decreased protein availability.

SERUM CHOLESTEROL INCREASED IN:

1. *Hyperlipoproteinemia,* with the direct cause-and-effect sequence unknown. Atherosclerosis and risk of coronary disease have been correlated with elevated lipoprotein levels, and more specifically with elevated cholesterol levels. Persons with increased cholesterol levels tend to have myocardial infarctions at an earlier age than do those with elevated triglycerides alone. Although the causes of hyperlipidemia are generally unknown, Harvey believes that it must "result from either increased synthesis or diminished removal of serum lipoproteins and their constituent lipids" (Harvey et al., 1976).
2. *Cancer of the head of the pancreas* due to blockage of excretion by biliary obstruction and/or interference with the circulation of cholesterol in the form of bile salts or neutral sterols. Elevations occur in obstructive jaundice as well, and for the same reasons. Levels can increase to 250 to 500 mg/100 ml. Greater elevations should be considered as being intrahepatic cholestasis rather than posthepatic obstruction (Davidsohn and Henry, 1969). Increased levels are sometimes found in pancreatitis due to secondary biliary obstruction.
3. *Moderate amounts in uncontrolled, or inadequately managed, diabetes mellitus,* due to a decrease in carbohydrate metabolism which causes increased utilization of lipids, increasing their serum levels as they travel to the liver. Hyperlipoproteinemia may be a contributory factor in the development of the diabetic complications of the peripheral vascular system.
4. *Hypothyroidism,* which may reflect the overall metabolic depression. The serum level is increased in spite of a decrease in cholesterol synthesis. The increased blood levels probably reflect the decrease in tissue utilization, storage, and excretion of cholesterol.
5. *Nephrotic syndrome,* a consistent feature of this disorder, due to a compensatory increase in hepatic synthesis to make up for the loss of protein through the kidney. Most plasma protein levels are decreased, but the lipid-binding proteins are not thought to pass into the urine; hence they, including cholesterol, increase in

the serum. Persons with the lowest serum albumin levels in this disorder often have the highest lipid levels (Harrington and Brenner, 1973).

6. *The third trimester of pregnancy;* the elevation remains until well after the delivery. The reason for this increase is not known.*
7. *Individuals on diets high in saturated fats.* Exogenous cholesterol will increase serum cholesterol in variable degrees. Factors that influence the amount of cholesterol absorbed include the total amount in each feeding, how frequently the feedings occur, the other types of dietary fats fed with the cholesterol, the past dietary intake, and the age of the person (Howard and Herbold, 1978). The liver tends to compensate by synthesizing less cholesterol with the additional intake. However, ingestion of *saturated* fats increases the synthesis of cholesterol.
8. *Early starvation,* probably due to mobilization of peripheral deposits.
9. *Individuals who have had a hypophysectomy* possibly linked to the loss of ACTH, which tends to decrease serum cholesterol, as well as possible decreased amounts of other hormones which tend to decrease synthesis (Faulkner et al., 1968).

IMPLICATIONS FOR NURSING

1. *To provide the most accurate data possible,* a serum lipid analysis should be done when the individual is at a stable weight, on his or her usual diet, and taking the same amount of alcoholic beverages as is his or her custom. No food or drink other than water should be given for 8 to 12 hr prior to having blood drawn for this test.
2. *Prevention of secondary problems,* or limiting the severity of the initial disorder associated with increased cholesterol and other lipids, is a major responsibility for nursing through the nursing role of health maintenance and nursing management of populations at risk. The cornerstone for nursing intervention is the precise identification of risk factors operant and adequate explanation of these factors to the individuals involved.
   a. In children who have a family history of premature cardiovascular disease (e.g., a myocardial infarction before age 50),

*For some interesting theories as to cause, the reader is referred to Pritchard and MacDonald (1976, pp. 125, 180-181).

encourage and facilitate screening tests for triglycerides and cholesterol by the age of 5.

b. All siblings of hyperlipoproteinemic persons should also be tested, regardless of age.
c. High-risk individuals, especially children, should be on low-saturated-fat diet (saturated fats in the diet being primarily coconut oil, butter fat, and animal fats). The nurse can counsel and assist in dietary planning.
d. The nurse should also supply assistance to high-risk individuals and their home caretakers in dietary planning to include increased use of polyunsaturated fats (corn, cottonseed, soy, and safflower oils as well as margarine).
e. Dietary planning should also aim to reduce total fat content in the diet to approximately 35% of dietary intake. The average diet in the United States consists of 40 to 50% fat intake. To reduce the total absorption of cholesterol, intake in the diet needs to be reduced from the usual 600 to 1200 mg/day to 100 to 300 mg/day (Howard and Herbold, 1978).
f. Water intake should be increased, unless contraindicated, to help eliminate waste products and to decrease the viscosity of the blood. A high-fat meal causes an increase in the coagulability of the blood for several hours after ingestion.
g. One of the major precipitating factors in the occurrence of hypertension is obesity. Weight loss to within one's own normal range for body build should be encouraged with dietary counseling. This should include the rationale and assistance in long-term planning for change in eating habits. Such counseling is most effective if the counselor is seen personally to follow the precautions suggested. Use of community resources (e.g., the American Heart Association) and referral to them can help the individual comply with the diet by providing additional support and assistance.
h. Yet another risk factor is that of smoking. The individual needs to be informed as to the cause-and-effect relationship and its hazards. Again, teaching is most effective when that which is taught is seen to be valued by the teacher.

3. *Assess all persons in your care,* those over the age of 30 especially, for evidence of the presence of risk factors for coronary artery disease.

   a. Presence of xanthomas (cholesterol deposits in the skin or tendons), frequently found in the achilles tendons, on the knuckles, and along the arm tendons.
   b. Family history of hyperlipidemia.

c. Personal history of alcohol abuse. Ingestions of large amounts of alcohol is felt to predispose to coronary artery disease in some types of hyperlipidemia (Howard and Herbold, 1978). Alcohol has been shown to depress ventricular performance, which causes less uptake of fatty acids leading to myocardial cell injury (Jones et al., 1978). The important factor is the amount ingested.

d. Personal smoking history, of particular importance in the occurrence of angina because of its vasoconstrictive effect.

e. Evidence of atherosclerotic arterial disease: for example, intermittent claudication; change in skin color, temperature, sensation; pain at rest; history of slow healing; easy infection and edema in the peripheral extremities, particularly the legs; faint or absent peripheral pulses (check bilaterally for comparison); bruits in peripheral arteries; trophic changes in skin on extremeties.

f. Premature arcus senilis. When it occurs with xanthomas, it is almost always indicative of familial hypercholesterolemia (Harvey et al., 1976).

g. Increased blood pressure. For persons over 50 a blood pressure of 160/95 indicates the need for further screening. Elevation of the diastolic pressure is more significant than elevation of the systolic pressure.

h. Significant glycosuria, or a fasting serum glucose of greater than 120 mg/dL, indicates a twofold risk of coronary heart disease.

i. Increases in uric acid levels greater than 7.5 mg/dL also contribute to coronary artery disease risk.

j. Increased serum sodium levels can indicate a potential for increased blood pressure and may need further examination as a risk factor.

4. *If any of the foregoing indicators are positive,* collaborate with the physician—or suggest that the individual confer with his or her physician—in order to obtain both serum cholesterol and triglyceride determinations if no recent test results are available. Any increase in normal levels should be followed seriously. If serum cholesterol and triglycerides are within normal limits, a primary lipid metabolic disorder is usually ruled out (Davidsohn and Henry, 1969).

5. *Increased cholesterol levels found in women around the menopausal age* should be investigated further on the possibility of the existence of hypothyroidism. Onset at this age is frequent in women and is easily mistaken for part of the menopausal syn-

drome (Spenser, 1973). Rather typical of hypothyroidism is an asymptomatic and concurrent increase of cholesterol, uric acid, and SGOT with normal liver function. Given the occurrence of increased cholesterol in women as described above, thyroid function should be checked.

6. *Gallstones should be suspected* in the individual with elevated cholesterol levels, accompanied by a history of gastrointestinal symptoms and/or fatty intolerance. With increased synthesis of cholesterol, the cholesterol contents of bile become supersaturated in relation to the other two components of bile, leading to cholesterol precipitation and stone formation.
7. *Persons being treated for primary biliary cirrhosis* with elevation of cholesterol levels, due to retention of bile, may show a drop toward normal in the cholesterol level, which can be secondary to liver failure. This decrease in cholesterol could easily be misinterpreted as a positive response to treatment (Frolich, 1976). Locate available liver function tests and examine the person for signs and symptoms of liver failure when cholesterol levels have reduced but the evidence of biliary cirrhosis has not. Bear in mind that symptoms and signs of liver failure occur only when there is diffuse parenchymal damage. Look for jaundice, bleeding tendencies, ascites, generalized edema, lortal hypertension, hepatomegaly, and skin changes.
8. *Knowledge of the action and uses of medication* to decrease serum cholesterol is basic in giving adequate nursing care.
   a. A trial of diet therapy and/or weight reduction is usually performed before medications are started because of the possible side effects of medication and, in some cases, because the medication is very distasteful when given orally (Govoni and Hayes, 1978).
   b. Drug therapy should be accompanied by an initial determination of serum cholesterol and triglycerides levels and the tests repeated at least at monthly intervals during treatment.
   c. The effectiveness of therapy—diet or medication—should be assessed by noting any changes in the size of xanthomas, return of pertinent laboratory values to normal range (see above), change in weight, and/or reduction in blood pressure.
   d. Dextrothyroxine sodium (Choloxin), an isomer of thyroxine, cannot be given to persons with known heart disease or those with familial increase in cholesterol. It tends to increase the body's metabolic rate, and signs and symptoms of coronary artery disease are known side effects. The purpose in giving

the drug is to prevent extension of atherosclerosis as well as to decrease cholesterol levels.

(1) Determination of protein-bound iodine is useful in validating effectiveness of the drug. Increased levels indicate drug absorption and transport.

(2) Can cause iodism and signs and symptoms (e.g., acneiform rash, itching, runny nose, brassy taste in mouth) should be reported immediately so that the drug can be discontinued.

e. Cholestyramine resin (Questran) is used as an adjunct to diet. It combines with bile salts, forming a nonabsorbable and insoluble compound that is excreted in the feces. It has many side effects. Prevent and/or alleviate them by:

(1) Providing a high-bulk diet and adequate fluids to prevent constipation.

(2) Reporting the occurrence of constipation and adjusting dosage as ordered.

(3) Observing for signs and symptoms of fat-soluble vitamin deficiency with long-term use: for example, observe for bleeding tendencies.

(4) Scheduling other oral medications and meals (e.g., 1 hr prior to giving Questran) so that their absorption is interfered with as little as possible. Questran can be given concurrently with Choloxin.

9. *Persons with nephrotic syndrome* are often placed on high-protein diets, which is not usual in other persons with increased cholesterol levels. Their need for replacement of plasma proteins supersedes their need to decrease cholesterol levels (Kagan, 1979, p. 98).

1.12 SERUM ENZYMES

Enzymes are special chemical catalysts, invariably protein, of biological origin. All living organisms synthesize enzymes. They are rapidly degraded and replenished. Enzymes are essential to life, enabling the many biochemical reactions in the body cells to occur. There is no test to measure the intracellular enzyme concentration *directly*. The serum measurements done are assumed to parallel enzyme concentrations and changes within the cells, much as serum potassium is believed to reflect intracellular potassium (Tietz, 1970).

Over 700 enzymes have been isolated and because of the increasing number and the increasing application to clinical laboratory work, a standard classification system was produced for general use. Of importance to nursing is an awareness that this system provides for more than one term to be used in dealing with an enzyme. For example, the test frequently referred to as serum LDH is also known as (1)L-lactate:NAP oxidoreductose—systemic name; (2) 1.1.1.27—International Union of Biologists code designation; and (3) lactate dehydrogenase—practical name. Enzymes named in recent years have suffix endings of "ase." Those named years ago may have names that do not now fit into the classification system but are retained as trivial or common names because of their familiarity (e.g., ptyalin for amylase). The classification system assists the clinical chemist in communication with other health team members, and vice versa (Tietz, 1970).

Intracellular enzymes have no known physiological function in the plasma and appear in much lower concentrations there than within the cell. Serum increases occur, their cause dependent on the physiologic mechanism of the enzyme involved. If an enzyme is present in fairly large concentrations in only one organ, a serum increase would help to determine the affected organ. Such enzymes are called *tissue-* or *organ-specific* enzymes, examples being acid phosphatase of the prostate gland or acetylcholinesterase of RBCs. *Non-tissue-* or *non-organ-specific* enzymes, when increased in serum levels, can be compared with levels of other such enzymes for information as to the affected organ, because the several enzymes are present in different tissues in different ratios. For example, damage to the liver cells will usually cause an increase in serum glutamic oxaloacetic transaminase (SGOT or AST), but many other cell injuries could cause the same rise. In comparing the SGOT to another enzyme, such as serum glutamic pyruvic transaminase (SGPT or ALt), more specific information is possible. If the SGPT is increased, liver damage can be fairly safely assumed because SGPT is more specific to liver cells while SGOT is more sensitive to change in the status of the liver cell. If SGPT were within normal limits, liver damage could almost be ruled out (Tietz, 1970). Therefore, a single test for a serum enzyme of a non-tissue or nonorgan-specific type is of limited diagnostic value in itself. Such a test can be most useful in following the course of a disease process once diagnosed, or following the response of the body to treatment. Isoenzyme fractionation of non-tissue- or non-organ-specific enzymes seems to be tissue-specific and can be used to follow up screening tests (Frolich, 1976).

Decreased serum enzyme levels happen infrequently and may or may not be of clinical importance. However, the absence in the serum of an expected enzyme is usually related to a single gene abnormality—an inborn error of metabolism—which results in the loss of services of tha enzyme [e.g., albinism, storage diseases (such as Gaucher's), Tay-Sachs disease, or phenylketonuria (PKU)] (Price and Wilson, 1978).

Units of measurement for serum enzymes can be a great source of confusion. International units (IU) of measurement are being adopted, but in the United States at least, other units of measurement are still in use. Thus Bodansky, King-Armstrong (KA), or Bessey-Lowrey units will be given in many lists of normal ranges. Conversion from one type of unit to another can produce results that are grossly in error even when International units are used, unless it is known that the exact methodologies were followed for the tests used, and that ambient conditions were identical in all laboratories. Therefore, the units given in this text (in International units, whenever available) do not reflect other measuring system units and the practitioner is *strongly* urged to work with the unit system given in the facility which has determined that client's serum levels. Efforts should *not* be made to translate results from one system of measurement to another.

This section deals with only three of the myriad of possible serum enzyme tests. These are the tests found to be used fairly consistently as screening tests. They provide a fairly broad, non-tissue- or non-organ-specific survey and offer information about several organs or systems within the body (e.g., cardiac, liver, skeletal, lung). This broad view makes them good screening tests.

1.12.1 Serum Alkaline Phosphatase

Synonyms: phosphatase, alkaline; ALP; alkaline phosphatase; SAP

Normal Ranges

Adult	
Male	19– 74 IU/L
Female	12– 63 IU/L (International units/liter)
Senior adult	
Male	19.0– 74 IU/L
Female	12.0– 63 IU/L
Pediatric	
Newborn	50–275 IU/L
Infant	100–330 IU/L
Child	90–230 IU/L
Adolescent	100–250 IU/L

Physiology and Pathophysiology. Serum alkaline phosphatase (SAP) is found in almost all body tissues. It is manufactured by bone (40 to 75%), liver, intestine, and placenta. It is called an enzyme of secretion. In the healthy person it is secreted constantly and rapidly from the cell into the interstitial area, and thence into the serum. Alkaline phosphatase is necessary for hydrolysis of organic phosphates and is, therefore, important to digestion and absorption through the mucous membrane of the gastrointestinal tract. The component produced by the liver is in greatest concentration in the serum of adults.

It is rapidly and constantly disposed of into urine, bile, and the gastrointestinal tract. There is some question as to the enzyme's actual pathway and, at one point, Tietz states that the enzyme found in the urine is that from kidney tissue only, and does not represent serum enzyme cleared by the kidney (Tietz, 1970). In any case, the constant secretion and excretion produces a relatively constant and low serum level. Should one of the excretory routes be blocked, the rate of production increased, or the rate of release from the cell increased, plasma levels will rise.

Activity of SAP gives important information about bone formation (osteoblastic activity) and is clinically useful as a test of liver function being the most sensitive test of common bile duct obstruction (Harvey et al., 1976). It is a more sensitive index of bile stasis than is the serum bilirubin level.

SAP is frequently the first enzyme to be studied in hepatic disease and is used extensively in differential diagnosis of jaundice. An increased serum level is said to reflect acute liver cell disease (given validation that it is the liver component that is elevated), or bile duct obstruction, but is not specific to any one liver disease. The mechanism of SAP increase with hepatobiliary disease is not clear. It is thought to be related to both impaired excretion with regurgitation of bile alkaline phosphatase, and to increased formation by, or release from, hepatic cells (Davidsohn and Henry, 1969). The mechanism for increase with bone formation is more straightforward in that the enzyme is formed by the osteoblast, so that increased numbers of osteoblastic cells will result in increased SAP concentrations.

SAP of bone origin can be differentiated from SAP of liver origin in a rough estimation by its response to heat: SAP of bone origin is heat stable whereas that of liver origin is not. As usually analyzed in most clinical laboratories, however, the activity of osseous alkaline phosphatase and hepatic activity are indistinguishable. There is often a significant overlap in the heat test and it has been found to be most useful in separating bone-liver SAP as a group from tumor-placenta as a group (SHMC, 1978). Isoenzymes are tissue-specific but seldom used.

Low levels of SAP are rarely encountered.

SAP INCREASED IN:

1. *Bone disease,* due to stimulation of osteoblastic activity secondary to bone destruction and remodeling, found in:
   a. Paget's disease (osteitis deformans), which demonstrates some of the highest known levels with localized bone destruction, absorption, and abnormal new formation.

b. Osteogenic sarcoma with increases 20 to 40 times normal. Other primary bone tumors will cause similar, but lesser, increases (e.g., chondrosarcoma).
c. Osteomalacia with moderate increases, due to low serum calcium stimulating parathyroid activity. Active rickets will present a similar picture for the same reason with increases two to four times normal.
d. Metastatic bone tumors from any primary site, but most commonly prostatic and breast cancer.
e. Healing fractures, frequently, but not always.

2. *Liver disease,* or hepatobiliary disease, such as:
   a. Biliary cirrhosis, or Laennec's cirrhosis, due to hepatic cellular damage and release of alkaline phosphatase, causing marked increases, but less than in biliary obstruction.
   b. Biliary obstruction, found secondary to a number of obstructive processes (e.g., gallstones, biliary atresia). Increases occur secondary to stimulation of, or injury to, epithelial cells of the liver or biliary tree (Sodeman and Sodeman, 1974).
   c. Toxic hepatitis (chlorpromazine hepatitis), due to a hypersensitivity response. Viral hepatitis often will not cause an increase in SAP.
   d. Space-occupying lesions or granulomatous diseases of the liver, such as amyloidosis, sarcoidosis, tuberculosis, and to a lesser degree, cancer. Primary hepatomas show no consistent elevation of SAP levels.

3. *Faulty calcium metabolism in kidney disease,* such as:
   a. Renal tubular acidosis, due to faulty calcium and phosphate reabsorption in the tubules, causing increased calcium reabsorption secondary to parathyroid stimulation and a reactive increase in SAP in an attempt to maintain normal calcium/phosphorus serum levels.
   b. Chronic nephritis, due to impaired calcium absorption secondary to the kidney's inability to form the active metabolite of vitamin D, causing decreased serum calcium, parathyroid stimulation, bone resorption, and an osteoblastic reaction.
   c. Chronic glomerulonephritis, due to decreased serum calcium. (Mechanism similar to that given in item b above.)

4. *Faulty or inadequate calcium absorption from the gastrointestinal tract,* causing a decrease in serum calcium levels which stimulates parathyroid activity, ultimately increasing osteoblastic activity

followed by alkaline phosphatase release into the serum. Found in:

a. Malnutrition.
b. Malabsorption syndromes in which calcium combines with the increased fats retained in the alimentary canal, forming an insoluble calcium soap, and decreasing absorption of fat-soluble vitamin D.
c. Hypovitaminosis D.

5. *Hyperparathyroidism* (rationale given above in item 3).
6. *Physiologic states* such as:
   a. Third trimester of pregnancy with increases two to three times normal, believed to be due to increased production from the placenta (Tietz, 1970).
   b. Periods of rapid growth and bone building.
   c. Aging. Normal values in healthy adults over age 70 may be one to one and one-half times the standard normal values (Carnevali and Patrick, 1979).

SAP DECREASED IN (Tietz, 1970; Collins, 1975):

1. *Kwashiorkor,* due to protein deficiency.
2. *Congenital hypophosphatasia,* due to lack of production.
3. *Dwarfism.*
4. *General debility and anemia;* exact mechanism not clear.

IMPLICATIONS FOR NURSING

1. *Serum for testing* must be free from hemolysis because of the large concentrations of alkaline phosphatase in RBCs. No special patient preparation is necessary.
2. *Serial determinations of SAP* are necessary for any conclusions as to dysfunction or response to treatment.
3. *An increase in SAP* without a rise in any other intracellular enzyme is probably due to bone enzyme serum increases. Other enzymes are not present in bone to any great extent.
4. *Correlation with clinical and laboratory data* helps to determine the importance/impact of an increased SAP level, and to indicate progress and prognosis.

a. Check serum calcium and phosphorus levels.
   (1) Increased SAP with a normal serum calcium and phosphorus occurs in osteogenic sarcoma. A dramatic rise in SAP in patients with Paget's disease may indicate a common complication of the disease—osteogenic sarcoma.
   (2) Imbalance in serum calcium, either increased or decreased levels, can ultimately cause an increase in SAP. (See "SAP Increased in," item 3.)

b. Check serum bilirubin.
   (1) Serum bilirubin and serum cholesterol can be expected to be elevated, together with the SAP in toxic hepatitis.
   An increase in bilirubin and cholesterol with the clinical picture of hepatitis, but without increases in SAP, may indicate viral hepatitis.
   (2) A normal serum bilirubin and an increased SAP may be suggestive of liver metastasis, given a known primary site or may suggest other space-occupying lesions, such as sarcoidosis or amyloidosis (Harvey et al., 1976).

c. Check x-ray films of long bones for demineralization.

5. *Comparison of an individual case* of increased SAP with others of the same diagnosis is not a fruitful exercise, as there is considerable variation in serum levels from patient to patient.

6. *Correlate with changes in jaundice.*
   a. A rise in SAP usually parallels the degree of jaundice.
   b. Higher levels are more likely an indicator of posthepatic jaundice than viral hepatitis.

7. *Correlate with therapy*
   a. Administration of vitamin D for osteomalacia should cause a slow drop in the SAP.
   b. SAP is the best indicator of the extent and change in bile stasis; it is more specific and sensitive than serum bilirubin.

8. *Prevent progression of liver disease in infants.* Prevent neonatal hepatitis due to a variety of congenital infectious agents, (e.g., rubella, herpes simplex, syphillis, cytomegalovirus) by thorough prenatal assessment, care, and teaching. In turn, the prevention of neonatal hepatitis prevents cirrhosis development in the infant, which is extremely debilitating and often fatal. Infectious hepatitis is also thought to influence the development of biliary atresia in the fetus (Whaley and Wong, 1979).

1.12.2 Serum Glutamic Oxalic Transaminase

Synonyms: aspartate aminotransferase; AST; GOT; SGOT

Normal Ranges

Adult	0–41 IU/L
Senior adult	8–33 IU/mL
Pediatric	
Newborn	2–55 IU/L at 31° C
Over 2 years	10–30 IU/L at 31° C

Physiology. GOT, an intracellular enzyme, is an enzyme of cellular metabolism with no known function in the plasma. Serum values for females are lower than for males (e.g., at ages 20 to 29, the males' range is 0.0 to 40.6, females from 0.0 to 31.8) and increase slightly with age, becoming almost equal with male values (Carnevali and Patrick, 1979). Very high concentrations of enzyme are found intracellularly; very low concentrations are found in serum and the enzyme may be totally absent when all cell membranes are intact.

The function of transaminase is to catalyze transfer of an amino group from one amino acid to a keto acid, thus forming another amino acid. GOT is widely distributed in the body tissues and is found in particularly high concentrations in those tissues with high metabolic activity. In descending order of enzyme concentration, these tissues are cardiac, hepatic, renal, skeletal muscle tissue, and red blood cells. The enzyme is present, but in lesser concentration in the cells of the lung, brain, and pancreas (SHMC, 1978).

Because of its wide distribution, GOT is considered a nontissue- or non-organ-specific enzyme and is, therefore, most helpful when its serum level is compared with the levels of several different serum enzymes (Tietz, 1970). Little is known of the production, regulation, or excretion of the transaminases. Very little SGOT is excreted in the bile because of the blood-bile barrier, and it is not known whether the small amount found in bile is from the blood or directly from the liver cells (Collins, 1975).

Pathophysiology. When body cells containing GOT are damaged, or their activity impaired or destroyed due to deficient oxygen or glucose, the cell membrane becomes permeable, or may rupture. The GOT, together with other cell contents, finds its way to the plasma, increasing the serum concentration of GOT (Tietz, 1970). The greater the intracellular concentration of the enzyme, the higher, and the more rapid, the rise in serum levels with cell damage. For example, damage to as little as 1% of the liver cells can rise the serum level of GOT because of the relatively high intracellular enzyme concentration as well as the large number of hepatic cells the 1% represents (Sodeman and Sodeman, 1974). Damage to cardiac tissue produces a rather rapid rise of SGOT; the degree of elevation correlates closely with the size of the infarct. Increases of over 500 units are unusual with solely cardiac involvement. In cardiac failure (congestive heart failure) elevations of over 1000 may occur. This extreme elevation is apparently due to the secondary congestion and necrosis of the liver rather than cardiac cell injury per se (Collins, 1975). In liver disease higher levels are produced. The release of GOT from the liver cells does not reflect liver function, which may well be normal even in the face of high SGOT levels. SGOT reflects the cells response to injury and greater cell membrane permeability.

Functional change of the liver occurs only after cell necrosis. Prolonged SGOT elevation in liver disease may be the first indication of a nonresolving or chronic active hepatitis. A rapid drop may indicate total liver failure (Harvey et al., 1976). SGOT also increases with cellular damage to skeletal muscle, but is the least sensitive indicator of muscle involvement. Although not specific to any one organ or system, SGOT changes are thought to be more sensitive to change in liver status than the more specific liver enzymes (e.g., SGPT). (See Appendix E for definitions of test sensitivity and test specificity.)

Since the normal range of SGOT includes complete absence of the enzyme in body serum, decreases in the serum level are of interest only insofar as the speed with which the drop occurs (liver failure), or as an indicator of disease progress and response to treatment.

SGOT INCREASED IN:

1. *Conditions causing injury to cardiac muscle cells,* as in:
   a. Myocardial infarction. Serum levels may increase to 500 IU (from a norm of 10 to 40 IU) within 24 hr (Phipps et al., 1979) and will return to normal in 4 to 7 days if further cell damage does not occur.
   b. Cardiac failure (congestive heart failure). Serum levels are frequently increased, but the amount of increase varies, depending on concomitant liver involvement (see "Pathophysiology" above).
2. *Conditions causing injury to hepatic tissue cells,* as in:
   a. Viral hepatitis. Serum levels are often high (greater than 100 IU) (Harvey et al., 1976). The major rise occurs in the prodromal-preicteric stage.

b. Hepatitis due to ingestion of toxic substances. Serum levels of 30,000 IU/mL are seen in carbon tetrachloride poisoning (Collins, 1975).
c. Obstructive jaundice. Elevations are relatively modest, usually under 300 IU/mL (Frolich, 1976).
d. Cirrhosis, metastatic malignancy of the liver and, less commonly, primary hepatomas, all of which can product hepatic necrosis and a clinical picture somewhat similar to that of hepatitis (Collins, 1975).
e. Acute pancreatitis due to posthepatic obstruction.
f. Morphine administration, which decreases biliary secretions and increases the tone of gastrointestinal and biliary sphincters (Govoni and Hayes, 1978).

3. *Conditions causing injury to skeletal muscle cells,* as in:
   a. Dermatomyositis. [Included among the group of collagen diseases. Can be acute, subacute, or chronic. Characterized by constant inflammation of muscles, leading to decomposition and atrophy (Spenser, 1973).] Since GOT is so widely distributed in the body, serum elevations are highly nonspecific in muscle disease and creatine phosphokinase (CPK) or aldolase are more specific and useful tests.
   b. Progressive muscular dystrophy, due to the cellular injury caused by the replacement of muscle cells with fat and connective tissue and an inflammatory process.
   c. Muscular trauma, due to overuse or external injury.
   d. Trichinosis, possibly due to cellular inflammation and injury resulting from the lodging of the larvae in body tissues such as the heart, lung, and striated muscle.

4. *Any condition that causes red blood cell lysis,* which releases GOT into the serum (e.g., hemolytic anemias).

5. *Later stages of pulmonary thromboembolism* (Harvey, 1976); see "Implications for Nursing," item 3a, in Section 1.12.3.

6. *Infectious mononucleosis* at times. Possibly due to liver involvement, which occurs in 8 to 10% of all cases and which resembles infectious hepatitis. May also be due, rarely, to involvement of the heart and lung.

7. *Hepatoxicity* secondary to administration of many drugs [e.g., narcotics (see item 2f above), analgesics, antibiotics, and steroids] (Danovitch et al., 1971).

SGOT DECREASED IN:

Not clinically significant.

1.12.3 Serum Lactic Dehydrogenase—Total

Synonyms: lactic acid dehydrogenase; LDH-L; LDH

Normal Ranges

Adult	60–220 IU/L
Senior adult	71–207 IU/L
Pediatric	
Newborn	300–500 IU/L
Thereafter	
Male	50–150 IU/L
Female	41–140 IU/L

Physiology. As with SGOT, LDH is an intracellular enzyme of cellular metabolism, present in very high concentrations within the cell, comparatively low in serum concentration—although higher than that of SGOT—and always present in the serum in some amount. The enzyme has no known function in the serum. LDH is involved in the end reaction of the anaerobic phase of carbohydrate metabolism, reducing pyruvic acid to lactic acid and, in the presence of oxygen, oxidizing lactic acid to pyruvic acid. As with SGOT, LDH is non-tissue- or non-organ-specific and is present in widely distributed body cells. It is found in substantial amounts, in decreasing order, in the following tissues; skeletal muscle, liver, heart, pancreas, spleen, and brain (SHMC, 1978). It is also present in varying concentrations in lymph nodes, thyroid, adrenal, and lung tissue. Its isoenzymes are more tissue-specific, and although not used as screening tests, are frequently employed to validate a diagnosis (see Part III). Tissue specificity in the isoenzymes by American classification follows the following pattern: LDH, heart; LDH_2, kidney and heart; LDH_3, adrenal and lung; LDH_4, lung; LDH_5, liver. In British classification the series is reversed in mirror image.

Pathophysiology. The mechanism for release of LDH from the cells is the same as that described for SGOT with increasing cell permeability, or rupture, in response to injury. The resulting increases in serum levels are proportionate to the extent of tissue damage and the degree of intracellular concentrations of the enzyme in a given tissue. The elevations of LDH occurring after a myocardial infarction stay increased much longer than those of other intracellular enzymes. LDH is considered highly sensitive in determining myocardial infarction and is more specific than CPK.

LDH is the least specific of enzymes in liver disorders and probably the most specific for pulmonary emboli. However, some 50% of all pulmonary emboli show no abnormality of serum enzymes; thus the LDH specificity is, at best, only 50% (Danovitch et al., 1971). Therefore, pulmonary embolism cannot be ruled out in the absence of serum enzyme elevations. LDH may also increase in renal disorders, neoplastic disease, and liver disease. Isoenzymes increase long before the total LDH (Widmann, 1979).

LDH INCREASED IN:

1. *Conditions causing cardiac cell damage,* as in:
   a. Myocardial infarction. Increase occurs 12 to 24 hr after injury and remains elevated for a prolonged period—up to 2 weeks, or as long as active inflammation persists (Harvey et al., 1976).
   b. Congestive heart failure, only when there is liver involvement as with SGOT. Values will be normal in congestive heart failure alone. Isoenzyme elevated will be LDH_5.
2. *Acute hepatitis* with large serum concentration increase. Only LDH_5 rises. Most liver diseases causing increased levels have increases in LDH_5 (Tietz, 1970).
3. *Approximately 50% of patients with a diagnosis of carcinoma.* This is a nonspecific change of no particular diagnostic value.
4. *Untreated pernicious anemia,* especially when hemoglobin is less than 8 g/dL (Wallach, 1970), due to hemolysis. A slight increase occurs in severe hemolytic anemias.
5. *Cardiac valve prosthesis postoperatively* (Holloway, 1979).
6. *Renal infarct occasionally,* but the increase is not clinically useful.
7. *Pulmonary infarction* with a rise in LDH_2 and LDH_3, but if hemolysis occurs due to hemorrhage about the infarct, LDH_1 may also rise.
8. *Skeletal muscle disease* with increases in isoenzymes 3, 4, and 5. This very lack of specificity makes the test of little value in evaluating the muscle disease (Streeten, 1971).
9. *The period following severe exercise* with a rapid rise and fall.

LDH DECREASED IN:

Not clinically significant.

IMPLICATIONS FOR NURSING FOR SGOT AND LDH

1. *No specific preparation* is usually required for the person having these tests, except in cases of suspected hepatic disease. If possible, any hepatotoxic drugs should be withdrawn for about 12 hr prior to testing (Danovitch et al., 1971). The person drawing the blood should assure that the sample is free from hemolysis. Care should be taken to avoid shaking the container and the sample should be sent promptly to the laboratory (Holloway, 1979).

2. *Intramuscular injections* should be avoided to prevent increases in serum levels in any person being followed with enzyme determinations for indication of disease progress or response to treatment.

3. *Because these serum enzyme tests are non-tissue- or non-organ-specific,* relationships among the enzymes tested should be explored. Nursing care can then be planned, based on the nurse's and/or physician's interpretation of those relationships, to support the organ or system threatened as well as the individual's ability to cope with the physiologic and psychologic changes occurring. SGOT and LDH changes very generally indicate dysfunction of either the heart, the lung, the liver, or skeletal muscle.

   a. Indications of lung dysfunction—generally limited to pulmonary embolism—differentiated from myocardial infarction. Enzymes are not totally reliable in pulmonary embolism and can often be normal, especially with smaller infarcts.
      (1) SGOT will be normal in 60 to 75% of all patients with pulmonary embolism or only slightly increased some time after infarct (Harvey et al., 1976).
      (2) LDH usually increased (isoenzymes LDH_2 and LDH_3) on the day of the embolism.
      (3) CPK will be normal.
      (4) Other laboratory data confirming status:
         (a) WBC increased with increased neutrophils.
         (b) Erythrocyte sedimentation rate (ESR) increased.
         (c) Serum bilirubin frequently increased to greater than 5 mg/dL.
         (d) Chest film or lung scan showing infarct shadow.
         (e) Serum aldolase slightly increased (Wallach, 1970).

b. Indications of myocardial infarction:

(1) SGOT increased. Not usually increased in pulmonary embolism. SGOT is the least useful of enzyme tests for diagnosis or prognostic application.

(2) LDH increased. Isoenzyme LDH_1 and LDH_2 elevated—LDH_1 greater than LDH_2, which is of specific diagnostic value (Holloway, 1979); see Part III.

(3) CPK increased. It is *not* increased in lung injury or liver disease. For further information regarding CPK isoenzymes, see Section 12.3.1. Enzymes are helpful not only in prognosis, but as a "clock" to tell when an infarct actually occurred. (See Fig. 1.2 as to amount and duration of increase.) Any noticeable deviation from the expected curve of enzyme activity indicates a pathologic change and must be reported promptly.

(4) Other laboratory data conforming status:

(a) Technetium pyrophosphate scan for circulatory perfusion changes of the heart.

(b) 12-lead ECG.

(c) Ultrasound imaging (echograms).

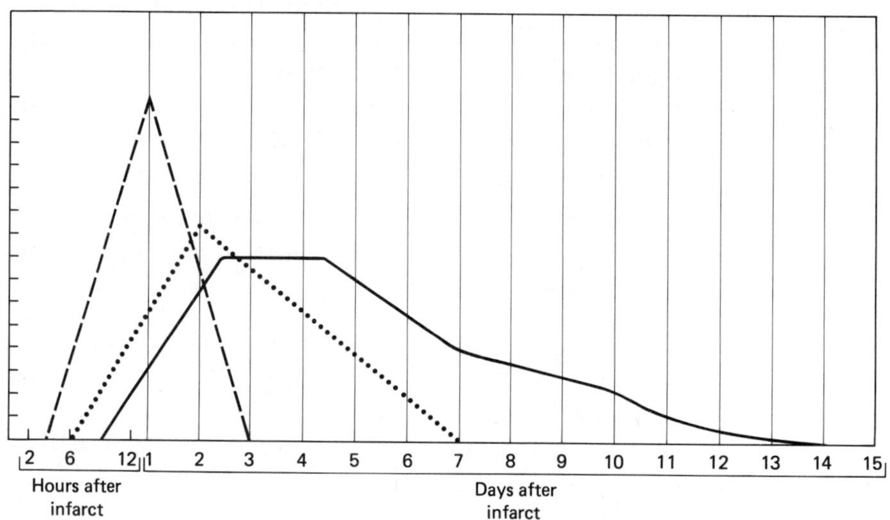

— — CPK : Increases within 2 to 5 hours; peaks during first 24 hours at 5 to 15 times normal; returns to normal by 2nd or 3rd day.

—— LDH : Increases in 6 to 12 hours after infarction; peaks in 42 to 72 hours at 2 to 8 times normal; returns to normal 5 to 6 days later, but can persist to 10th day – or two weeks after infarct.

•••••• SGOT : Increases within 6 hours after infarction; peaks in 24 to 48 hours at 2 to 15 times normal value; returns to normal after 3 to 7 days.

FIGURE 1.2 Elevation of enzymes in myocardial infarction.

c. Indications of liver dysfunction:
   (1) SGOT.
      (a) Values greater than 500 IU are more likely related to liver dysfunction than cardiac.
      (b) Values usually increase prior to the occurrence of jaundice in hepatitis.
      (c) Read, or obtain if not available, a medical and social history for any person whose SGOT levels reach concentrations in excess of 500 IU with some signs or symptoms of liver involvement (e.g., increased SAP, jaundice), to determine possible contacts with viral heptatitis.
      (d) Those with levels over 1000 IU should have a careful investigation of recent history to identify any possible toxic ingestants.
   (2) LDH is not usually increased in viral hepatitis or in posthepatic obstruction. Increase will occur with an associated malignancy.
      (a) Slight to moderate increase in LDH in cirrhosis.
      (b) LDH is less useful than SGOT or SGPT in the diagnosis or evaluation of liver disease.
      (c) Serial alterations follow a characteristic pattern; deviation indicates relapse or complication (see Fig. 1.2).
   (3) CPK normal.
   (4) Other laboratory data confirming status:
      (a) Increased serum bilirubin in posthepatic and intrahepatic obstruction.
      (b) Increased SAP.
      (c) Increased SGPT (more specific to liver disease than LDH or GOT).
      (d) Increased gamma glutamyl transferase (GGT) in hepatobiliary and pancreatic disease.
      (e) Decreased serum albumin, increased serum globulin, in long-term cirrhosis particularly. Total protein may be normal or decreased. Rarely increased.

d. Indications of skeletal muscle disorders:
   (1) Enzyme tests should be taken at a time of maximum muscle tenderness and fever.
   (2) SGOT and LDH usually elevated in myositis.
   (3) CPK, aldolase, and SGOT increase first in acute myopathies (12 to 24 hr); LDH increases after 48 hr.
   (4) Abnormal CPK activity (increased levels) occur in some asymptomatic carriers of muscular dystrophy (Duchenne's disease) (Danovitch et al., 1971).

(5) Other laboratory data confirming status:
  (a) Muscle biopsy.
  (b) Electromyographic studies.

1.13 THYROID FUNCTION DETERMINATION AS A SCREENING TEST

Normal Ranges	
T_4 RIA	4.5–12.5 μg/dL
TSH	2.0–10.0 μg/dL

IMPLICATIONS FOR NURSING

Newborns are frequently screened for disorders in serum chemicals other than those discussed thus far (see Section 1.14). Tests included in such screening of newborns are, among others, evaluation of the level of thyroid stimulating hormone (TSH) and thyroxine (T_4) (see Section 8.3 for further information on these tests). There exist other groups at risk for thyroid dysfunction which should be screened as carefully as are newborns. Further, *any* physical examination done by any health practitioner should include palpation of the thyroid as well, and a history and physical examination that is sensitive to manifestations of thyroid disorders.

A. Identification of groups at risk

The Most Commonly Screened Group—Newborns. Hypothyroidism is one of the most common endocrine problems of childhood. If the diagnosis is delayed past early infancy, the chance of permanent mental retardation is great, and the neonate does not usually exhibit obvious signs of hypothyroidism (Whaley and Wong, 1979). Despite the fact that congenital hypothyroidism occurs in only approximately 1 of 5000 live births (SHMC, 1978), the significant risks of mental retardation and failure in physical development indicate a strong need for such screening.

Males over 50 Years of Age. This group of individuals has been found to more likely present with a masked form of hyperthyroidism (apathetic hyperthyroidism) in which the epinephrinelike effects are not prominent. The lack of these characteristic signs and symptoms, such as tremor, hyperkinetic behavior, tachycardia, and heat intolerance, make the likelihood of accurate diagnosis and treatment of the thyroid imbalance highly unlikely (Harvey et al., 1976). Single-system predominance of hyperthyroid symptoms also occurs more frequently in this age/sex group. Hyperthyroidism should be suspected, and tested for, when such individuals present with unexplained congestive heart failure or arrhythmias such as atrial fibrillation/flutter, first-degree block, or multifocal premature ventricular contractions (PVC). Also suspect would be a new onset, or accentuation of previous, angina pectoris, or when there is a lack of response to, or requirement for, unusually high doses of digitalis for control of cardiac symptoms.

Other systems can produce the major number of systemic symptoms in masked hyperthyroidism: for example, the person presenting with skeletal muscle wasting and weakness; profound weight loss without muscle wasting; unexplained severe abdominal cramps—with or without pernicious diarrhea, which, when it occurs, is unaccompanied by blood or pus—or profound depression or marked emotional lability (Harvey et al., 1976).

Individuals with Psychiatric Problems. Masked hyperthyroidism should be screened for, and ruled out, in all newly diagnosed psychiatric patients. Although it has been suggested that the presence of thyroid increase can precipitate frank psychosis in persons with latent psychiatric problems, it is also possible that hyperthyroidism presenting only as profound depression or marked emotional lability can be misdiagnosed as a purely psychiatric problem.

Previously diagnosed psychiatric patients who suffer an unexplained decompensation in their condition should also be evaluated for thyroid imbalance.

Both hyperthyroidism and hypothyroidism may present with single system predominence and signs and symptoms of the imbalance may be overlooked, or treated as a totally different problem, for weeks, months, even years.

Menopausal Women. This group is less readily defined by age, but as a group women in general have a higher incidence of almost all endocrine disorders and might benefit from closer attention to the possibility of thyroid disorders.

Women of menopausal age, especially those showing an increase in serum cholesterol, should be considered with a high index of suspicion for a decrease in thyroid function (Spenser, 1973).

The Elderly (over 70 Years of age). This population was once thought to be at particular risk for hypothyroidism. More recent investigation makes the concept of routine senile hypothyroidism less easy to accept. The gland does atrophy with age, and function does decline—there is a decrease in circulating T_3—but it is more logical to assume that the decrease in normal thyroxine turnover is due to reduced peripheral need (Carnevali and Patrick, 1979; Groer and Shekleton, 1979). However, hypothyroidism can and does occur in the elderly and should be assessed.

Individuals with a History of Low-dose Irradiation to the Head, Neck, or Superior Mediastinum (usually over age 25). Although thyroid cancer may be associated with euthyroidism, hyperthyroidism, or hypothyroidism, so that evaluation of the hormone is not specifically useful in the diagnosis of neoplastic changes, the incidence of thyroid nodules occurrence increases with each decade of life, and the probability of malignancy increases when there is a history of low-dose irradiation to the head, neck, or superior mediastinum (Harvey et al., 1976).

Low-dose irradiation was used fairly extensively two to three decades ago to reduce the size of the thymus gland or to treat acne.

The major rationale behind the need for laboratory screening tests for thyroid dysfunction in these risk populations is that early and accurate diagnosis of thyroid imbalance cannot be made without laboratory tests (Steffes, 1979).

B. Related action

1. *The nurse needs to attain a thorough knowledge* of the signs and symptoms of thyroid imbalance (increase and decrease), so that awareness of the existence of such clues is enhanced, and the probability increased that such clues will be picked up and acted upon.
2. *Any nursing assessment should include* pertinent investigation for thyroid disorders. The skill of physical appraisal (palpation) of the thyroid should be one of the talents of the nurse, as should the ability to seek out information pertinent to the existence of thyroid disorder in history taking.
3. *Individuals in the risk groups* should be urged to request thyroid evaluation from their physicians.
4. *When examining the individual born and raised two to three decades ago,* the nurse should inquire into the possibility of low-dose irradiation having been used on the thymus gland or to treat acne.

1.14 NEWBORN SCREENING TESTS

1.14.1 Test for Phenylketonuria

Synonyms: phenylpyruvic acid; Guthrie test

Normal Ranges

Less than 4 mg/dL phenylalanine: reported as negative.
Levels of 4-8 mg/dL: reported as presumptive positive.

Generalized systemic screening tests of all newborn infants for phenylketonuria (PKU) is mandatory in 43 states of the United States. The remaining states offer voluntary screening. PKU causes a hereditary type of mental and physical retardation, but is one of the few hereditary diseases in which the negative effects can be prevented by early recognition and treatment (Ravel, 1973), thus the widespread, and even mandatory, screening of newborns.

The Guthrie test is the most widely used screening test. It is sensitive and accurate enough to detect definitely abnormal blood levels (4 mg/dL or greater) and is the most reliable test available for screening purposes, as well as being relatively inexpensive. It is a bacterial inhibition test. Fresh capillary blood is obtained by a heel-stick, and three areas of blood are placed on a special filter paper, which in turn is placed on a special culture medium of *Bacillus subtilis*. The bacterium's growth is inhibited by the special culture medium but is stimulated by the presence of sufficient concentrations of phenylalanine—greater than the normal plasma level of 2 mg/dL or less. Therefore, a growth of bacteria indicates a positive reaction and the presence of PKU. With a positive response, further tests are done to confirm and investigate further in order to rule out false positives. A typical PKU plasma concentration of phenylalanine is usually greater than 15 mg/dL, and tyrosine levels are lower than 5 mg/dL (Ravel, 1973).

Urine screening tests are available but are not usually of value until the infant is over 2 weeks of age, since the serum level of phenylalanine must exceed 10 to 15 mg/dL for phenylpyruvic acid to present in the urine (Whaley and Wong, 1979). By that time irreversible mental deficiencies may have already occurred. Therefore, the more sensitive test, responsive to lower plasma concentrations, such as the Guthrie test, is necessary for early diagnosis. Carriers can be identified by a phenylalanine loading, or tolerance, test, similar to a glucose tolerance test (Harvey et al., 1976).

Physiology. The metabolism of the essential amino acid phenylalanine, and subsequently that of the amino acid tyrosine, is extremely complex and not yet fully understood. Phenylalanine cannot be synthesized by the body but is required by it to function. Usually, dietary phenylalanine, which is found in all protein, is acted upon by the hepatic enzyme phenylalanine hydroxylase, converting it to yet another amino acid, tyrosine. Tyrosine is needed for the formation of the pigment melanin and the hormones epinephrine and thyroxin (Howard and Herbold, 1979).

Pathophysiology. The primary defect in PKU is the absence or deficiency of the enzyme phenylalanine hydroxylase. In its absence phenylalanine cannot be converted to tyrosine, nor can the subsequent conversions take place. This defect can be noted only after the infant has ingested foods (usually milk) containing protein, since the amino acid is not synthesized by the body. With the administration of protein phenylalanine, plasma concentration rises and "alternate catabolites" accumulate in the blood to be excreted in urine once plasma concentration levels reach the renal threshold (greater than 4 mg/dL, usually 10 mg/dL or more). In infants, or children, with still maturing central nervous system (CNS) structures, mental development is retarded, either due to the increased levels of plasma phenylalanine and its increased levels in the spinal fluid, or to the presence of various phenylketones in the blood. Brain development is abnormal; nerve sheath myelinization is defective; cystic degeneration of the gray and white matter occurs; and cortical lamination is disturbed. CNS destruction, and therefore possible mental retardation, occurs before the abnormal metabolites (the phenylketones) begin to be excreted in the urine (Whaley and Wong, 1979).

The decreased production of melanin is thought to be responsible for the phenotypical appearance of PKU victims. They routinely have blond hair, fair skin, and blue eyes (Ravel, 1973).

Because the excess presence of phenylalanine is the single defect, and because it occurs in the body only by exogenous administration, the disease can be successfully treated by extremely strict diet manipulation. If begun in the first month of life and carried out faithfully, it can prevent mental or physical retardation. It has not been established with any certainty just how long the diet must be maintained. Some authorities believe that it can be terminated at school age—the rationale being that the brain has achieved maximum growth by then. Others recommend dietary management indefinitely (Howard and Herbold, 1978). Most authorities recommend the former course, continuing treatment until age 6 or 8.

PKU FALSE-POSITIVE RESPONSES CAN OCCUR IN:

1. *Liver disease,* due to defective metabolism, resulting in increased levels of precursors.
2. *Galactosemia,* due to secondary liver disease.
3. *Transient states of hyperphenylalanemia,* or variants of PKU that do not require dietary treatment.

PKU FALSE-NEGATIVE RESPONSES CAN OCCUR IN:

1. *Testing done before 4 days postbirth.*
2. *Testing done in premature infants* due to delayed maturation of enzymes required for phenylalanine catabolism (Harper, 1971).
3. *Testing done before the infant has ingested sufficient quantities of protein.* May be due to insufficient feedings secondary to the infant's refusal to eat because of anorexia or vomiting. Infants with PKU tend to vomit and refuse to eat more than do normal infants.

IMPLICATIONS FOR NURSING

1. *Prior to having the Guthrie test done,* it is important that the infant ingest at least two high-protein feedings. Since normal plasma values of phenylalanine are related to both age and protein intake, the test is usually done just prior to the infant's discharge from the nursery, approximately 4 days after birth, and a retesting is ordinarily done on all infants within 1 to 2 weeks. False negatives can occur if the test is done before 4 days, or before enough protein has been ingested (SHMC, 1978).
2. *Case finding* is a shared responsibility among all health care workers. The nurse can assist in the process by:
   a. Validating that all newborns in the nurse's care are tested before leaving the hospital.
   b. Being alert for any "mousey, musty, horsey" odor in urine from any infant or child in the nurse's care and immediately doing a urine or diaper test for PKU.
   c. Reinforcing the need for a recheck test, usually within a month of birth, with the parents. This can be done by:
      (1) Being sure that the parent fully understands the purpose of the test.

(2) Informing the parents of the correctable nature of the defect and the essential role that only the parents can play in the future well-being of the infant.

(3) Helping the parents deal with feelings of blame and guilt that often occur in reaction to a positive test. Since there are a number of false positives with the initial Guthrie test [some reports state that the majority of initially positive Guthrie tests are not due to PKU (Ravel, 1973)], this possibility can be mentioned, but should not be stressed, in helping encourage the return for the second test, and in dealing with feelings.

3. *Follow-up support and guidance in management of the child* as he or she grows is an important area for nursing intervention, especially in a clinic or home setting.

   a. Whereas complete dietary control is possible with the infant, the older child is likely to rebel, particularly as children become more independent and can find their own food, or as the attitude of their peer group becomes important.

   b. The philosophy of approach to a handicapped child applies in this instance. Helping the child to be as well socialized as possible given the restrictions necessary, placing the responsibility of dietary control increasingly with the child as he or she matures, and understanding and dealing realistically with the child's negative feelings, are all concepts to be applied to the child with PKU.

   c. Helping the family to deal with other possible effects of the illness in the child is equally important. These can include failure to thrive, frequent vomiting, irritability, hyperactivity, unpredictable or erratic behavior, fright reactions, bizarre behavior, screaming episodes, unusual posturing, and eczema and other dermatologic problems. Any of these would require major adaptation and coping on the part of the parents. The nurse might assist the parents to:

      (1) Arrange and accept relief time from child care without guilt feelings.

      (2) Reinforce the knowledge that the behavior is due to the disease and may be temporary and reversible. Consult with the physician about this.

   d. The need for careful and systematic follow-up must be reinforced at frequent intervals and the parents assisted with the process. Changes will be necessary in the diet to cope with growth spurts and developmental changes of the child. The nurse can help with the necessary teaching and support to provide for:

(1) Monitoring changes in behavior that indicate inadequate phenylalanine intake (e.g., anorexia, rash, listlessness, failure to grow).
(2) Monitoring growth by keeping daily (infant) or weekly (child) records of height and weight, which records can provide positive reinforcement for the child and the parents.
(3) Using an exchange equivalent list to provide for more flexible, less cumbersome diet planning (Howard and Herbold, 1978). If the parent does not have such a list, consult with the dietician to provide one or to update it to make it more suitable to the age of the child. Free access to a dietician is a high-priority need for parents of PKU children.
(4) Establishing a schedule for blood phenylalanine determinations (Guthrie test) usually twice weekly during the initial diet stabilization period, weekly for infants, at 2 to 3-week intervals for toddlers, and monthly thereafter as long as the diet is continued.
(5) Routinely testing urine, especially if the child has not been adhering closely to the diet.
    (a) Diaper test using 10% ferric chloride solution in drops, which is inexpensive and easy to do.
    (b) Phenistix Test—more accurate but more expensive; not useful until the child is 6 weeks old or older.
    (c) DNPH (dinitrophenylhydrazine)—a more complex process, but the least expensive and accurate. Might be suggested for use if a parent or health care worker is accustomed to dealing with testing.

4. *Special counseling* is indicated for adult carriers who plan to marry and for the female adult with PKU who plans pregnancy.
    a. Refer those planning marriage, or motherhood, for genetic counseling if necessary and/or possible.
    b. Acquire sufficient knowledge and understanding of the genetic pattern to be able to reinforce and elaborate on the genetic counseling given, or in the absence of such a service, to provide accurate and necessary counseling.
    c. Women with PKU who wish to bear children should be placed on a phenylalanine-restricted diet regardless of their serum levels at the time. The outcomes of such pregnancies are as yet unknown.

1.14.2 Test for Galactosemia

> *Synonym:* UDP-galactose transferase utilization test
>
> *Normal Range:* 2.5-9 IU of enzyme activity per gram of hemoglobin

This is a semiquantitative measurement of the amount of enzyme activity which is deficient, or totally absent, in the inherited disease of galactosemia. The enzyme measured is one of the three needed for the conversion of galactose to glucose in the body, and is the one deficient or absent in this disease (galactose-1-phosphate uridyl transferase) (Davidsohn and Henry, 1969). This blood test is considered to be a better screening test for the condition than is the older approach of urine testing (e.g., Clinitest) because it will yield a positive result whether or not the child has been eating, whereas the urine test depends on the ingestion of lactose. As in PKU, the infant with galactosemia may refuse milk, or may be vomiting.

Not all infants are tested routinely. Usually, those that are suspected of having the disease (e.g., both parents known carriers) have the cord blood tested at birth. Others are often picked up by a combination of physical findings and urine testing. Such a case finding is confirmed by further testing using the red cell utilization test or blood galactose determination. Galactosemia is of sufficient importance, although rare, to be included among the general screening tests, in that case finding can mean lifesaving or markedly increasing the future quality of life. The disease is treatable so as to eliminate the negative consequences and is often "outgrown" (Ravel, 1973).

Physiology. Following is a diagram of the metabolism of galactose.

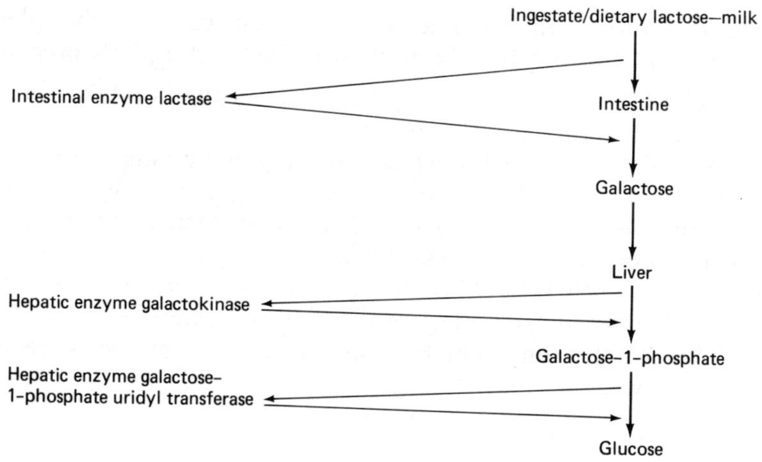

Pathophysiology. Galactosemia is a hereditary autosomal recessive disease. At birth the child appears nornal. After feeding the infant usually vomits and weight loss ensues. There is an absence or deficiency of the final enzyme in the metabolism of galactose (see "Physiology" above). Increased amounts of galactose-1-phosphate accumulate in the plasma; at the same time, a state of hypoglycemia exists, since galactose is not processed to glucose. The hypoglycemic state can lead to convulsions and mental deficiency. Proteinuria and aminoaciduria also occur.

By an unknown mechanism the accumulation of galactose-1-phosphate causes cerebral damage, aminoaciduria, and liver damage in the form of a cirrhotic process and enlargement. Jaundice can occur by the second week of life. Splenomegaly follows the liver damage, secondary to portal hypertension. Recognizable cataracts appear by the end of the first or second month if untreated. The excessive galactose is excreted in the urine.

Carriers are asymoptomatic but may show a spontaneous dislike for, or avoidance of, galactose-containing food, primarily milk, milk products, and legumes (Whaley and Wong, 1979; Howard and Herbold, 1978).

IMPLICATIONS FOR NURSING

1. *No special preparation* is necessary for the test.
2. *As galactosemia is a genetic and treatable disease,* genetic counseling is encouraged.
3. *Since not all children are routinely screened* for the disease, the nurse needs to be alert for signs and symptoms of its presence. Many of these signs and symptoms are similar to PKU and the nurse must be able to recognize differences if they occur.
   a. Initial signs and symptoms are vomiting and failure to gain, or actual loss of weight below birthweight. Drowsiness, failure to feed well, failure to thrive, and diarrhea often follow. None of these symptoms differ substantially from those of infants with PKU.
   b. The child with galactosemia frequently develops an enlarged liver or spleen and has aminoaciduria and proteinuria. None of these problems is normally found in children with PKU.
   c. Independent testing of urine (positive Clinitest versus negative strip or dipstick tests indicate galactosemia), and urinalysis results should be checked.

4. *Dietary teaching* is of major importance since dietary manipulation is the primary treatment.
   a. The diet ordinarily totally eliminates *all* milk and milk products (e.g., cream, cream soups, butter, cheese, ice cream, sherbert, yogurt).
   b. The family/patient need to be especially aware of the inclusion of lactose in many prepared foods and need to be advised to read the labels of such foods very carefully.
   c. The family should also be instructed to read labels on patent medicines with care. Many contain lactose as a filler. They also need to consult with their pharmacist when obtaining prescription drugs so as to eliminate drugs containing lactose as filler.

5. *It is generally easier to get compliance with the therapeutic regime* for galactosemia than for PKU. The substitution of soybean formula is usually well accepted by the child, although the odor may be objectionable to the parent, and the probability of being able to include milk and milk products some day adds to the ease with which the diet is accepted by the growing child. Such compliance does not eliminate the need to stress the importance of compliance and the potentially harmful effects, as well as irreversible effects, of noncompliance. Follow-up should be consistent and supportive.

1.14.3 Sickledex

Synonyms: sickle cell solubility; sickle-turbidity test

Normal Range: Negative

The Sickledex is a highly specific screening test since it is used to screen for only one form of bleeding disorder, hemoglobin S (Hb-S). This variant form of hemoglobin produces sickle cell anemia, or sickle cell trait, which occurs almost exclusively in blacks. It will detect both homozygous (sickle cell anemia) and heterozygous (sickle cell trait) but does not differentiate between them (SHMC, 1978).

The principle underlying the test is that deoxygenated hemoglobin S is virtually insoluble in certain media (e.g., high phosphate buffer solution) and will form a cloudly, or turbid, mixture when mixed in the solution. All other forms of hemoglobin (A, A_2, F, C, D) produce a clear suspension (Ravel, 1973). The test is felt to be reliable as a screening test despite some false positive and negative results (listed below), and it can be quickly done using blood obtained from a finger stick. Hemoglobin electrophoresis (see Section 1.14.3.1) is often necessary after a positive Sickledex to differentiate between trait, disease, or false positive due to other hemoglobinopathies (Whaley and Wong, 1979). It is included as a routine screening test for newborn blacks in many hospitals.

Physiology. See "Physiology" in Section 2.1.2.

Pathophysiology. Sickle cell anemia (or trait) is a recessive, hereditary blood dyscrasia which is characterized by the presence of hemoglobin S (Hb-S) in place of hemoglobin A (Hb-A) in the RBCs. This variant hemoglobin differs from normal hemoglobin only in that one of the 574 amino acids making up its structure is different (valine instead of glutamine). Such a small alteration in the hemoglobin molecule causes remarkable changes in the characteristics of the RBCs containing it. The hemoglobin is markedly decreased in its solubility. When it is exposed to decreased environmental pH and/or decreased oxygen, the hemoglobin forms long slender crystals which deform the RBC into a crescent, or sickle, shape. This causes the blood to become more viscous as the cells tend to become sticky and adhere to each other. Sickling will also occur when there is inadequate fluid–dehydration states–which enhances the viscosity. The situation readily progresses to thrombosis, following venous stasis. Thrombosis further decreases oxygenation locally; hypoxia is increased; more sickling results. Cells with Hb-S are more fragile and hemolyze readily, their life span is 26 to 35 days compared to a normal of 120 days, and anemia results despite increased production of RBCs. The defective Hb-S also has a greatly reduced ability to transport oxygen, which increases the body's hypoxia.

The disease is characterized by symptom-free periods interspersed with acute crisis episodes, most frequently related to vascular occlusion, which is accompanied by excruciating pain in the area or organ affected. The severity and site of the crisis episodes are not predictable (Groer and Shekleton, 1979).

The person afflicted with the trait (genetic inheritance from only one parent) rather than the disease (genetic inheritance from both parents) does not usually have symptoms unless severely stressed, since the majority of his or her blood has normal hemoglobin.

The disease is not evident in infants until they are approximately 6 months of age because of the high percentage of hemoglobin F (Hb-F) found in the newborn. Once the infant replaces the Hb-F with the defective hemoglobin, symptoms will appear. Pathologic changes throughout the body can include:

1. *Spleen:* enlargement, ultimately fibrotic changes ("autosplenectomy").

2. *Blood:* hemolysis, anemia (normocytic, normochromic), hyperplastic bone marrow, decreased hemoglobin (7 to 10%), bilirubinemia, reticulocytosis.
3. *Kidney:* ischemia, causing an inability to concentrate urine, enuresis, hematuria.
4. *Skin:* chronic leg ulcers, due to decreased peripheral cirulation and thrombosis.
5. *Liver:* enlargement secondary to circulatory stasis; cirrhosis may occur secondary to capillary obstruction, necrosis, and scarring. Hemosiderosis (increased storage of iron) secondary to hemolysis. May also occur in spleen, bone marrow, kidney, and lymph nodes.
6. *CNS:* possible CVA secondary to thrombosis, signs and symptoms of minor brain hypoxia—headache, weakness, convulsions, and visual disturbances, including loss of vision from progressive retinopathy and retinal detachment.
7. *Heart:* potential congestive heart disease secondary to chronic anemia.
8. *Bones:* osteoperosis secondary to bone marrow hyperplasia and congestion, skeletal deformities secondary to weakening of bone (especially lumbar and thoracic regions), arthralgia secondary to erythrostasis in joints, hand-foot syndrome secondary to infarction of short tubular bones (swelling and pain), aseptic necrosis of femoral head secondary to chronic ischemia (Whaley and Wong, 1974).

SICKLEDEX FALSE NEGATIVES OCCUR IN (Ravel, 1973):

1. *Persons with a hemoglobin concentration of 10 g/dL or less.*
2. *Infants less than 6 months of age,* due to the presence of Hb-F.

SICKLEDEX FALSE POSITIVES OCCUR IN:

1. *Non-S-sickling hemogloinopathies* (rare occurrence) [e.g., hemoglobin C (Harlem, Georgetown, and perhaps Alexandria)] (SHMC, 1978).
2. *Dysglobulinemias,* such as Waldenstrom's, myeloma, cryoglobulinemia.

IMPLICATIONS FOR NURSING

1. *No special patient preparation* is necessary.

tests is not met in the use of the Sickledex for identification of the trait, which helps provide a rationale for opposing its use. The unmet criterion is that the test be used for the purpose of uncovering a serious, or common, disease that *is treatable* (see the introductory essay to Part I). Hb-S trait is treatable only through selective reproduction, which can easily be viewed as racial genocide by the most affected race, the blacks. The nurse needs to be aware of this point of view to understand and deal tactfully and effectively with negative responses to "routine" screening tests.

3. *The nurse will need to acquire knowledge in the area of genetic transmission* so as to correctly reinforce genetic counseling or to provide such when necessary. For example, it is well to know that *each* child born to parents both carrying the sickle trait has a 25% chance of having the disease.

4. *Implications for nursing applicable for hyperbilirubinemia* may also apply in this instance. Monitor blood levels of bilirubin as well as urinary bilirubin and urobilinogen.

5. *Assess* gently *for enlargement of the liver and/or spleen.* If a physician is doing this on a routine basis, there is no need to subject the patient to a second palpation. Decrease in size is, of course, a favorable sign, and vice versa.

6. *Following the list of potential pathological changes* given under pathophysiology, do an initial assessment of each area as a baseline for future comparisons to determine the effectiveness of therapy and/or progress of the disease.

7. *The major nursing goal* in the care of the individual with sickle cell disease, not in crisis, is to prevent sickling by preventing hypoxia and providing adequate hydration. This is done not only by implementing a well-conceived plan of care, but by teaching that plan of care to the patient/family/home caretaker with an adequate and compelling rationale to increase compliance. Some possible interventions are given below.

   a. Provision of adequate hydration for hemodilution by:
      (1) Calculating the child's intake based on a minimum of 100 to 125 mL/kg/day.
      (2) Providing highly specific instructions for intake in terms of numbers of glasses, bottles, or cups per day rather than in mL/day.
      (3) Listing and using high-fluid-content foods particularly enjoyed by the patient (e.g., fruit with high water content, popsickles, soups).

(4) Arranging patient/family access to a variety of fluids for "self service."
(5) Offering a small amount of a different fluid on each contact with the patient—encouraging the family to do the same.

b. Evaluating for adequate hydration by:
(1) The absence of physical signs and symptoms of sickling [e.g., complaints of severe pain, evidence of increased hemolysis (jaundice, hematuria)].
(2) Moist mucous membrane.
(3) Intake and output balanced when corrected for insensible losses.
(4) Infant fontanels full, not sunken.
(5) Weight either increased or at baseline.
(6) The urine will be dilute because of the kidney's inability to concentrate; therefore, urine specific gravity is not a good criterion for measurement.

c. Prevention of fluid loss by:
(1) Preventing perspiration by control of ambient temperature:
(a) Avoid undue exposure to the sun.
(b) Avoid excessive clothing/bedding.
(c) Look at or check with the patient rather than assuming that the temperature is correct.
(2) Enuresis frequently occurs even in adults, due to the kidney defect.
(a) If dehydration threatens, weigh bedding dry and then wet for better calculation of loss.
(b) Use of diapers when appropriate—weighing them.
(c) Arrange ready access to toilet during day and night; instruct in urine measurement.
(d) Take to toilet during night if sleep patterns not disturbed.
(e) Adapt toilet training in youngsters to allow for blameless lack of success. Psychological problems occur readily with enuresis.
(3) Monitoring lab reports and signs and symptoms for electrolyte loss. Loss of potassium in urine can precipitate acidosis, which enhances sickling.

d. Prevention of hypoxia by preventing increased cellular oxygen demand through:
(1) Preventing infection (see "Implications for Nursing" in Section 1.9.2 and items 2c and 3a and c in Section 2.2.3).
(2) Monitoring lab reports for evidence of acidosis (see Appendix A) (e.g., decreased venous CO_2 with SMA profiles).

(3) Preventing overheating [see item c(1) above].
(4) Monitoring RBC count, hematocrit, and hemoglobin for changes in oxygen-carrying capacity.
(5) Limiting physical activity based on results of item (4) above plus evidence of fatigue, complaints of dyspnea on exertion, and the acceptance of the limitations by the patient without emotional stress.
(6) Identifying, and preventing as possible, emotional stressors. Work independently with the patient/family in positive management of stressors.
(7) Providing analgesia promptly with pain (other than aspirin, which promotes bleeding). Giving oxygen if pain is due to sickling, but with judicious restraint, recalling that prolonged use of oxygen will decrease the stimulus for erythropoietin production, thus increasing the anemia and hypoxia.
(8) Providing passive range of motion (ROM) to prevent thrombus formation as well as to maintain muscle mass for later active exercise, while decreasing immediate oxygen demand.
(9) Providing a nutritious diet with adequate nutrients necessary for replacement of lost blood cells and provision of energy (see "Implications for Nursing" in Section 1.8).
(10) See also Section 2.1.6.

1.15 SMA PROFILES—AUTOANALYZER

The SMA is not a test in itself, but rather the name given an instrument used for different assortments of tests. SMA stands for sequential multiple analyzer; the initials are usually followed by numbers (e.g., SMA-12/60). The first of the number groups indicates the number of analytical procedures performed by the particular instrument on one sample; the second group of numbers, following the slash, refers to the sample frequency, the rate at which individual samples can be handled: 20, 40, or 60 per hour (Tietz, 1970). AutoAnalyzer is the trade name given the first of these multiphasic, automated instruments marketed by Technicon in 1957, as well as to subsequent machines. The instrument has been applied singly and in combinations to a large number of different chemical determinations. Information about this particular testing method is included because the group of tests done by a particular machine are often ordered as a unit (e.g., SMA 12). The process is still in use and the nurse should be familiar with the terminology, if only to know what tests have been ordered or to understand the method of reporting and to be able to utilize the results.

When first developed, the instrument was widely used to screen apparently healthy people, without clinical signs or symptoms, for early disease, as a logical outgrowth of the technical capability, and of both medical and governmental interest in preventative care. The cost per test was markedly less than was the cost for individual nonautomated methods, or even the cost of automated, but individual, testing methods. The process has other advantages. The results are available quickly and give a comprehensive, chemical profile of each patient. The volume of tests done by one laboratory was markedly increased, and the dependability and accuracy of the tests improved immensely. Studies done on the outcomes of its use reported discovery of significant, unsuspected disease in a sufficient number of persons—4% of hospitalized patients screened—and excellent leads to diagnosis in sufficient numbers of persons with vague symptoms—20 to 30% of all patients screened—to be an excellent and productive procedure (Collins, 1975). However, as mentioned in the introduction to this chapter, attitudes, particularly of government and private insurance carriers, changed and the SMA is now used less frequently as a wide-sweeping screening process on apparently healthy individuals, or on all hospital admissions, but *is* used in those patients with vague signs and symptoms.

The SMA-12 is made up of 12 blood chemistry tests. These vary among institutions but two patterns frequently seen are listed in Table 1.3.

Reporting. The 12 (or whatever number is included on a given profile) chemistries are usually listed horizontally on the automatic printout. The ranges of concentrations (in mg, g, or IU) are given numerically on the vertical axis above the test title. Normal ranges

TABLE 1.3 *SMA-12 survey and hospital models*

Survey model	
1. Total protein	7. Glucose
2. Albumin	8. Uric acid
3. Calcium	9. Creatinine
4. Inorganic phosphorus	10. Total bilirubin
5. Urea nitrogen	11. Alkaline phosphatase
6. Cholesterol	12. SGOT
Hospital model	
1. Sodium	7. Urea nitrogen[a]
2. Potassium	8. Glucose[a]
3. Chloride	9. Calcium[a]
4. CO_2	10. Total bilirubin[a]
5. Total protein[a]	11. Alkaline phosphatase[a]
6. Albumin[a]	12. LDH (may be SGOT)

[a]Tests that occur in both series.

are shaded in gray on this axis and the recorder traces the patient's concentrations across the graph, usually in red. Abnormalities are detectable at a glance, as are the relationships among test results, and the results are ready rapidly, without the potential for error inherent in having to retranscribe.

SMA-4 analyzes whole blood samples for RBC, WBC, hemoglobin, and hematocrit.

SMA-7 includes the hematology given in SMA-4 with the addition of the other blood indices—MCV, MCH, MCHC.

SMA-6 includes 6 of the 12 tests from the hospital model above. They are: sodium, potassium, chloride, bicarbonate (or CO_2), glucose, and urea nitrogen (Brand and Tollins, 1979).

NOTE TO THE READER

Blood chemistry screening tests often include calcium and inorganic phosphorus, as well as venous CO_2 (carbon dioxide, a measurement of the body's base content). These three tests have been placed in Part 3 because calcium and phosphorus are unique measurements for parathyroid funciton and coverage in that section seemed most appropriate; CO_2 is intimately related to the arterial blood gas levels and respiratory function and thus is presented in Chapter 11.

Hematology Screen

chapter 2

Hematology is the study of the blood. Hematologists are concerned with all aspects of blood, such as blood volume, blood flow, and tests done on the blood for the diagnosis of disease of other organs. This chapter is limited to tests done on the major cellular components of blood, particularly tests done primarily for diagnosis of diseases of the blood itself. Because there is a close relationship among the cellular blood components, all those components should be tested so that the relationships can be explored.

Blood consists of both fluid and solid elements. The fluid portion is called *plasma* and is made up predominantly of water. When the fibrinogen is removed from plasma, the resulting fluid is called *serum.* The cellular components consist largely of white blood cells, platelets, and red blood cells. Red blood cells normally outnumber white blood cells by a ratio of at least 700:1 (Greisheimer and Wiedeman, 1972).

Complete Blood Count and Differential. The *complete blood count* (CBC) traditionally includes the following tests: red blood corpuscle (cell) count, hemoglobin, hematocrit, white cell count, and white cell differential.

Frequently included in the CBC are the Wintrobe blood indices (mean corpuscular volume, MCV; mean corpuscular hemoglobin, MCH; mean corpuscular hemoglobin concentration, MCHC). A platelet count, or estimation, is usually done as a part of the differential or smear evaluation. The presence of reticulocytes and nucleated red blood cells is noted and red blood cell morphology (determination of variance in size, shape, or pigmentation) is described. The sedimentation rate has been included in this writing, although is not usually done as a part of the CBC because of its nonspecificity. This nonspecificity makes it a screening test in the true sense of the word, and as such it is therefore of interest.

The CBC is probably one of the more important laboratory tests. A great percentage of all hematologic disease can be diagnosed from the CBC findings. It is frequently part of the routine laboratory work included on a hospital admission and has the advantage that it can be performed on either venous or capillary blood.

2.1 TESTS RELATED TO THE RED BLOOD CELL

2.1.1 Red Blood Corpuscle Count

Synonyms: RBC; red blood cell count

*Normal Ranges**

Adult	
Female	4.0–5.3 million (mil) cubic millimeters (mm^3)
Male	4.4–5.7 mil/mm^3
Senior adult	3.0–5.0 mil/mm^3
Pediatric	
Newborn	4.8–7.1 mil/mm^3
Neonate	4.1–6.4 mil/mm^3

*When counts are reported from the Coulter automated counter, only the numerals are reported (e.g., 4.0 to 5.3). To get the total figure, multiply the reported total by 1 million (10^6).

The red blood cell count is simply that—a count of the red blood cells in a given sample of either venous or capillary blood, venous blood being preferred. The count can be done individually "by hand," using a counting chamber or by an automated process. The automated process is more accurate and is used more frequently.

Physiology. There are several theories on the origin of the cellular blood components, including red blood cells, the most commonly accepted being the monophylectic, or fixed stem cell, which is outlined in Fig. 2.1. The red blood cell becomes progressively smaller as it matures and loses its nucleus, at which point it is more correctly called a corpuscle than a cell. Reticulocytes (young RBCs; see Fig. 2.1) are found in the peripheral blood in small numbers and are grossly indistinguishable from normal red cells. They are identified by special staining of the blood smear.

Blood cells are formed in red bone marrow (ribs, sternum, vertebrae, and pelvis of the normal adult). In infants, and children through adolescence, all bone marrow produces blood cells, later some marrow being replaced with fat—yellow marrow. RBC production depends on a number of things, such as adequate intake of protein, carbohydrate, fat, minerals (especially iron), and vitamins [especially vitamin B_{12}, folic acid, vitamin B_6 (pyrodoxine) and vitamin C (ascorbic acid)]. Vitamin B_{12} also requires the presence of intrinsic factor, produced by the cells of the stomach lining, to be absorbed.

Erythrocytes are carried by the blood, which is propelled by heart beat and somatic muscle "pumps" (peripheral muscle action that propels blood by contraction, squeezing the vasculature). RBCs function only within the vasculature, as opposed to the white blood cells, which migrate into tissue when needed. The major function of the red blood cell is to carry hemoglobin, which in turn carries oxygen, in a weak bond, to the body tissues, and carbon monoxide, in a strong bond, from the tissues to the lungs (Davidsohn and Henry, 1969). It also has a function in acid-base balance (see Section 1.2 on the chloride shift).

RBCs survive about 120 days. This fairly long survival is due in great part to their unique shape, being thin in the center and thick at the edges once the nucleus is lost—a biconcave disc (Frolich, 1976). They are flexible and elastic, so they can slip through the smallest vessels by deforming, then returning to functional shape. As they speed through the blood vessels, they take on the shape of tiny parachutes, with their central portion well in advance of a thicker edge (Greisheimer and Wiedeman, 1972). As the RBC ages, it becomes more fragile and ultimately will rupture. If the cell does not disintegrate spontaneously, it will be broken down by the spleen or other parts of the reticular-endothelial system, which also picks up the debris and degrades it to bilirubin (see Fig. 1.1).

Regulation of the RBC production is dependent on several factors. The primary factor for production and termination of production seems, at present, to be the level of tissue oxygenation, tissue hypoxia causing increased production. Tissue hypoxia is believed to stimulate the kidney to release a hormone called erythropoietin, which increases

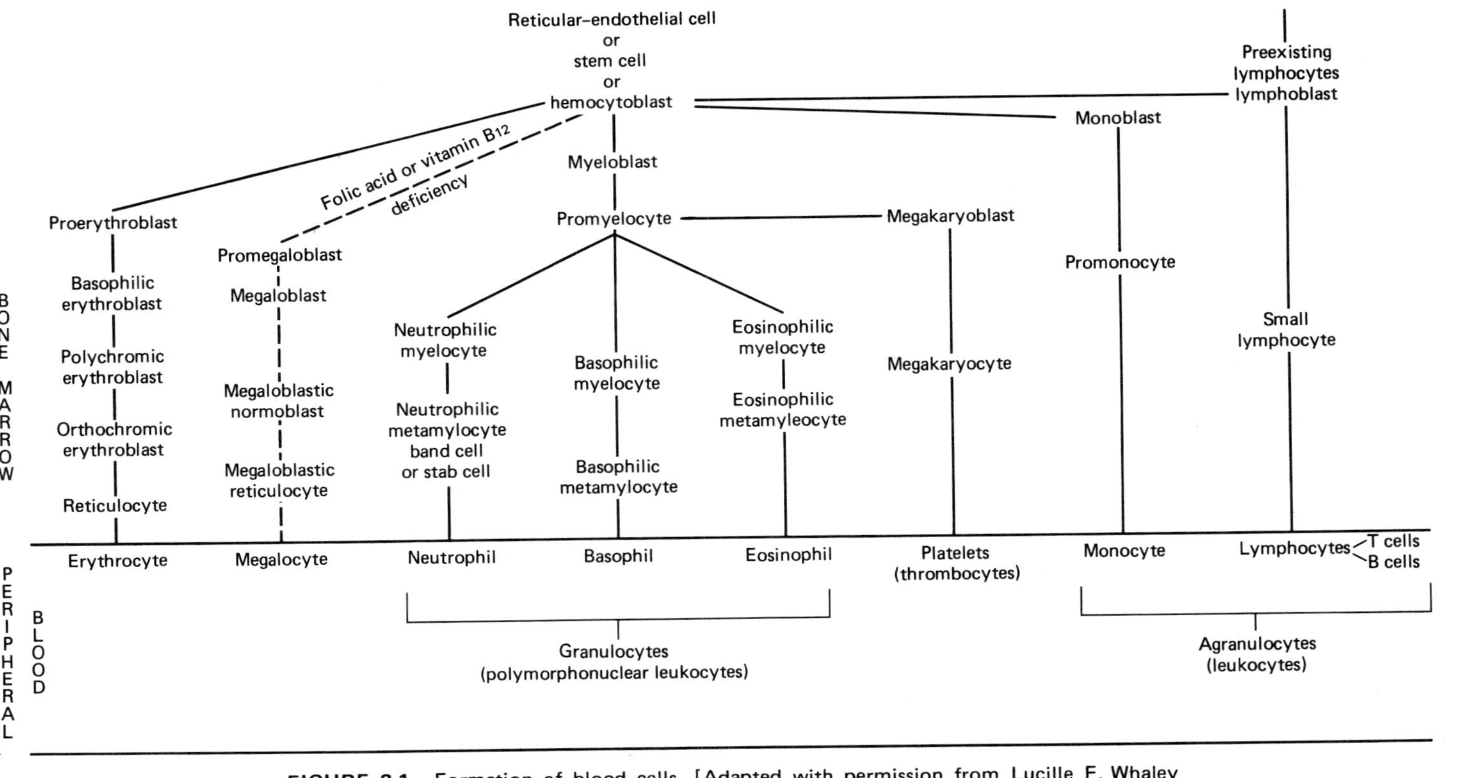

FIGURE 2.1 Formation of blood cells. [Adapted with permission from Lucille F. Whaley and Donna L. Wong, ***Nursing Care of Infants and Children*** (St. Louis, Mo.: The C. V. Mosby Company, 1979), p. 1367.]

both red blood cell mitosis and rate of RBC release from the bone marrow. When tissue oxygen reaches normal levels, erythropoietin production ceases (Collins, 1975).

A significant percentage of RBCs are in the spleen at any one time, not in storage but rather in a dynamic equilibrium with the circulation (Nordin, 1980). Epinephrine released into the system, usually secondary to stress, will alter that equilibrium and increase the number of circulating RBCs as a physiologic compensatory measure.

Physiologic variations. In the elderly, ranges of normal are wider than the adult norm, not only for RBCs but for hemoglobin and hematocrit as well. In general, values are lower. At one time the so-called "anemia of the aged" was considered a function of aging. It is now thought to be due to the generally poor nutritional state among the elderly, due to a variety of factors (Carnevali and Patrick, 1979).

Blood volume, and consequently the RBC count, in the neonate depends on the amount of blood transfer from the placenta at the time of birth. Also, few new RBCs are produced for the first 8 to 10 weeks of life, causing a physiologic anemia (Whaley and Wong, 1979).

Pathophysiology. When the balance of red blood cell production and destruction is lost, blood disorders occur. Production can be decreased if the mechanisms of control are lost, such as in deficits of erythropoietin due to kidney disease. Disease can occur as well through the endocrine system relationships with cell production, which may account for anemias accompanying thyroid or adrenal disorders (hypothyroidism, Addision's disease) (Collins, 1975). Blood disorders can occur due to defects anywhere along the process of cell production (i.e., differentiation, proliferation, and maturation). Such defects are most commonly due to deficiency states, which are frequently congenital in origin or secondary to drug administration.

An increased rate of destruction occurs in some hereditary diseases: for example, spherocytosis, some acquired diseases (e.g., liver failure), or with an abnormal environment for the red blood cell (e.g., transfusion reactions).

Increased production of RBCs occurs as a compensatory response seen in adaptation to high altitude, or in pathology causing tissue hypoxia (respiratory or cardiac disease). It can also be secondary to pathologic states in which there is an increase in erythropoietin without tissue hypoxia as a stimulus, such as in tumors of the kidney or polycythemia vera (Frolich, 1976) (see Table 2.3 for definition of abnormal cells).

RCB COUNT DECREASED IN:

1. *Conditions related to defects in regulatory mechanisms,* such as loss of adequate erythropoietin in:
   a. Chronic renal disease, due to decreased secretion of erythropoietin and possibly depression of the bone marrow itself by the uremia. This causes a normocytic (cell normal in size and shape), normochromic (cells normal in hemoglobin content) anemia. The anemia is roughly proportional to the uremia; the hemoglobin rarely falls below 6 g/dL (Harrington and Brener, 1973). Recall that with an increase in the BUN greater than 200 mg/dL, the RBC life span is shortened to about half of normal (see "Implications for Nursing" in Section 1.6).
   b. Addison's disease, by a mechanism that is unclear, causing a normocytic, normochromic anemia.
   c. Hypothyroidism, due to multiple factors and most frequently causing a normocytic, normochromic anemia. Achlorhydria is present in some cases, which increases the problem of poor intestinal absorption often present with hypothyroidism, and causes a macrocytic (cells larger than normal) anemia.*
   d. Chronic inflammatory disease, causing a normocytic, normochromic anemia with shortened red blood cell life.

2. *Conditions related to defects in cell differentiation,* proliferation, or maturation, such as:
   a. Defects in stem cells leading to aplastic anemia. True aplastic anemia demonstrates suppression of all myeloid (bone marrow) elements; or red cell aplasia/hypoplastic anemia (which usually refers to a depression of the RBCs only); or Fanconi's syndrome (a familial hypoplastic anemia or pancytopenia—depression of all cellular production); or Blackfan-Diamond syndrome (a congenital purely red cell anemia). Besides familial or hereditary defects, there are defects secondary to the administration of toxic substances (irradiation) or drugs (chemotherapy), or to an autoimmune/allergic process.
   b. Defects in nuclear development (DNA-RNA), due to deficiencies in folic acid or vitamin B_{12}, two critical coenzymes of nuclear development (Frolich, 1976). This causes macrocytic (cells larger than normal) anemia (see Fig. 2.1). This anemia

*Hypothyroidism and pernicious anemia appear together more frequently than could be due to chance. This link between the two is believed to be on the basis that both may have, at least in part, an autoimmune cause (Nordin, 1980).

can be secondary to inadequate intake (malnutrition) or inadequate absorption (idiopathic steatorrhea–lack of intrinsic factor from inherent defect = pernicious anemia–lack of intrinsic factor after gastrectomy); or the use of certain drugs [diphenylhydantoin/Dilantin, Methotrexate (a folate antagonist)]; or in greatly increased requirements for RBC production (hemolytic anemias, pregnancy).

3. *Conditions causing increased erythrocyte destruction,* such as:
   a. Abnormalities of the corpuscle, due to membrane defects found in:
      (1) Hereditary spherocytosis, which causes rapid hemolysis of the RBCs.
      (2) Acquired paroxysmal noctural hemoglobinuria (PNH), which has many of the characteristics of an inherited disease, and causes repetitive intravascular hemolysis with morning hemoglobinuria and potential thrombotic problems (Harvey et al., 1976).
      (3) Hereditary nonspherocytic hemolytic anemias caused by enzyme defects.
   b. Ingestion of and intoxication by heavy metals (e.g., lead, copper).
   c. Abnormalities in the erythrocyte's environment as found in:
      (1) Microangiopathic hemolytic anemia [anemia believed to be caused by the mechanical and perhaps chemical effects of vascular lesions on RBCs, resulting in red cell abnormalities (e.g., schistocytes and irregularly contracted cells such as Burr cells) and often associated with disseminated intravascular clotting (D.I.C.)] (Davidsohn and Henry, 1969; Harvey et al., 1976) secondary to gas gangrene, malaria, prosthetic heart valve replacements, vasculitis, malignant hypertension, disseminated carcinoma ecclampsia, hemolylic-uremic syndrome in children, sepsis, and renal homograft rejection.
      (2) Intoxication with chemical agents (e.g., arsenic).
      (3) Antibody responses secondary to transfusion reactions (including erythroblastosis fetalis), and certain drug reactions (e.g., quinine, quinidine, penicillin, phenacetin).
      (4) Autoantibody responses in certain disease states:
         (a) Malignant lymphomas.
         (b) Chronic lymphocytic leukemia.
         (c) Lupus erythematosus.
         (d) Infectious mononucleosis.
         (e) Most viral infections.

RCB COUNT INCREASED IN:

1. *Physiologic compensatory states* (see "Physiology" and "Physiologic variations" above) occurring in response to:
   a. Blood loss due to hemolysis or hemorrhage. Occurrence of an actual numerical increase other than just an increase in RBC production is dependent on the severity and duration of blood loss.
   b. Tissue hypoxia:
      (1) Relatively long-term existence at high altitudes.
      (2) Cardiorespiratory insufficiency (e.g., mild, chronic congestive heart failure, emphysema and some forms of congenital heart disease).
2. *Pathophysiologic responses* in:
   a. Tumors (unilateral) of the kidney, liver, adrenals (Cushing's syndrome), lung, and cerebellum, causing excessive release of erythropoietin or erythropoietin-like substances.
   b. Myeloproliferative disease without relative increase in erythropoietin activity (e.g., polycythemia vera), which increases not only the RBC count but also all cellular elements formed in the bone marrow—leukocytes (increased number of immature neutrophils), and platelets—a total increase in marrow activity (Frolich, 1976).

2.1.2 Hemoglobin

Synonyms: Hgb; Hb

Normal Ranges

Adult	
Female	12.0–15.0 g/dL
Male	13.0–17.0 g/dL
Senior adult	10.0–17.0 g/dL
Pediatric	
Newborn	14.0–24.0 g/dL
Neonate	11.0–20.0 g/dL*
Infant	10.0–15.0 g/dL
Child	11.0–16.0 g/dL

*During the neonatal period capillary blood values are 2 to 3 g/dL greater than venous blood values (Whaley and Wong, 1979).

Hemoglobin is the main component of the RBC, and determination of that content is one of the most frequent tests done in clinical laboratories and is one of the oldest and most important tests done (Tietz, 1970). The test has been found to be more helpful in terms of diagnosis and management of therapy in anemia than is the RBC count because it is the simplest means available for detecting anemias and their severity. It can be used as an index of the oxygen-carrying capacity of the blood.

Before automation the hemoglobin test was one of the most inaccurate of blood tests, and results were reported in terms of a percentage of a norm. There is too much variation within the normals of age and sex for that method of reporting to be accurate. Hemoglobin is more accurately reported in grams per deciliter (or in grams per 100 mL).

Physiology. Hemoglobin is produced by the immature red blood cells, which are nucleated. Mature cells lack the nucleus and thus cytoplasmic protein-synthesizing ability. Hemoglobin is a red pigmented protein that is found only in erythrocytes, giving them their characteristic color. Iron is essential to the formation of hemoglobin, the heme molecule being made up of a protoporphyrin globulin, and iron, and is one of the few proteins whose structure is relatively well understood. Physiologically normal red blood cells contain the maximum amount of hemoglobin (Tietz, 1970).

The main function of hemoglobin is the transport of oxygen to body cells from the lungs. The hemoglobin molecule contains four heme molecules, each one of which can react with, and bind, one molecule of oxygen—the oxygen binds directly to the iron (oxyhemoglobin). The amount of oxygen that can be carried by a hemoglobin molecule is influenced by three major factors:

1. *Oxygen partial pressure.* When that pressure is increased, the amount of oxygen combining is increased, and vice versa. The changes in oxygen's ability to be bound by hemoglobin at varying oxygen tensions is frequently described graphically by the *hemoglobin dissociation curve.* This curve shows the percent saturation of hemoglobin to be expected (given the stability of factors 2 and 3 below) at different partial pressures of oxygen in the blood. It emphasizes the relatively high oxygen saturations with fairly low partial pressures of oxygen (e.g., 75% at pO_2 of 40 mm Hgb), as well as the rapid drop in saturation below that pressure.
2. *pH (Bohr effect).* If the other factors (partial pressure and temperature) are constant, oxygen saturation is less with a low pH and greater with a high pH (Groer and Shakleton, 1979).

3. *Temperature.* Increased blood temperature causes the blood pH to fall, thus decreasing the oxygen saturation of the hemoglobin, and vice versa. This phenomenon partially explains the metabolic acidosis that occurs with hyperthermia (Danovitch et al., 1971).

In muscle, myoglobin, a protein similar to hemoglobin but found only in muscle cells, conveys the oxygen from the blood and interstitial fluid to the cell. Heme can also bind with carbon monoxide (carboxyhemoglobin–reduced hemoglobin), and the binding is much stronger than with oxygen. Thus carbon monoxide is removed from body cells by hemoglobin (Griesheimer and Wiedeman, 1972).

Hemoglobin concentration is high at birth, a carryover from fetal life when it was necessary to provide adequate oxygen *in utero;* it drops rapidly until well into the second year of life. Newborn hemoglobin consists of 40 to 70% fetal hemoglobin (hemoglobin F), which is produced by the fetus, but is abnormal in the adult in amounts greater than 1 to 2% (Whaley and Wong, 1979). Erythropoiesis is also decreased in the newborn, virtually ceasing for a period after birth and the infant's red blood cells are fragile and readily destroyed (Ziegel and Van Blarcom, 1972). However, once erythropoiesis is established, the hemoglobin rises slowly, with female values stabilizing at puberty and males at about the seventeenth year of life (Tietz, 1970).

Compensatory Physiologic Mechanisms:

1. Intravascular hemolysis takes place all the time, yet free hemoglobin is found in the plasma in only minute amounts (less than 1 mg/dL). The levels are kept low by the binding of free hemoglobin with haptoglobin, the levels of which decrease in response to increased amounts of free hemoglobin. This mechanism works only until free hemoglobin levels reach 7 to 14 mg/dL. Above that, free hemoglobin is excreted in the urine.
2. Decreases in environmental atmospheric pressure (high altitudes) will increase hemoglobin concentration by increasing the numbers of normal red blood cells. Levels rise to 16 to 23 g/dL in the adult.

Pathophysiology. Abnormalities in hemoglobin levels are most frequently related to decreases and can be due to a number of causes; for example, decreased production due to lack of necessary materials (iron, protein); increased loss (acute or chronic bleeding–there needs to be an acute loss of 1000 mL of blood before hemoglobin decreases); or conditions that interfere with red cell production (see "Pathophysiology" in Section 2.1.1) since hemoglobin concentration depends mostly on the number of RBCs present, although decreased amounts of hemoglobin per cell do occur (hypochromic anemia). Abnormal forms of hemoglobin, hemoglobin variants, may prevent what appears to be a normal hemoglobin level from being effective in its major function, that of gas transport and exchange. Abnormal forms are identified by hemoglobin protein electrophoresis (Tietz, 1970).

The mechanism for synthesis of hemoglobin protein is inherited from both parents. When an abnormal characteristic is inherited from only one parent (heterozygous) the condition may be without clinical signs or symptoms except for the "trait" found on examination of the blood (e.g., sickle cell trait). A great change in hemoglobin function occurs when even a single amino acid of its four polypeptide strands is altered, and it is possible to have several abnormal hemoglobins at one time. Abnormalities in hemoglobin synthesis are usually accompanied by abnormal variations in red blood cell size (anisocytosis) and shape (poikilocytosis).

Acquired dysfunction of hemoglobin also occurs. An example would be the formation of methemoglobin in heavy smokers, which replaces as much as 6 to 10% of total hemoglobin. Heavy-metal intoxication has the same effect (Tietz, 1970).

Compensatory mechanisms for pathologic change. The body is able to compensate in part for blood loss. Early response to massive changes in blood volume is hemodilution. This helps maintain circulating blood volume but cannot replace the RBCs, so that a drop in RBC count, hemoglobin, and hematocrit will occur, noticeable only after 6 to 24 hr when hemodilution is complete. Immediately after massive hemorrhage the RBC, hemoglobin, and hematocrit will be normal (Harvey et al., 1976). Bone marrow response is indicated by the release of an increased number of immature red blood cells into peripheral circulation (reticulocytes). If the loss is massive or the duration prolonged, the bone marrow will undergo hyperplasia. Fetal sites of red bone marrow production can revert to cell production. An increase in nucleated RBCs will be found in peripheral circulation (Collins, 1975).

Gradual changes in blood volume can be compensated to the extent that no acute symptoms may be noted and diagnosis is unlikely unless red blood cell tests are undertaken (Harvey et al., 1976).

HEMOGLOBIN INCREASED IN:

Severe dehydration.

HEMOGLOBIN DECREASED IN:

1. *Conditions causing a decrease in absolute number of RBCs* (see "RBC Count Decreased in" in Section 2.1.1).
2. *Conditions related to impaired cytoplasmic red cell development,* such as:
   a. Defective heme synthesis found in:
      (1) Iron deficiency anemias secondary to inadequate intake or absorption of iron, chronic bleeding, or pregnancy, with its increased need for iron.
      (2) Chronic disorders, causing impaired release of iron from stores in reticuloendothelial cells (the anemias of chronic disease).
      (3) Sideroblastic anemia, in which the pathogenic factors are not understood.
      (4) Heavy-metal (lead, copper) intoxication, which also causes ineffective erythropoiesis.
   b. Defective globin synthesis found in:
      (1) Thalassemia major (Cooley's anemia), secondary to a defect in total hemoglobin synthesis with the presence of fetal hemoglobin, which affects the rate of synthesis of the amino acid chains (Harper, 1971).
      (2) Hemoglobinopathies secondary to structural changes of the amino acid chains, affected by the genetic coding of their sequence [e.g., hemoglobin H; hemoglobin Bart; hemoglobin M; hemoglobin G (Gun Hill)].*

2.1.3 Hematocrit

Synonyms: Hct; "crit"; packed cell volume; PCV

Normal Ranges

Adult	
Female	36–45%
Male	39–51%
Senior adult	
Female	30–54%
Male	36–56%
Pediatric	
Newborn	44–64%
Neonatal	35–49%
Infant	30–40%
Child	31–43%

*More recent nomenclature is the addition of the original geographic origin of the

Traditionally, the hematocrit is defined as the percentage of RBCs per volume of whole blood. It is currently defined as the calculated value MCV/RBC (mean corpuscular volume) from the automated cell counter and does not include "trapped plasma." PCV (packed cell volume) is the "spun" (centrifuged to separate cells from plasma) hematocrit and does contain trapped plasma. PCV values average 2 to 3% greater. The PCV gives an indirect estimate of hemoglobin present in the blood, whereas the automated value is a calculated one. As a rule of thumb, the hematocrit is usually about three times the hemoglobin value (*Lab, Drugs, and Nursing Implications,* 1979).

The hematocrit is considered a fundamental diagnostic test in anemia as a measure of the size, capacity, and number of cells present in a person's blood. This test, together with the hemoglobin value, establishes the presence and severity of an anemia. There is close agreement between hematocrit determinations done on either venous or capillary blood; therefore, either can be used (Davidsohn and Henry, 1969).

Physiology and Pathophysiology. In general, the physiology and pathophysiology underlying the hematocrit determination is the same as that described for RBC count and hemoglobin. Some data concerning the significance of changes in the hematocrit are worth inclusion here.

The hematocrit is not considered a good measure of water (not saline) deficit as it shows relatively little change during development of a pure water deficit, even when the loss is great enough to be life threatening. A loss of 20% of body water would elevate a hematocrit of 42% only one percentage point, to 43% (Harvey et al., 1976).

Blood viscosity shows little variation within the hematocrit's normal range, but the increase in the hematocrit from the highest range of normal in an infant (40%) to 70% will double the relative viscosity, as well as doubling the resistance to blood flow (Frolich, 1976).

Changes in hematocrit, although dependent mostly on the numbers of RBCs present, are also sensitive to changes in size, shape, and density of the RBCs. As with hemoglobin, changes do not occur in the hematocrit until several hours (6 to 24) after massive hemorrhage, and an acute drop in hematocrit is usually accompanied by acute symptoms of anemia (e.g., extreme fatigue, weakness, shortness of breath, dyspnea, dizziness). Also, as in changes in RBC count and hemoglobin values, the

---

variant. Normal hemoglobin is hemoglobin A with alpha, beta, or gamma chains, and it will be found written to identify that information. That is, normal hemoglobin can also be identified as $\alpha_2 \beta_2$ (Harper, 1971).

signs and symptoms of anemia secondary to slowly advancing losses—chronic blood loss—are less evident and therefore harder to diagnose.

HEMATOCRIT INCREASES AND DECREASES:

See increases and decreases in hemoglobin in Section 2.1.2.

2.1.4 Erythrocyte Indices

Synonyms: Wintrobe red cell indices; blood indices

The word "indices" is a plural form of the word "index" and refers to something that points out, indicates, manifests, or directs attention. The erythrocyte indices point out the characteristics of size and hemoglobin content of the red blood cells and the relationship of these characteristics to the number of red blood cells. A rough idea of such elements can be determined by looking at a stained smear of peripheral blood. Wintrobe introduced the indices calculations to substitute objective quantitative standards for the subjective impressions produced by such observations of stained smears. It is well to bear in mind that complete accuracy of these indices depends on the accuracy of the values given for RBC count, hemoglobin, and hematocrit.

The indices are useful in determining the morphologic type of anemia (e.g., microcytic, macrocytic, hypochromic, hyperchromic), which in turn helps decision making about further diagnostic or treatment needs. Knowledgeable evaluation of the results of the erythrocyte indices can prevent the need for a bone marrow examination.

The values given in the erythrocyte indices are an average, not a precise, value.

A. Mean corpuscular volume (MCV)

Definition. The average, or mean volume, or size, of a single RBC.

Normal Ranges

Adult	78– 95	fL*
Senior adult	90.5–105.5	fL†
Pediatric		
Newborn	96–108	fL
Thereafter	82– 91	fL

*fL = femtoliter(s) = cubic microgram(s) (μg^3 or Cμg).

†Calculated from an average of normal values given ± 5 fL (Davidsohn and Henry, 1969).

Calculation

$$\frac{\text{hematocrit} \times 10}{\text{RBC millions/mm}^3} = \text{MCV}$$

Significance. Increases above 103 fL in the adult indicate a macrocytic (cells larger than normal) anemia. Values above 120 fL are found in the adult with a folate and B_{12} deficiency. Decreases below 78 fL in the adult usually indicate a microcytic (cells smaller than normal) anemia; values below 64 fL are found with iron-deficiency anemias and thalassemia. These findings should be correlated with RBC morphology (smear).

Discussion. If the average size of the RBC is increased, as in premature forms, the same number of RBCs will have a slightly larger cell mass, and thus an increased hematocrit, which in turn will increase the MCV, and vice versa (*Lab, Drugs and Nursing Implications,* 1979).

B. Mean corpuscular hemoglobin (MCH)

Definition. An expression of the amount (weight) of hemoglobin per average, single red blood cell.

Normal Ranges

Adult	27–33 pg*
Senior adult	28–32 pg†
Pediatric	
Newborn	32–34 pg
Thereafter	27–31 pg

*pg = picograms = (10^{-12} g) = micromicrograms (μμg) (Davidsohn and Henry, 1969).

†Calculated from an average of normal ranges given for men and women ±2 pg (Davidsohn and Henry, 1969).

Calculation:

$$\frac{\begin{array}{c}\text{Hemoglobin in g/L}\\ (\text{or g/dL} \times 10)\\ (\text{or g\%} \times 10)\end{array}}{\begin{array}{c}\text{RBC} \times 10^{-6}/\mu\text{L of blood}\\ (\text{or RBC millions/mm}^3)\end{array}} = \text{MCH}$$

Significance. High values are found in macrocytic (large cell size) anemias; low values are found in microcytic (small cell size) anemias. Results usually parallel MCV values.

Discussion. Increases in MCH may be also found in some stages of hemolytic anemias, due to an increase in immature, and therefore macrocytic, cells and large-"shift" erythrocytes (Harvey et al., 1976). (See "Pathophysiology" in Section 2.2.1 for information on "shift to the left.")

C. Mean corpuscular hemoglobin concentration (MCHC)

Definition. The average amount of hemoglobin in each red cell, expressed as a percentage of the volume of the red blood cell.

Normal Ranges	
Adult	30–40%
Senior adult	29–33%*
Pediatric	
Newborn	32–33%
Thereafter	32–36%

*Calculated from an average of normal values given ±2% (Davidsohn and Henry, 1969).

Calculation:

$$\frac{\text{Hgb in g/dL blood (or g/L} \times 10)}{\text{Hct}} \times 100 = \text{MCHC}$$

Significance. A higher-than-average concentration is not possible. Values in megoblastic (macrocytic) anemias are usually normal. A decrease will occur in iron-deficiency anemias, indicating a hypochromic state (an abnormal decrease in the hemoglobin content of the RBC). (SHMC, 1978).

Discussion. The MCV and MCH depend on the accuracy of the RBC count. The MCHC does not. Thus the MCHC can be reliable when automatic methods are not available to ensure the accuracy of the RBC.

2.1.5 Sedimentation rate

Synonyms: erythrocyte sedimentation rate; ESR; SR; "sed" rate

Normal Ranges

Adult	
Male	1–10 mm/hr
Female	1–20 mm/hr
Senior adult	
Male	15–20 mm/hr
Female	20–30 mm/hr
Pediatric	
Newborn	0–2 mm/hr
Neonatal to Puberty	3–13 mm/hr

This is a highly nonspecific test, done on anticoagulated whole blood. The blood is allowed to stand in a calibrated tube. The corpuscles (cells) will settle and the plasma will displace upward. In the healthy individual the rate of settling is constant. The sedimentation rate is determined by measuring the plasma layer 1 hour after the blood sample is placed in the tube. The test is more often increased (e.g., the rate of settling is faster) than decreased and may not increase consistently in any given disease process. It is of value, then, in those disease processes in which it has been found to be elevated. Changes in the degree of increase of the sedimentation rate can be a useful guide in assessing the progress and activity of the disease.

Pathophysiology. The sedimentation rate is a rough measure of abnormal concentrations of fibrinogen and serum globulins; the cause of the increased concentrations is not clear. With elevations of fibrinogen content, and to a lesser degree elevations of globulin content in the plasma, there is increased rouleaux formation of the RBCs (rouleaux = clumping together of RBCs in piles, like rolls of coins) (Greisheimer and Wiedeman, 1972). Such formation tends to increase the weight of the RBCs and, thereby, the speed of sedimentation (Davidsohn and Henry, 1969).

SEDIMENTATION RATE INCREASED IN:

1. *All inflammatory diseases,* such as:
   a. Chronic infectious disease (e.g., tuberculosis). An increase in the sedimentation rate usually parallels an increase in the disease activity.

   b. Diseases of the connective tissue (e.g., rheumatic fever and rheumatoid arthritis).
   c. Acute localized infection in which the increase is seen with an accompanying increase in white blood cells.

2. *All diseases associated with tissue degeneration or necrosis,* such as cancer, in which the increase in ESR often parallels the extent of the malignancy.

3. *Multiple myeloma,* due to the presence of abnormal immunoglobins which increase the formation of rouleaux (Nordin, 1980).

4. *Most anemias,* due to a change in the erythrocyte/plasma ratio which favors rouleaux formation of erythrocytes.

5. *Normal pregnancy* after the third or fourth month of pregnancy. The mechanism is not clear and the ESR usually returns to normal about one month postpartum.

SEDIMENTATION RATE DECREASED IN:

1. *Conditions causing increased serum albumin* (see "Serum Total Protein Increased in" in Section 1.8).

2. *Sickle cell anemia.*

3. *Unexpectedly within normal limits, hypogammaglobinemia* in the presence of serious infection (Meuwissen, 1979).

2.1.6 Implications for Nursing Related to Tests of RBCs and Hemoglobin

1. *Data from related tests of importance,* depending on the diagnosis —or probable diagnosis—should be gathered and compared to known results of tests on the RBCs.

   a. Stool for occult blood. To detect gastrointestinal bleeding in known history of bleeding, clinical indications of bleeding, and in anemias of unknown origin.
   b. White blood count (WBC). Decreased with total marrow depression; decreased in macrocytic anemias.

      Differential. Neutrophils are multilobulated (hypersegmented—extra lobes in the nucleus) in idiopathic steatorrhea and pernicious anemia—macrocytic anemias. Neutrophils are increased in polycythemia vera but usually not increased in compensatory polycythemia.
   c. Platelets. Decreased with total marrow depression. Increased in polycythemia vera but not increased in compensatory polycythemia.

d. Serum iron. Decreased in nutritional anemias; useful to check for this decrease before doing any diet teaching so as not to overload the person with iron and/or unnecessary and confusing information. The test results will not be valid if done shortly after a blood transfusion or when the patient has been on oral iron therapy.
e. B_{12} and folate levels. Checked with any macrocytic anemia.
f. Shilling test. Checked in macrocytic anemias—a test for vitamin B_{12} absorption. Done when vitamin B_{12} and folate levels do not respond to dietary supplementation (Nordin, 1980).
g. Gastric analysis. Rarely used now. No free acid is present in pernicious anemia.
h. Bone marrow examination. Indicated when there is increased immature forms of all myeloid cells in peripheral circulation.
i. Reticulocyte count. To determine positive marrow response in the face of decreased RBC count. Absence of increased reticulocytes after blood loss indicates poor marrow function.
j. Serum bilirubin and/or urobilinogen. To validate presence of intravascular hemolysis. Hemoglobin breakdown serves to increase serum bilirubin and/or urobilinogen (see Fig. 1.1).
k. Red blood cell morphology. (See Section 2.3.1.)
l. Serum haptoglobin. Decrease or absence may indicate intravascular hemolysis.
m. Increased free hemoglobin. Indication of intravascular hemolysis.
n. Urine hemosiderin. Indication of intravascular hemolysis.
o. Sickledex. Screening test for potential hemoglobin S carriers (trait) or sickle cell anemia.

2. *Check for increased values of hemoglobin, hematocrit, and RBC* in response to treatment of anemias.

3. *Prevent changes in RBC tests* because of technical errors in obtaining blood.

a. There is no special patient preparation for tests of RBCs other than the usual instruction in preparation for venipuncture. Capillary blood is frequently used for children.
b. For capillary samples particularly, there should be no excessive massage of the ear lobe, fingertip, or heel to improve blood flow. Massage can increase the total number of cells in the sample over the true number, or can cause mechanical injury to the cell resulting in cell destruction and dilution of the sample by tissue fluid, thereby decreasing values. Capillary blood must also be handled more carefully than venous blood, as it will coagulate more rapidly (Davidsohn and Henry, 1969).

c. With venous samples, the tourniquet should be removed, *circulation restored,* then the tourniquet reapplied when there is difficulty locating the vein. This will prevent hemoconcentration, which would invalidate the test.
d. The sample must be sent to the laboratory as quickly as possible. Standing causes changes in the character of the blood and the distribution of the cells in the plasma (sedimentation).
e. Timing of sample taking should be observed by the nurse. Unless specifically ordered for that time, samples should not be drawn following a transfusion, nor shortly after the person has acted as a blood donor. If the sample must be taken in spite of such invalidating circumstances, the nurse should note the circumstances on the request slip and in the nursing records. The presence of IV infusions or evident dehydration, especially in children and the elderly, should also be noted on the request slip and nursing record.

4. *Identify risk groups for anemia:*
   a. Persons having had gastric resections (loss of intrinsic factor), intestinal resections or bypasses, especially with loss of the terminal ilium (where vitamin B_{12} is absorbed).
   b. Persons with problems with alcohol (liver disease impairs synthesis and storage of RBC materials).
   c. The elderly, mentally retarded, or poor, especially those who are living alone (inadequate diet).
   d. Persons with long-term or chronic gastrointestinal disease (decreased absorption of necessary material for RBC production).

5. *Identify high-potential groups for secondary polycythemia:*
   a. Persons with chronic respiratory or cardiac disease.
   b. Persons who have been living in areas of high altitude.

6. *Because the patient problems* related to both an increase in RBCs and above-normal hemoglobin, when symptomatic, as in polycythemia vera, and a decrease below normal are remarkably similar, they will be treated together. Both dysfunctions are based on inadequate oxygenation of body cells; anemia because of inadequate oxygen-carrying capacity of the blood; polycythemia vera because of ineffective transport of oxygen secondary to a slowed circulation; and hemoglobinopathies because of ineffective or decreased RBC hemoglobin content. The major goal of the nursing plan of care is to equalize oxygen demand and available oxygen at the tissue cell level.

7. *Common nursing problems* related to abnormal laboratory findings in tests of the RBC and suggested nursing actions are listed in Table 2.1.

TABLE 2.1 *Abnormal RBC test results and corresponding nursing actions*

Test result	Problem(s) to observe for	Nursing actions
Decreased RBC count	Fatigue; SOB; DOE; dyspnea at rest; increased heart rate (HR); precordial pain (myocardial hypoxia); decreased level of consciousness (LOC)	Decrease metabolic needs by decreasing physical activity, (e.g., passive rather than active ROM), preventing stress by preventing infection and determining stressful situations in environment and controlling as possible Provide adequate environmental oxygen: O_2 per cannula as indicated; O_2 should be given judiciously because (1) elimination of all hypoxia effectively eliminates erythropoiesis; (2) SOB, etc., may be due to a primary pulmonary problem (COPD) and depend on low O_2 for respiratory drive; should be an independent nursing judgment, but may require an order Open windows can decrease subjective dyspnea by psychological impact on the patient Position of comfort, arms and shoulders supported, for adequate lung expansion Change of position to permit equal lung expansion and prevent pooling of fluids Deep breathe, cough, turn, and instruct patient in procedure and rationale Provide for safety with decreased LOC: No smoking, or only when observed Accompany patient when out of bed Use of side rails Infections should be prevented even in simple anemias, especially in children because of cellular dysfunction caused by hypoxia

TABLE 2.1 *Abnormal RBC tests results and corresponding nursing actions (cont.)*

Test result	Problem(s) to observe for	Nursing actions
Decreased hemoglobin	Potential oliguria (blood flow to kidney decreased by 50% when Hgb less than 7–8 g/dL); complaint of cold; cool pale skin due to decreased peripheral perfusion; absence of cyanosis when Hgb less than 5 g/dL	Measure input and output; report change; keep health team informed Monitor IV carefully, maintain access; adequate clothing and bedding, preferably several light layers to decrease weight and effort in moving In patients with cyanotic cardiac respiratory disease use other parameters than presence of, or changes in, degree of cyanosis in evaluating level of oxygenation in response to activity. In dehydrated patient, hemoglobin should be above normal limits; otherwise, anemia is present
Increased RBC count	Engorged color of face and extremities due to capillary sludging and stasis of blood; potential thrombus; precordial pain due to increased cardiac effort	Check peripheral circulation and venous return; assist venous return as practical (e.g., posture change), encourage leg exercises to increase action of "somatic pump"; provide adequate hydration (within limits of primary pathology) to decrease blood viscosity
Poikilocytosis (spherocytosis) (sickling)	Decreased capillary flow; potential thrombus; joint pain; intravascular hemolysis; potential jaundice; misdiagnosis of pain secondary to vascular occlusion at sites other than joints (symptoms do not occur in newborns up to 6 months of age—protected by presence of hemoglobin F)	See "Implications for Nursing" in Section 1.14.3 Adequate hydration (as above) to decrease blood viscosity Provide, or refer for, genetic counseling when both partners have the "trait" and plan a family Immobilize painful joint Provide analgesics and rest No aspirin should be given because of its effect on platelet function Practice and teach prevention of crisis: Avoid chilling, contact with persons with infectious disease Avoid high altitudes Avoid physical fatigue Identify and avoid stressful situations

TABLE 2.1 *Abnormal RBC tests results and corresponding nursing actions (cont.)*

Test result	Problem(s) to observe for	Nursing actions
		Assure intake of adequate, balanced diet Assure intake of adequate fluids Undertake total immunization program and updates Institute good dental hygiene/ checkups
Increased MCV and MCH	Increased numbers of immature RBCs or macrocytic cells in peripheral circulation, causing potential hemolysis; lemon yellow jaundice; glossitis; stomatitis	Protect from bleeding of mucous membrane: Use soft toothbrush Monitor diet to eliminate caustic, spicy, or tart substances Avoid extremes of temperature in food Stress intake of protein vitamins Provide and teach need for mouth care prior to meals and after meals: Provide cool midly alkaline mouthwashes Provide comfort measures if jaundice causes itching (see "Implications for Nursing" in Section 1.10)
Decreased MCV, MCH, MCHC	Possible iron deficiency/ nutritional anemia	Do diet history Teach management of adequate diet [e.g., iron-rich foods (liver, red meat, raisins, kidney beans, peas, dried apricots, fortified cereals and breads, molasses) Observe patients with anemia of unknown origin for ice eating (pagophagia), which has been observed in some iron-deficient individuals Administer iron as ordered: prevent and teach prevention possible constipation secondary to its use; inform patient of expected change of stool color to black Label any stool specimens with information that patient is on iron Iron given intramuscularly (Imferon, Jectofer) must be given by Z-track technique to prevent staining (see Govoni and Hayes, 1978, p. 372)

TABLE 2.1 *Abnormal RBC tests results and corresponding nursing actions (cont.)*

Test result	Problem(s) to observe for	Nursing actions
Increased ESR	Inflammatory or degenerative process; potential signs and symptoms of acute infection, fever, chills, etc.	Provide measures to prevent further cross-infection or infection of others Consistent decrease in the ESR can be used as one index for increasing activity levels after systemic or chronic inflammatory processes
Decreased haptoglobin	Intravascular hemolysis Potential jaundice and pruritis	Monitor bone marrow effectiveness by checking reticulocyte response Provide comfort measures in cases with pruritis
Pancytopenia	Potential infection; potential bleeding	Protective isolation may be necessary Provide protective measures to prevent or minimize bleeding (see increased MCV, MCH), e.g.: Give all medications orally if possible Give all injectables with smallest-gauge needle possible

Source: Data from Frolich, 1976; Howard and Herbold, 1978; and Whaley and Wong, 1979.

2.2 TESTS RELATED TO THE WHITE BLOOD CELL

2.2.1 White Blood Cell Count

Synonyms: WBC count; WBC; total white count; leukocyte count

*Normal Ranges**

Adult	4.0 – 10.0 thousand (th)/cubic millimeter (mm^3)
Senior adult	
Male	4.25–14.0 th/mm^3
Female	3.1 – 12.0 th/mm^3
Pediatric	
Newborn	9.0 – 30.0 th/mm^3
4 weeks	5.0 – 19.5 th/mm^3
6 months to 1 year	6.0 – 17.5 th/mm^3
2–5 years	5.0 – 10.0 th/mm^3

*Automated reports by single number only. Multiply by 1000 for total count.

Normal Ranges for Different Count:

	Adult	Senior adult	Pediatric	
Neutrophil	2.0–7.5 th/mm^3 or 32–62% of 100 counted WBCs	As for adult with slightly wider variation in range*: 43-79% (Fowler results)	Newborn: 4 weeks: 6 months to 1 year: 2-5 years:	61% 35% 32% 30%
Eosinophil	0.4–0.44 th/mm^3 or 2.2%	0.0–10.0%	Newborn: 1 week: 2 weeks and after:	2.3% 5% 2–3%
Basophil	0.0–0.3 th/mm^3 or 6%	0.0–0.3%	Not available	
Monocyte	0–1.4 th/mm^3 or 0–4%	1.0–15.0%	Newborn: 2 weeks: 3 months: 6 months to 1 year: 2 years to adult:	6–12% 8–9% 7% 5% 5–8%
Lymphocyte	1.0–4.5 th/mm^3 or 31 ± 5%	11–48%	Newborn: 4 weeks: 6 months to 1 year: 2–5 years:	31% 56% 61% 30%

*Automated reports by single numbers only. Multiply by 1000 for total count.

A total white count is one of the routine tests done as a screening test for leukocyte disorders. Evaluation of the other myeloid cells (red blood cells, platelets) is also routinely ordered with the white count because leukocyte disorders rarely occur alone. They are more usually associated with changes in the other myeloid cells. A white blood count is done on almost every patient admitted to the hospital regardless of disease. By itself it is of little value as an aid to diagnosis. It must be related not only to other clinical tests, but also to the clinical condition of the patient.

No patient preparation is necessary for the test. It is subject to errors of random distribution of the cells, however, and is only as accurate as the laboratory worker involved. Most laboratories now rely on automation for the white cell count, which increases the accuracy of the test. A larger volume of blood must be examined than that used for red cell counts because white blood cells are far fewer in number in the blood. An increase in the total number of white blood cells is referred to as leukocytosis. A decrease is termed leukopenia.

Physiology. White blood cells are found in the bloodstream at approximately a 1 : 500 to 1000 ratio to the number of red blood cells present. Less than 1% of the body's total white cells are in the peripheral blood. The remainder are in the marrow as developing and mature cells, lining the capillary walls, and in extravascular areas throughout the body, especially the lungs, liver, and spleen. WBCs are nucleated cells which become smaller as they mature, the nucleus taking up a smaller portion of the cell space (Harvey et al., 1976). They are separated into two major categories: granulocytes (polymorphonuclear leukocytes or polys) and agranulocytes. Granulocytes are further divided into neutrophils, basophils, and eosinophils, based on their staining properties. Agranulocytes (without granules in cytoplasm and with an unlobulated nucleus) are made up of monocytes and lymphocytes.

Production. The monocytes and granulocytes are produced from the bone marrow, and, it is generally accepted, originate from the same stem cells as do erythrocytes (see Fig. 2.1). Lymphocytes are formed in lymph nodes and lymphoid tissue found in the spleen and intestines. Recent evidence suggests that they originate from the same stem cell as the other formed elements of the blood. They are subdivided into two major systems. The T-cell system requires a functioning thymus for normal development and is responsible for cell-based immunity. The B-cell system is responsible for antibody production (humoral immunity) (Nordin, 1980).

Regulation. It is postulated that the human body produces a "colony stimulating factor" from monocytes and some lymphocytes. This factor appears to have properties closely resembling those described for erythropoietin in red blood cell production, thus a granulopoietin. The substance, a glycoprotein, has been produced under laboratory conditions and is found in many body tissues (e.g., bone marrow, urine) ("Lithium. . . " 1979). It is thought to be produced in response to granulocyte breakdown rates and to endotoxemia. Granulocytes are produced at about the same rate as RBCs (Frolich, 1976) in response to an antigen process (Harvey et al., 1976).

Storage. The 99% of white blood cells not circulating are stored in bone marrow, temporarily adhered to the capillary walls, or migrated into tissues until needed or until they die. Since white blood cells do not function within the bloodstream itself, but rather when they migrate into the tissues, those cells circulating in the bloodstream could be considered a storage pool as well.

Life span. Granulocytes live for 10 to 14 days. They remain in the bloodstream only 6 to 10 hr and survive in the tissues for 4 to 5 days under normal conditions. Lymphocytes survive for a longer period, over 100 days. In healthy tissues the macrophage form of monocytes can survive for months.

Function. Leukocytes are considered a part of the reticulo-endothelial system and their function, as a group, is to protect the body against bacterial and protein invasion. They do this by phagocytosis (granulocytes–monocytes), antibody production (B-cell lymphocytes), and delayed hypersensitivity response (T-cell lymphocytes) (Greisheimer and Wiedeman, 1972). Granulocytes are stimulated to migrate to areas containing necrotic tissue and bacteria, where they recognize foreign objects, then phagocytize and digest them. This characteristic of stimulus/response is called "chemotaxis." Mature granulocytes enhance the migration of monocytes. Monocytes, after entering tissues, can be converted to macrophages with enhanced phagocytic and digestive ability. Plasma cells are normally not found in the blood of well persons and originate from B lymphocytes after antigenic stimulation of that tissue. Their chief function when present is antibody synthesis (Harvey et al., 1976).

Pathophysiology. When an infectious process occurs, neutrophils are mobilized early in the inflammatory reaction. As with RBCs, the appearance of additional immature, or juvenile neutrophils (band cells) indicates that there is stimulation of neutrophil production. This state of increased numbers of juvenile neutrophils in circulation is termed a *shift to the left.* The term originated because the table of cells used for differential counting in the laboratory indicates the immature forms of neutrophils toward the left of the table. Neutrophilia (a relative increase in the percent of neutrophils in a differential count) is usually accompanied by some degree of shift to the left in acute infections. (At times, the appearance of hypersegmented polymorphonuclear cells, as with pernicious anemia, is called a "shift to the right," but this term is much less commonly used.)

With a generalized infection the leukocytes respond in three phases:

1. *Acute, progressive.* Relative neutrophilia (increased percentage of neutrophils), may or may not have leukocytosis, shift to the left, appearance of some toxic granulation in the *mature* neutrophils' cytoplasm (presence in immature neutrophils signals marrow exhaustion). A white blood count that exceeds 100 th/mm^3 has a markedly increased viscosity, which can impair circulation in the small vessels of the brain, kidney, lungs, or retina.
2. *Recovery phase.* Neutrophils decrease, monocytes increase, and eosinophils appear.

3. *Convalescent.* Neutrophils return to normal percentage, lymphocytes increase, shift to the left disappears.

Phagocytic activity of granulocytes is increased in anemic persons and those with fever, but is impaired in malnourished persons, or those with high blood glucose concentrations, such as uncontrolled diabetes mellitus, or the malnourished person on prolonged concentrated glucose infusion via hyperalimentation.

WBC INCREASED IN (ABSOLUTE WBC COUNT INCREASE: LEUKOCYTOSIS):

1. *Acute infections,* particularly those produced by pyogenic organisms (e.g., streptococci, staphylococci, pneumonococci).
2. *Chronic infections* (e.g., tuberculosis).
3. *Administration of hydrocortisone,* which decreases the rate at which neutrophils leave the blood; administration of epinephrine, which stimulates release of white blood cells in the marginal pool of the capillaries.
4. *Myeloproliferative disorders* (defined as all disorders that involve the uncontrolled proliferation of bone marrow cells) (e.g., chronic lymphatic leukemia, polycythemia vera).
5. *Tissue necrosis and extreme stress,* as in acute myocardial infarction, burns, gangrene, convulsions, and paroxysmal tachycardia.
6. *Acute hemorrhage.*
7. *Metabolic intoxications,* such as uremia, acidosis, and acute gout.
8. *Physiologic states,* such as:
   a. Physical exercise
   b. Obstetrical labor
   c. Response to cold
   d. Response to pain
   e. Response to massage
   [States (c) to (e) are probably due to release of cells from bone marrow.]
   f. Emotional Stress
   g. Menstruation
   [(f) and (g) are probably due to increased release from capillary walls.]
   h. Diurnal variation (increased in afternoon)

WBC DECREASED IN
(ABSOLUTE WHITE BLOOD COUNT DECREASE: LEUKOPENIA):

1. *Response to ionizing radiation* as treatment or accidental exposure.
2. *Certain diseases of the blood* (e.g., pernicious anemia), due to a disordered DNA synthesis.
3. *Response to certain infecting agents* [e.g., viral infections, rickettsial infections (Rocky Mountain spotted fever, typhus) or protozoan infections (malaria)].
4. *Hypersplenism,* as in hereditary spherocytosis and idiopathic thrombocytic purpura.
5. *Physiologic states,* such as prolonged rest (basal conditions decrease WBC count and production) and aging.
6. *Response to administration of drugs,* especially chemotherapeutic agents (e.g., Cytoxan) or drugs with similar action (e.g., antithyroid propylthiouracil). WBC depression has been reported as a rare and not expected response to many other drugs, perhaps as an idiosyncratic response on the part of the individual.

2.2.2 Differential White Count

Synonyms: differential; blood smear; smear evaluation

Normal Ranges: see Section 2.2.1

This test identifies the relative proportions (percentages) of the different types of white cells that make up the total white cell count. Frequently, the differential count is reported in percentages.

Increases or decreases in the WBC may be due to increases or decreases in one or more of the categories of leukocytes. A white cell differential gives the percentage of each category in a particular sample of blood. This differential must always be interpreted *with* the total white count for the blood sample being examined. An increase in the percentage of any particular category may be secondary to a true increase in the number of cells in that category, or secondary to a decrease in one or more of the other categories. A true increase is termed an *absolute increase,* whereas that secondary to a decrease in other categories is termed a *relative* increase. To avoid possible misinterpretations, several laboratories report the differential count in absolute numbers for each category rather than as a percentage, thereby circumventing interpreting the percentage in light of the total count (Nordin, 1980).

Differential counts are done as chamber counts or on stained blood smears as part of the peripheral blood smear evaluation, but we treat them separately in Table 2.2 because of their importance as an individual test. Each leukocyte seen is identified and classified and the percentage of each cell type observed is calculated. When "hand-counted," 200 to 1000 leukocytes should be counted for accuracy. Percentages are based on 100 cells counted, giving the percentage distribution of the several different types of leukocytes. The differential count often yields more helpful information than any other single procedure used to examine the blood. As with the WBC count, the differential must be related to the clinical condition of the patient and to other hematological tests for correct and useful interpretation.

For individual white blood cells' function and causes for change, see Table 2.2, pp. 162-166.

(See Section 2.2.1 for related physiology and pathophysiology.)

2.2.3 Implications for Nursing Related to Tests of White Blood Cells

1. No special patient preparation is necessary. Since the major function of the WBCs as a group is to protect the body from bacterial and foreign protein invasion, it is obvious that the major nursing goal in caring for a person with abnormalities of any or all of the WBCs would be *to provide protection from such invasions.* This goal can be reached by the following steps.
   a. Assess for risk populations.
      (1) Primary immunodeficiency due to genetic defects, or unknown causes, is rare and presents in many different ways–identification is a primary responsibility of the physician.
      (2) Secondary immunodeficiency is very common, particularly in the hospitalized patient or the person being treated for a chronic disease.
         (a) Review available data for possible immunosuppressive factors.

            Presence of severe infections.

            Presence of severe trauma (e.g., burns) or emotional stress.

            Presence of malnutrition.

            Presence of malignancy.

            Presence of a collagen disease.

            Presence of an enlarged spleen or history of splenectomy (check for surgical scar). [Continues on p. 167.]

TABLE 2.2 *Differential white counts*

White cell	Function	Causes of increases or states in which increases are found	Causes of decreases or states in which decreases are found
Neutrophil (polymorphonuclear)	1. Phagocytosis 2. Major phagocyte in first 12 hr of inflammatory response 3. After death, rupture, release enzymes that digest tissue, to excavate the inflamed site and stimulate appearance of more phagocytes *Major role:* to dispose of invaders, foreign bodies and debris	*Pathological* 1. *Acute infections,* especially in localized cocci infections (e.g., tonsilitis, otitis media); in some *general infections* (e.g., rheumatic fever, diptheria) 2. *Intoxicants:* a. Metabolic: diabetic acidosis, uremia, burns b. Chemical/drugs: lead, mercury/especially with nephrotoxic and hepatotoxic drugs, digitalis, epinephrine, ACTH, hydrocortisone 3. *Acute stress* (e.g., severe hemorrhage, surgery) 4. *Tissue necrosis:* MI, gangrene, neoplasm 5. *Myeloproliferative disease:* polycythemia vera, myelocytic leukemia 6. Thrombosis 7. Acute hemolysis, especially intravascular (DIC) *Physiological* 1. (See increased absolute WBC) 2. Newborn 3. Neutrophilia response more rapid and intense in children	1. Acute viral infections, (e.g., rubeola, viral hepatitis, viral pneumonia) 2. Utlimately in all grave infections of prolonged duration (due to increased rate of destruction or sequestration into tissues?) 3. Nutritional deficiencies, especially folic acid and vitamin B_{12} 4. With splenomegaly 5. Marrow aplasia secondary to ionizing radiation, antimetabolites

Discussion: The splenic vasculature contains only a small portion of the body pool of granulocytes. Its role in leukopenia is not clear. It is altogether likely that the spleen's role in the disappearance of granulocytes from the circulation when it is enlarged is a very minor one.

TABLE 2.2 *Differential white counts (cont.)*

White cell	Function	Causes of increases or states in which increases are found	Causes of decreases or states in which decreases are found
Eosinophil	1. Weak phagocytic action 2. Specific function not known. *Theory:* Detoxification of proteins (would explain the increases seen in allergic and parasitic conditions) *Theory:* Production of a substance that digests fibrin, thus could dissolve clots	1. *Allergic reactions* (e.g., hay fever, asthma, exfoliative dermatitis, erythema multiforma) and drug reactions 2. *Parasitic infections:* intestinal (hook and round worms), tissue (toxicara, trichina) 3. *Skin disorders* (e.g., pemphigus vulgaris, dermatitis herpetiformis) 4. *Neoplasms* 5. *Myeloproliferative disorders* (e.g., Hodgkin's disease, metastatic cancer, polycythemia vera) 6. Following ionizing radiation 7. *Other:* pernicious anemia, polyarteritis, Addison's disease due to decreased glucocorticoid production)	1. Increased circulating glucocorticoids 2. In pancytopenia, for whatever cause

Discussion: Presence of eosinophils in sufficient numbers after a rise in neutrophils secondary to an infection indicates resolution and healing of inflammatory reactions.

TABLE 2.2 *Differential white counts (cont.)*

White cell	Function	Causes of increases or states in which increases are found	Causes of decreases or states in which decreases are found
Basophil	1. Actual function is unknown 2. Contains both heparin and histamine and releases histamine on contact with antigen/allergic reactions, which increases local vascular and capillary permeability 3. Bears a close resemblance to mast cells[a]; may therefore be of some help in chronic infections in the prevention of agglutination, which is part of the chronic inflammatory response	1. Infrequently increased 2. When elevated, most often associated with a myeloproliferative disorder (e.g., chronic myelocyte leukemia) 3. Increased during healing phase of inflammatory response and in chronic inflammation	Not seen except in states of pancytopenia

Discussion: Since the function of the basophil is not really known, its variation with disease and infection are, as yet, of no help in management or prognostication of disease.

[a]Defined as a connective tissue cell containing heparin and believed to be instrumental in immune reactions, anaphylactic and atopic.

White cell	Function	Causes of increases or states in which increases are found	Causes of decreases or states in which decreases are found
Monocyte	1. Phagocytosis: may be converted into large macrophages in tissue with increased phagocytic and digestive	1. *Certain bacterial infections* (e.g., brucellosis, Tbc, subacute bacterial endocarditis) 2. *Certain protozoal and rickettsial diseases* (e.g., malaria,	Not seen except in states of pancytopenia

TABLE 2.2 *Differential white counts (cont.)*

White cell	Function	Causes of increases or states in which increases are found	Causes of decreases or states in which decreases are found
	capacity; in presence of tubercular bacillus, characteristically forms into this epitheloid, multinucleated giant cell 2. Processes antigen, interacts with antigen-antibody-complement complexes to promote phagocytosis	Rocky Mountain spotted fever, typhus) 3. Recovery phase of inflammatory response 4. Recovery phase after marked neutropenia 5. *Other:* monocytic leukemia; Hodgkin's disease	

Discussion: There is a special relationship between the monocyte and the tubercle bacillus, and an increase in monocytes not otherwise explained should alert the practitioner to the possibility of an active tuberculosis process. Disseminated Tbc may be indicated by the appearance of promonocytes in the peripheral blood. The monocyte is the chief cell in the formation of the tubercle of tuberculosis.

White cell	Function	Causes of increases or states in which increases are found	Causes of decreases or states in which decreases are found
Lymphocyte	1. May be the first leukocyte to enter virally infected tissue. 2. Closely involved in the body's immune response and antibody formation	1. *Certain acute viral infections* with early increase (e.g., pertussis, infectious mononucleosis, rubella) 2. *Large numbers of chronic infections* (e.g., brucellosis, syphilis) 3. *Collagen disease* (e.g., systemic lupus erythematosis, rheumatoid arthritis, scleroderma, dermatomyositis, polyarteritis nodosa)	1. Increased circulating ACTH causes immediate decrease; in time, lymphocytosis may occur 2. Thymoma 3. Congential immunodeficiency in children 4. Hypogammaglobulinemia 5. Stress, physiological and psychological

TABLE 2.2 *Differential white counts (cont.)*

White cell	Function	Causes of increases or states in which increases are found	Causes of decreases or states in which decreases are found
		4. *Other:* chronic granulomatous disorders, chronic lymphatic leukemia, lymphosarcoma, Addison's disease (due to loss of glucocorticoid production) 5. *Relative increases* occur with hyperthyroidism and with neutropenia, for whatever cause 6. *Physiological increases:* a. Relative increase at expense of neutrophils at high altitudes b. Relative increase closely related to degree of tanning of the skin, thus seen more often in warm-weather areas c. Relative and absolute increase in infants and children	

Discussion: A progressive increase in the lymphocyte percentage is considered a favorable prognostic sign in pulmonary tuberculosis, and vice versa. Increases not usually of diagnostic significance unless at 40% or more, unless baseline level available. Percentage can vary from 14 to 45% in apparently healthy persons.

Source: Data from Collins, 1975; Davidsohn and Henry, 1969; Faulkner et al., 1968; Greisheimer and Wiedeman, 1972; Groer and Shekleton, 1979; Hall, 1972; Harvey et al., 1976; Jones et al., 1978; Kintzel, 1977; *Lab, Drugs and Nursing Implications,* 1979; Whaley and Wong, 1979.

Presence of any myeloproliferative disorder.

Lack of breast feeding in newborn.

Administration of immunosuppressive drugs (see "WBC Count Decreased in," item 2, in Section 2.2.1 for a partial list).

Treatment of malignancy with radiation or chemotherapy.

Check family history for inheritance pattern of immunodeficiency (e.g., death of young child due to unknown cause).

Uncontrolled diabetes mellitus with high serum glucose (phagocytic activity is impaired in such states).

(b) Assess the person at risk for a pattern of immunodeficient response.

Presence of unexpectedly severe infection.

Presence of infection secondary to ordinarily benign organisms (see Appendix F).

History of recurrent infections.

Presence of eczema or candidiasis.

Impairment of growth and development.

Absence of palpable lymph nodes or visible tonsils in children over 6 months of age. The presence of local lymphodenopathy (palpable enlargement of lymph glands) is a reassuring sign of adequate body immune response to an infecting agent (Groer and Shekleton, 1979).

Lymphocyte count (not just a relative percentage figure) less than 2000 per mm^3 in a child, or less than 1500 per mm^3 in an adult. If count is this low, look for (request, if necessary) a repeat count. Assess patient with a low lymphocyte count for possible stressors that would decrease the count temporarily (e.g., viral infection, severe emotional stress, even in an immunologically healthy person).

Absence of pus in sites infected by pus-forming organisms.

Absence or decreased numbers of granulocytes in biopsy of pyogenic infection site.

History of frequent URI without evidence of pneumonia or purulent otitis media in children over 12 months of age.

Failure to thrive in infants and very young children.

Recurrent staphylococci skin infections.

Presence of chronic diarrhea, especially in children.

b. Assume that any individual who is malnourished, has uncontrolled diabetes mellitus, is on high glucose concentration hyperalimentation, is elderly, or has any change in the absolute WBC to be a person at risk for immunodeficiency.

2. *Provide protective, anticipatory care to risk populations.*
   a. Since WBC production decreases at rest, activity, carefully graded to the capacity of the individual, should be an integral part of the nursing care plan, as should education of both patient and family as to the purpose of each nursing measure instituted and the rationale behind the measure.
   b. Review "Implications for Nursing" in Section 1.9.2 with regard to serum globulin disorders. All are applicable for persons with disorders of the white blood cell as well.
   c. Isolation of any type should be instituted only with adequate knowledge of the individual's resistance, potential for infection, and mode of transmission of potential pathogens. Strict isolation, or protective (reverse) isolation, can produce emotional stress, further decreasing the individual's immunoresponse, and tends to decrease the patient's activity, which can decrease WBC production, decreasing immunoresponse. Further, improper isolation is often worse than no isolation because it can breed false confidence and important assessments for evidence of infection may not be done.

3. *Assess for, and prevent as possible, specific complications* in persons with disorders of the WBCs.
   a. White counts of 100,000 and greater (as in leukemias) increase the risk of circulatory sludging and thrombosis due to increased blood viscosity.
      (1) Provide adequate fluids within the limits of the primary pathology. Fluids are of particular importance in acute lymphatic leukemia (ALL) because of the tendency in that disease to high uric acid levels and urate nephropathy.
      (2) Provide measures to prevent peripheral stasis (e.g., ROM, frequent position change, frequent inspection of skin color and temperature).

(3) Be alert for indication of thrombus formation of vital structures (e.g., flank pain, alteration in urine output = possible kidney occlusion; complaints of blurring of vision, visual cuts = possible retinal occlusion; possible pulmonary emboli) (see "Implications for Nursing" in Sections 1.12.1 and 1.12.3).

b. Persons with relative or absolute decreases in granulocytes are at risk for development of septicemia. Localized infections will not form abscesses since pus does not form. The infection is thus less likely to remain walled off locally and septicemia results. The occurrence of fever may be the first indication of the problem.

(1) Inspect the body daily for indications of infection, especially in those areas most susceptible to infection (e.g., mucous membranes, skin folds with high moisture levels—axilla, perineum, etc.).

c. Children frequently tend to develop URI even when not immunodeficient.

(1) Provide excellent mouth care and pulmonary toilet.

(2) Auscultate chest for diminished breath sounds or evidence of rales.

d. Inspect frequently for evidence of fungal infections (e.g., white patches on mucous membrane); report and obtain treatment order as rapidly as possible.

4. *Monitor repeated white blood counts and differentials* for response to therapy and/or changes in status.

a. Changes in absolute white blood count:

(1) Increase can signal occurrence of superimposed infection or other severe stress.

(2) Increases almost always accompany hereditary anemias.

(3) Increases in patients with subacute bacterial endocarditis could signal an embolic complication (Sodeman and Sodeman, 1974).

(4) Decreases can indicate either a positive response to treatment or bone marrow exhaustion. Check differential for more useful information as to what is occurring.

(5) Decreases below the normal range indicate the possibility of bone marrow exhaustion or suppression.

b. Changes in differential counts:

(1) The presence of some band cells or even metamyelocytes (immature white blood cells), coupled with an increase in neutrophils and total white count (leukocytosis), in-

dicates a healthy bone marrow response to infection (shift to the left).

(2) A shift to the left without the accompanying leukocytosis indicates an overworked and potentially exhausted bone marrow (Hall, 1972).

(3) The appearance of "blast" cells in the lymphocyte or monocyte series (see Fig. 2.1) also indicates a stressed bone marrow.

(4) The presence of toxic granules (large, deeply stained granules thought to consist of enzymes rather than phagocytized material) in *immature* neutrophils, an increasing number of juvenile forms in circulation, and a fall in total white count indicates inadequate marrow response—marrow exhaustion (Groer and Shekleton, 1979).

(5) The appearance of significant numbers of immature forms of WBCs, especially metamyelocytes and myelocytes, coupled with a decrease in total WBC, indicates probable bone marrow exhaustion. This occurrence must be reported to the health care team and the individual must be carefully protected from infection and injury.

(6) Eosinophil increase indicates healing or recovery in inflammatory states.

(7) Lymphocytes and eosinophils will be decreased in acute stress responses.

(8) Monocytes should be expected to increase relative to the decrease in neutrophils in the recovery phase of inflammatory diseases.

(9) Increase in monocytes alone, and independent of acute infection, may indicate onset, or reactivaton, of tuberculosis.

2.3 PERIPHERAL SMEAR

Synonyms: smear evaluation; blood smear; stained blood film

Defined, this test is an examination of the cellular contents of the blood under a microscope, using a variety of stains. Basic dyes (blue) and acid dyes (red) are used. Certain structures take up only the acid dyes and are therefore called *acidophilic* (or oxyphilic, or eosinophilic). Others take up only the basic dyes and are called *basophilic.* Those that take up both dyes are referred to as *neutrophilic.* Modern hematology began with the recognition and use of these staining properties.

Much information of great importance is available from this test. It allows for the determination of blood cell morphology (form and arrangement of structure), which can identify cell origin and maturity as well as the ratio of various cell types to each other. These data, sometimes alone, more often combined with information from the history, physical, and other laboratory tests, provide the medical diagnosis, much as would a histologic tissue section. The information can also be used as a guide to treatment, or as an indicator of harmful effects of chemotherapy or radiotherapy. The differential can be a part of this examination or a totally separate count.

2.3.1 Red Blood Cell Morphology

To an experienced laboratory worker the peripheral smear can give a fair indication of the amount of hemoglobin present, as well as the number of red cells (see Table 2.3). Hemoglobin can be roughly estimated by the depth of staining present. This quantitative analysis is of help in characterizing a number of conditions, such as microangiopathic hemolytic anemia, iron-deficiency anemia, pernicious anemia, sickle cell anemia, and hereditary spherocytosis.

No special patient preparation is necessary. Either venous or capillary blood can be used, but if a platelet count is to be done, venous blood should be used (Davidsohn and Henry, 1969).

(For related physiology and pathophysiology, see Section 2.1.1.)

TABLE 2.3 *Analysis of RBC abnormalities*

Morphology abnormality	Definition	Possible causes
Anisocytosis	Variations in size	
Microcytes	5 μm or less in diameter	Nutritional iron-deficiency anemias.
Macrocytes	10–20 μm in diameter	Presence of increased number of reticulocytes; pernicious anemia; folic acid or vitamin B_{12} deficiency; pernicious anemia rarely found in other conditions
Megalocytes	12–25 μm in diameter	
Poikilocytosis	Variations in shape; can be oval, pear-shaped, saddle-shaped, club-shaped, irregularly shaped	Common occurrence, multiple causes
Burr cells	Irregular projections from RBC; also called acanthocytes or spur cells	Liver disease: albumin deficiency; kidney disease
Fragmented cells	Small fragments of RBC debris, schistocyte	Metastatic malignancy: angiopathic disease

TABLE 2.3 *Analysis of RBC abnormalities (cont.)*

Morphology abnormality	Definition	Possible causes
Sickle cells	RBC bent in crescent or sickle shape	Sickle cell anemia
Spherocytes	Globular rather than usual biconcave cell without central pallor of normal RBC; slightly smaller in diameter than normal	Hereditary spherocytosis: some types of hemolytic anemia
Ovalocytes	Elliptic-shaped cell	Found in normal healthy persons as an inherited trait, or associated with many anemias
Target cells	RBCs with a dark peripheral rim of hemoglobin and dark central ring, separated by an unstained ring; abnormally thin cell	Chronic anemias: hemoglobinopathies (sickel cell anemia; HbC): thalassemia; lead intoxication; severe iron deficiency; liver disease; absence of spleen
Variations in staining		
Polychromatophilia	Residual RNA picks up blue stain, which is mixed with usual red stain of hemoglobin	Further staining will reveal reticular structure of the reticulocyte; 1% occurrence normal in peripheral blood; increased in hemophiliac anemias and in response to blood loss; hemolytic anemias
Basophilic stippling	Variable-sized granules staining blue, found in the RBC due to degenerative changes in cytoplasmic RNA of young cells	Present after exposure to lead, no direct relationship between degree of stippling and degree of toxicity; present in some serious blood diseases (e.g., severe pernicious anemia, leukemia)
Malarial stippling	Fine granular appearance of RBC (Schuffner's granules), staining purplish red; cells larger than normal	Found in RBCs that harbor the malarial parasite in tertian malaria
Variations in structure (see Fig. 2.1)		
Megaloblast	Markedly larger RBC; does not divide normally	Vitamin B_{12} or folic acid deficiency, pernicious anemia; megaloblastic anemia in liver disease
Megaloblastic normoblast	Juvenile form of megalocyte	Occurs in same series as above; when coupled with presence of a shift to the left (immature neutrophils in peripheral circulation) may indicate space occupying lesion of marrow (e.g., metastatic cancer, leukemia, multiple myeloma, Gaucher's disease)
Howell-Jolly bodies	Nucleus broken up into segments; may be singular or multiple	*Singular:* megaloblastic anemias; hemolytic anemias; postsplenectomy; leukemia; *multiple:* indicative of megaloblastic anemia (multilobulated nucleus)

TABLE 2.3 *Analysis of RBC abnormalities (cont.)*

Morphology abnormality	Definition	Possible causes
Cabot's ring	Ring, figure of 8 or loop-shaped structure in RBC	Occurs rarely; found at times with pernicious anemia or lead poisoning
Variations in degree of color		
Hypochromia	Enlargement of central pale area of the RBC; area is also paler than normal	Nutritional and iron-deficiency anemias
Hyperchromia	Deep staining of outer ring of RBC; usually lack the pale center entirely	Pernicious anemia

Source: Data from Davidsohn and Henry, 1969.

IMPLICATIONS FOR NURSING

See Section 2.1.6.

2.3.2 Platelet Estimation

Synonym: thrombocyte estimation

Normal Range: on smear estimation, usually reported as adequate, increased, or decreased; normal or abnormal (for actual platelet count normals, see Section 3.11)

When a peripheral smear is examined, a comment regarding the platelets is considered a necessary part of the report. This comment usually simply describes the general impression obtained by the person doing the test. For instance, the platelets can be described as "adequate" and "normal," when found so, referring to their numbers and morphology, or "decreased" and "abnormal." Some laboratories will routinely provide an indirect count when the numbers do not appear normal with the gross examination. This semiquantitative assessment of platelets is an effective screening test for changes in the numbers of platelets present.

The indirect method of counting is a somewhat easier technique than the direct count (see Section 3.11). The results obtained tend to be higher than are those from direct methods of counting. Roughly, the procedure involves the platelets being counted simultaneously with the red cells. The number of platelets is then calculated on the basis of the RBC count.

Physiology and Pathophysiology. See Section 3.11.

IMPLICATIONS FOR NURSING

1. *The presence of a single abnormal platelet report* does not necessarily indicate a pathologic condition.
   a. Physiologic causes for changes in platelet levels:
      (1) Newborns have fewer platelets during the first few days of life.
      (2) Decreases occur for 2 weeks prior to menstruation. Decrease is progressive over that period and starts to rise again by the third day of menses.
      (3) Daily variations occur within one individual for unexplained reasons.
      (4) Increases are found at high altitudes.
      (5) Levels are higher in winter than in summer.
      (6) Increased following violent exercise, possibly due to distribution change.
   b. Platelets can be normal in number but deficient in function, so a report of adequate numbers and appearance does not indicate a *lack* of pathology either.
   c. The nurse should be aware that platelet counts from different laboratories using different methods will report different values. Because of this, there is difficulty in comparing various findings for platelet counts.

2. *Only great variations from normal* in platelet counts have clinical significance. Decreases in count are considered of more importance clinically than are increases. Differences less than 25% from normal are not considered significant (Davidsohn and Henry, 1969).

3. *When a platelet estimation causes suspicion* of ineffective platelet function, the nurse should assess the individual for physical signs of bleeding tendencies and for the history of, or presence of, conditions that might increase the probability.

a. Check skin of arms, legs, upper chest for ecchymosis (bruising) or petechiae (minute hemorrhagic areas under the skin).
b. Check mucous membrane of the nose and mouth for bleeding.
c. Inquire about history of:
   (1) Excessive menstrual bleeding (menorrhagia).
   (2) Nose bleed (epistaxis).
   (3) Tarry stools.
   (4) Recent viral infections. [Such infections have been found to cause temporary platelet production failure. This is of special importance in children ages 2 to 6, who tend to have acute idiopathic thrombocytic purpura–post infectious thrombocytopenia–more frequently than adults (Jones et al., 1978).]
d. Take a thorough and comprehensive history of drugs presently used and those taken over the previous week or two. Platelets affected by drugs do not "recover" and will remain ineffective until they disintegrate. The life span is variously reported, with a wide range of 4 to 11 days. Numerous drugs have been found to induce, or are suspected of inducing, thrombocytopenia by immune mechanisms. The best documented and most universal offender is aspirin.

4. *If the platelet variation from the norm* is greater than 25% of normal, or if bleeding tendencies are observed, or if the person is routinely taking drugs found to alter platelet function:

   a. Document significant findings in writing.
   b. Check repeat platelet counts. If not available, request that one be ordered.
   c. Institute nursing actions to prevent trauma and bleeding.
      (1) Provide a soft toothbrush and instruct client in its use and rationale for need.
      (2) Advise the use of an electric razor to minimize skin trauma with shaving.
      (3) Request that medication be given by mouth rather than parenterally if possible.
      (4) Use smallest-gauge needle possible if parenteral drugs must be given.
      (5) Apply pressure at injection site, or after venipuncture, for prolonged period, 3 to 5 min, or until bleeding stops.
      (6) Prevent as much trauma as possible related to venipuncture for blood samples.
         (a) Try to organize requests for blood work so that all can be done with one sample.

(b) The use of a heparin lock might be considered for repeated blood sampling. Although heparin has some effect on platelet aggregation, this is not its main physiologic function in coagulation disorders and the amount of heparin actually present in the blood tested would be miniscule, especially if first portion of blood drawn is discarded. Testing norms could be readily adjusted for the variance, should one occur.

(c) Do not prolong the use of a tourniquet when doing venipuncture.

(7) Maintain patent IV to prevent the need for repeated venipunctures. If the procedure of the facility requires automatic IV restarts after a certain period of time, consult with those responsible to arrange an exception for this individual. Then maintain diligent watch for irritation or inflammation at the needle site.

(8) Examine skin and mucous membrane daily for evidence of bleeding or changes in the amount or pattern of bleeding.

(9) Inflate blood pressure cuff no higher than the mean between previous baseline systole and diastole levels, unless a change in blood pressure is evident. Remove the cuff as soon as possible and try not to have to reinflate it.

(10) Inform the individual of the reason for the measures listed above and elicit his or her cooperation in preventing trauma (e.g., no forceful nose blowing or removal of crusts from nares). (Supply water-soluble gel for application to the nose to prevent crusting.) When up, wear slippers (hard) or shoes. Keep nails short and smooth.

d. Acquire knowledge of problematic platelet levels so as to anticipate, prevent if possible, or take immediate corrective action for bleeding or hemorrhage.

(1) Platelet counts from 100,000 to 50,000 per mm^3 usually have hemorrhagic tendencies (Davidsohn and Henry, 1969).

(2) Spontaneous hemorrhage usually does not occur until the count is less than 20,000 per mm^3 (Whaley and Wong, 1974).

(3) Platelet levels less than 10,000 per mm^3 may be life threatening (Jones et al., 1978).

(a) A patient demonstrating such low platelet levels requires intensive nursing care and may require a platelet transfusion.

(b) If a platelet transfusion is probable, the nurse is a logical source of information for the family and the patient for explanations about the process, and the role of donors.

(c) Although not strictly necessary, especially with a single transfusion, cross-matching is done on rare occasions.

e. If active bleeding occurs, independent nursing measures to control the bleeding should be instituted immediately.

(1) Local pressure at the site without disturbing clot formation. (Pressure must be continuous and at the same spot or the fibrin laid down to produce a clot will be mechanically moved and bleeding will resume.)

(a) With epistaxis, pinching the anterior nasal septum between thumb and forefinger is usually the best first step. If such pressure does not stop the bleeding after 10 minutes, packing may be necessary.

(b) Whaley and Wong (1979) suggest two intriguing hemostatic measures, both of which are inexpensive, logical, nontraumatic, and available in most homes. For epistaxis, use salt pork packs, cut to the size of the nostril. Serves as an astringent as well as a pressure pack. Since it is moist, this pack will not adhere to the clot formation when removed. For gingival bleeding, apply pressure with a finger over a dry tea bag.

(2) For epistaxis, have the patient sit in an upright position and breathe through the mouth.

(3) Whenever possible, the area of bleeding should be maintained at a position above the level of the heart to decrease hydrostatic pressure and enhance circulatory return.

(4) Decrease metabolic activity to decrease heart rate and blood pressure.

(a) Place the person in a position of rest.

(b) Reassure that bleeding is not a hemorrhage (if true). Provision of reassurance in the face of *any* bleeding is a difficult task requiring creative efforts on the part of the nurse, as well as knowledge of the individual's unique concerns. It is often useful to involve the patient and/or family members in active care of the problem.

f. The person with bleeding tendencies should not receive aspirin or phenacetin for pain. Substitution of products such as Tylenol is recommended. (See Section 3.11.)

Coagulation Screen

chapter **3**

The coagulation screen is not usually used unless there is reason to believe that a bleeding disorder exists, and is therefore not a true multisystem screen. However, portions of the screen are used for almost all preoperative patients, including at least a prothrombin time (PT), a partial thromboplastin time (PTT), and a platelet estimation (discussed in Section 2.3). It does look at more than just the bleeding problem in that blood vessel integrity, blood component integrity, and by implication, the integrity of the functions of other organs—such as the liver—all are involved in the pathogenesis of bleeding problems. The coagulation screen can determine, quickly and efficiently, the presence of a bleeding problem, the pathway involved, and to a lesser extent, the component(s) that are defective. Each laboratory selects a few procedures from the many available which will best serve the needs of its community. They are often chosen on the basis of relative simplicity (Davidsohn and Henry, 1969).

All coagulation tests, with the exception of whole blood clotting time, are done on plasma. Calcium, removed when the blood is anticoagulated, must be replaced at the time of testing (Wheelis, 1979).

TABLE 3.1 *Plasma coagulation factors*

Coagulation factor number[a]	Common synonyms
I	Fibrinogen
II	Prothrombin
III	Tissue thromboplastin; platelet factor III
IV	Calcium
V	Labile factor; plasma accelerator; A.C. globulin
VII	Stable factor; serum prothrombin conversion accelerator (SPCA)
VIII	Antihemophilic factor
IX	Christmas factor: plasma thromboplastin component (PTC)
X	Stuart-Prower factor
XI	Rosenthal's factor; plasma thromboplastin antecedent (PTA)
XII[b]	Hageman factor
XIII	Fibrin-stabilizing factor; Laki-Locano factor (LLF)

[a]There is no factor VI. Although it has been described, it is not currently believed to be a separate factor and has been deleted from the list (Harper, 1971).

[b]Deficiency of this factor is evident only in laboratory studies. The person with a deficiency will present no bleeding tendency (Harper, 1971).

Source: Data from Caprini, 1973, and Whaley and Wong, 1979.

3.1 PHYSIOLOGY OF COAGULATION

Coagulation is the process of changing fluid plasma of the blood to a solid gel by the ultimate conversion of fibrinogen to fibrin. Its central process is that of thrombin generation. Coagulation involves participation of at least 12 identified factors (see Table 3.1), as well as many cellular blood components. The factors are thought to circulate in an inactive form. When stimulated they become active in a sequential, not necessarily strictly numerical order which is often called the *coagulation cascade.* There are two introductory pathways which can initiate the process. The site of the stimulus determines the pathway (see Fig. 3.1). The extrinsic pathway is the most rapid because of the presence of tissue thromboplastin (factor III), while the intrinsic pathway must produce thromboplastin from the activation of platelets. Coagulation is most rapid in the child and adolescent because of the superb elasticity of their blood vessels.

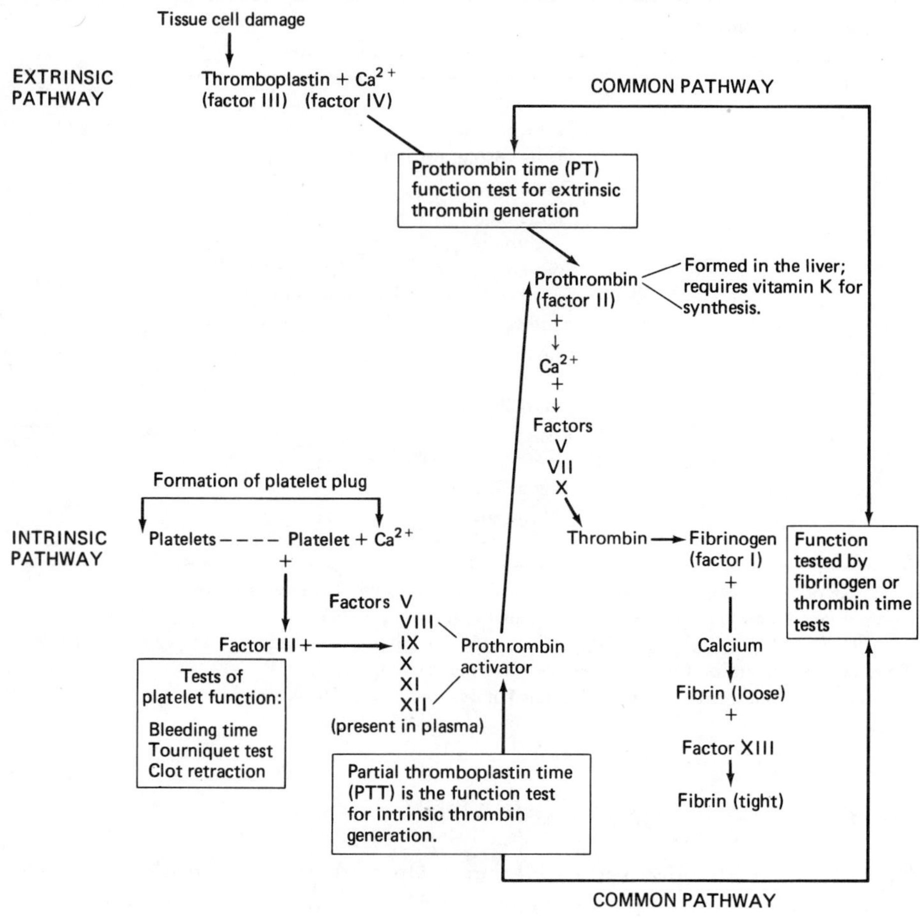

FIGURE 3.1 Blood clotting mechanism.

3.1.1 Formation of the Platelet Plug—Intrinsic Pathway

Damage to a blood vessel causes it to contract, an important hemostatic mechanism of the extrinsic pathway, but of lesser value in the intrinsic system. The platelet plug bridges the gap between vascular contraction and clotting. It is the self-sealing attribute for local vessel repair. It is a different process than that of clotting, since blood can clot without the presence of platelets, but the plug cannot form without them. A platelet plug can occur in the absence of clotting, but requires some thrombin for the process. The steps of the process are as follows:

1. *Disruption of vessel wall due to multiple causes* (e.g., antigen-antibody complexes, foreign contaminants, or products released from neutrophils).
2. *Exposure of collagen fiber.* Endothelium of blood vessels usually provides a nonwettable surface, not stimulating to platelets.
3. *Platelets activated by contact with collagen* (can also be stimulated by mechanical disruption of blood flow); change in characteristics—become sticky and adhere to collagen; spread out (pseudopods) to cover maximum surface.
   (a) Release adenosin diphosphate (ADP) and calcium (Ca^{++}).
   (b) Platelets in circulation begin to stick to platelets adhering to the wall in the presence of Ca^{++}—platelet aggregation.
   (c) Releases serotonin and epinephrine, which stimulate local vessel contraction, allowing platelets to anchor.
   (d) Release phospholipid (platelet factor III, thromboplastin), which triggers prothrombin—thrombin generation (see Fig. 3.1).
4. *Presence of thrombin* continues platelet activation and aggregation.
5. *Ultimately, if coagulation occurs,* fibrin strands produced by the activation of prothrombin-thrombin are deposited in the platelet plug.
6. *Platelet plugs* form less readily when blood flow is rapid (e.g., arterial vessels) and require sufficient blood loss to decrease flow pressure before the plug will occur. Thus pressure exerted on the exterior of the vessel wall will decrease local blood flow and enhance clotting.

3.2 PATHOPHYSIOLOGY OF COAGULATION PROCESS (Caprini, 1973)

1. Problems related to small vessels (vascular phase of hemostasis)
   a. Telangiectasia
   b. Purpura
2. Problems related to the platelet plug
   a. Thrombocytopenia—decreased number of platelets
      (1) Idiopathic thrombocytopenia purpura

(2) Systemic lupus erythematosus
(3) Drugs
(4) Tumors
(5) Consumptive coagulopathy [disseminated intravascular coagulation (DIC)]

b. Thromboasthemia–decreased platelet function; thrombopathy
(1) Glanzmann's thrombasthenia
(2) Congenital and acquired
(a) Combined defect (Von Willebrand's disease)
(b) Drugs: primarily dextran and aspirin
(c) Uremia

3. Problems related to thrombin generation

a. Factor depression VIII, IX, XI
(1) Hemophilia A (VIII)
(2) Hemophilia B (IX): Christmas disease
(3) Hemophilia C (XI)
All clinically indistinguishable except by laboratory test.)

b. Factor depression II, VII, IX, X (vitamin K–dependent factors)
(1) Coumarin therapy (vitamin K antagonist)
(2) Liver disease (factor VII first to decrease) (liver synthesizes vitamin K)
(3) Vitamin K deficiency (dietary malabsorption)

c. Factor depression common pathway
(1) Parahemophilia (V)
(2) Stuart-Prower (X)
(3) Calcium (IV) [very rare; unlikely as cause of clinical bleeding except *rarely* in instances of transfusion of ACD blood (almost all blood is now ACD blood); coagulation process can take place with less CA^{2+} than that necessary for usual physiologic function].

d. Antithrombin
(1) Heparin
(2) Endogenous–secondary to other disease process

e. Fibrin network
(1) Fibrin stabilizing factor
(2) Congenital hypofibrinogenemia
(3) Acquired hypofibrinogenemia
(a) Disseminated intravascular coagulation (DIC)
(b) Primary fibrinolysis

Defects in platelets and clotting factors are the most common causes of bleeding in children.

3.3 BLEEDING TIME

Synonyms: Ivy bleeding time; Duke bleeding time

Normal Ranges

Adult	
Ivy method	2.0–8 min (reported to nearest ½ min)
Duke method	Less than 3 min
Senior adult	As for the adult
Pediatric (Ivy method)	
Premature	1–8 min
Newborn	1–5 min
Thereafter	1–6 min

This is a simple and inexpensive test, thought to reflect the platelet function of aggregation and the vasoconstriction of the vessel. The platelet function measured is independent of the blood clotting mechanism. However, severe impairment of clotting might prolong the bleeding time (see Section 3.1.1). The time measurement reflects the interval needed for bleeding from a small superficial wound to cease.

Of the two methods usually employed, the Duke and the Ivy, the Ivy method is more popular and is considered the more sensitive of the two tests. It is performed by applying pressure to the forearm with a blood pressure cuff at 40 mmHg and making a small standardized cut in the forearm. The blood is then blotted at 30-sec intervals, care being taken not to touch the cut itself until bleeding stops. The Duke method involves a standardized cut on the earlobe with the same timed blotting until bleeding ceases.

BLEEDING TIME PROLONGED IN:

1. *Thrombocytopenia, thrombopathies* (see Section 3.2). Aspirin is a major offender. It is thought to affect platelet adhesiveness. Can increase bleeding time up to 21 min if given within 1 week preceding the test (SHMC, 1978).
2. *Parahemophilia, Von Willebrand's disease.*
3. *Fibrinolytic states.*
4. *Senile purpura,* due to the loss of elasticity and turgor of the vascular wall. It is clinically benign, the most serious consequence being cosmetic (Sodeman and Sodeman, 1974).
5. Scurvy

BLEEDING TIME NORMAL IN:

Hemophilia A and B. Hemophilia A is a disorder of factor VIII, as is Von Willebrand's disease, but Von Willebrand's has a defect in platelet adhesion which hemophilia A does not.

BLEEDING TIME DECREASED IN:

Not clinically significant.

IMPLICATIONS FOR NURSING

1. *The person having the test should be informed* of the possibility of scarring (Ivy method) from the small incision. He should also be informed if the usual practice consists of taking at least two, if not more, samples. Most labs now use a disposable device which makes two simultaneous standard cuts. In some facilities the test is repeated until two bleeding time values are not more than a minute apart when the Ivy test is used. Since the normal range is broad, and the test is quite variable, such repetition is recommended.
2. *A relevant history should be taken for drugs* affecting platelet function (see "Implications for Nursing" in Section 2.3.2).
3. *Note the administration of thrombocytopenic drugs* on the laboratory request slip for bleeding time. This is particularly important when aspirin is being given. Note date and time of last dose.
4. *If the patient's platelet count* is less than 25,000 per mm^3, a special, informed order for a bleeding test usually must be obtained from the physician.
5. *If the patient is on therapeutic heparin administration,* the test should not be done for approxlimately 4 hr after a dose is given. This precaution does not usually apply to heparin used in a heparin lock to keep it patent.
6. *Observe the skin of the arms carefully* after routine blood pressure taking for petechiae in any person with a prolonged bleeding time, as well as after venipuncture or the Ivy method of the bleeding test. A test sometimes used, which the nurse can employ as a nursing observation with the activities described above, is the *tourniquet test.* When the blood pressure cuff is inflated halfway between the systolic and diastolic pressures (about 40 mmHg)

for 5 min, petchiae will appear distal to the cuff. The normal person can form up to five petechiae. In the person with a platelet or vascular defects, petechiae formation is markedly increased.

7. *All nursing actions relevant to platelet estimation* may apply as well for the patient requiring a bleeding time (see "Implications for Nursing" in Section 2.3.2, as well as Section 3.12).

3.4 PROTHROMBIN TIME

Synonyms: protime; PT; quick prothrombin time; quick test

Normal Ranges (one stage)*

Adult	11–18 sec Mean of 13 sec
Senior adult	No change from adult value
Pediatric	
Premature	12–21 sec
Newborn/neonatal	12–20 sec
Thereafter	12–14 sec

*Normals are usually measured against a control. Therefore, there is variation in normals between laboratories. In many instances results are expressed as a percent of activity rather than elapsed time in seconds.

The prothrombin time test indicates the rapidity of blood clotting and is a good test of the extrinsic thrombin generation pathway. It does not measure the amount of prothrombin generated, rather the activity. The extrinsic prothrombin time is so short that any contribution to clotting from the intrinsic pathway is usually negligible.

In the past prothrombin time was thought to measure prothrombin activity only. It is now known that a normal test result depends on adequate levels of factors V, VII, and X as well—all factors of the extrinsic pathway (see Fig. 3.1). It is the *only* test that measures factor VII activity (Caprini, 1973).

The protime test is widely used for differential diagnosis in jaundice. Vitamin K administered parenterally usually restores a prolonged PT to normal in a patient with obstructive jaundice and will fail to do so in patients with intrinsic hepatic (parenchymal) disease (Davidsohn and Henry, 1969; see also Section 1.10). Probably its greatest uses are as a guide for anticoagulant dosage in the administration of coumarin (Wafarin), phenindione (Indon), or dicumarol; as a diagnostic test in bleeding disorders; and a measure of vitamin K deficiency (Wheelis, 1979).

Physiology and Pathophysiology. Prothrombin (factor II) is synthesized in the liver and is dependent on the presence of vitamin K. There are other precoagulation factors also dependent on vitamin K for synthesis: factors X, VII, and IX (Christmas factor). Vitamin K is synthesized primarily by intestinal bacteria and, being lipid-soluble, absorbed only if bile salts are present. Thus deficiencies in either of these substances, bile salts or fat, lead to deficiencies in vitamin K, and thus in the precoagulation factors noted, prothrombin among them. Prothrombin deficiency is almost always associated with other factor deficiencies.

In the absence of vitamin K, the protein normally activated by the vitamin may enter the bloodstream, where it acts as a competitive inhibitor of the vitamin K-dependent factors, enhancing their deficiency (Frolich, 1976).

The amount of prothrombin in the blood is actually less critical in clotting than is the availability of the other factors necessary for its conversion to thrombin. The amount of prothrombin usually available provides a wide margin of safety against its being deficient. Therefore, the two-stage prothrombin test, which actually measures the prothrombin, is not frequently used. The one-step method measures deficiencies in factors V, VII, X, and II (Davidsohn and Henry, 1969).

The stimulus for prothrombin generation via the extrinsic pathway is tissue damage, releasing tissue thromboplastin. Because fewer reactions are required to complete this pathway, the protime is about one-third that of the partial thromboplastin time (PTT).

PROTHROMBIN TIME PROLONGED IN:

1. *Inadequate intake of vitamin K,* as in:
   a. Hemorrhagic disease of the newborn, due to an inadequate supply of milk. Milk is the only source of vitamin K for the newborn since it lacks bacteria in the bowel for vitamin K synthesis (see Section 1.10).
   b. NPO states prior to surgery in persons who have had antibiotic bowel sterilization.
2. *Impaired intestinal absorption of vitamin K,* as in:
   a. Sprue.
   b. Ulcerative colitis or Crohn's disease.
   c. Obstructive jaundice.
3. *Parenchymal hepatic disease,* as in:
   a. Cirrhosis.
   b. Hepatitis.

4. *Persons being given certain drugs,* such as:
   a. Questran, due to binding of bile salts.
   b. Aspirin in large doses.
   c. Long-term antibiotic therapy, due to decreased vitamin K synthesis (or gut sterilization prior to surgery).
   d. Large amounts of laxative, due to decreased absorption of vitamin K.
   e. Wafarin or dicumarol, due to decreased vitamin K synthesis. The therapeutic level of prothrombin with these drugs is usually 1 to 1½ times the normal range.
5. *Disease states producing decreased fibrinogen values,* below 100 mg/dL (see Section 3.6).
6. *Disease states producing coagulation inhibitors,* such as lupus erythematosus, alcoholism, renal insufficiency, malnutrition, and scurvy.

PROTHROMBIN TIME SHORTENED IN:

1. *Response to treatment with certain drugs* (e.g., vitamin K, anabolic steroids).
2. *Persons on an excessively high fat diet,* or one with an excessive intake of vitamin K-rich foods.

IMPLICATIONS FOR NURSING

1. *No special patient preparation* is necessary.
2. *Small amounts of vitamin K* are frequently given to a mother prior to childbirth, or given to the newborn if necessary. The nurse needs to supply not only the drug, but also the reason for the injection and reassurance as to its effectiveness in preventing hemorrhagic disease of the newborn.
3. *Any person who has had prolonged antibiotic therapy* for more than 2 days, or intensive therapy for gut sterilization, should be supplied with foods to replace the intestinal flora as a regular part of the diet, or when feeding is resumed. Foods helpful in the repopulation of intestinal flora include yogurt, acidophilus milk, buttermilk, and soft natural cheeses. These individuals also need to be carefully observed for superimposed infections from nonsusceptible organisms. Candidias of the mucous membrane of the

mouth, or in women the mucous membrane of the vagina, is a frequent complication.

4. *Plasma taken for PT determination* must be tested promptly (within 6 hr of collection) or frozen for longer storage. Factor V activity is rapidly lost at temperatures of 37°C or greater.
5. *See* Section 3.12 for general nursing implications which also apply.

3.5 PARTIAL THROMBOPLASTIN TIME, ACTIVATED

Synonyms: aPTT; APTT; partial thromboplastin time; PTT*

Normal Ranges†

	Activated method	Traditional method
Adult	35–45 sec	60–85 sec
Mean	40 sec	70 sec
Senior adult	No change from adult values (Method not described in the literature; apparently activated)	
Pediatric		
Premature	Less than 120 sec	
Newborn	Less than 90 sec	
Thereafter	Less than 60 sec	
Range	39–53 sec	

*The only difference between partial thromboplastin time and the activated thromboplastin times is that the activated method uses the addition of a silica compound to standardize the initial, or activation, phase of the test, thus decreasing the length of time between the addition of calcium and visible clotting. It is felt to be the more reproducible test and almost as sensitive as the standard test (Sodeman and Sodeman, 1974).

†Reference ranges or "normals" for both PT and PTT are dependent on the commercial reagents used and vary from lab to lab (Nordin, 1980).

The partial thromboplastin time test is used as a screening test for deficiencies of coagulation factors in the intrinsic and common systems (see Fig. 3.1) of thrombin generation. Single deficiencies can be further isolated, especially if the deficiencies are severe. Such isolation is less useful in mild deficiencies, or where combined deficiencies exist, such as in intravascular clotting. Factor inhibitors can also prolong the PTT. There is a further simple test (1:1 mix with normal plasma) to differentiate inhibitors from factor deficiency, and it is usually done with a prolonged value (Wheelis, 1979). The PTT is sensitive to all factors except VII (stable factor or serum prothrombin converter accelerator).

The PT and PTT tests form the basis of screening tests for coagulation factor deficiencies.

The name "partial" thromboplastin is derived from the use of a thromboplastin which lacks the ability to compensate totally for the plasma defect of hemophilia, hence, a *partial* thromboplastin (Caprini, 1973).

Physiology and Pathophysiology. (See also "Physiology and Pathophysiology" in Section 3.4.) The intrinsic pathway of coagulation is stimulated by the release of factor III (platelet thromboplastin) and involves a longer period of time to reach its end point—the production of fibrin—than does the extrinsic pathway. It also requires a greater number of coagulation factors to complete its process. The PTT responds with prolongation primarily in persons with factor IX and VIII deficiences—hemophilia (Harvey et al., 1976).

PTT PROLONGED IN:

1. *Hemophilia,* due to factor VIII or IX deficiency.
2. *Von Willebrand's disease* (pseudohemophilia), although the increase may be slight.
3. *Persons receiving coumarin or dicumarol therapy,* although not consistently prolonged, and the increase is usually slight. The increase is due to the failure of the liver to synthesize factor IX.
4. *Heparin therapy,* due to the inhibition of the formation of thrombin from prothrombin. Heparin probably also prevents plasma thromboplastic activity. The PTT is commonly used to monitor heparin therapy. The dosage is adjusted to keep the PTT at 1½ to 2½ times normal.
5. *Disseminated intravascular coagulation* (DIC), due to consumption of platelets and decrease in factor VIII.
6. *Conditions requiring multiple doses of Narcan,* process unclear.

PTT DECREASED IN:

Extensive cancer, except hepatic cancer, due to the increasing amount of thromboplastin from the tumor content.

IMPLICATIONS FOR NURSING

1. *No special patient preparation* is necessary.
2. *Related to patients on heparin therapy:*
   a. A PTT test is usually done before each heparin dose when therapy is being started; therefore, the nurse must check that the blood sample has been collected before giving the medication.
   b. PTT determination is done 4 hr postdose if heparin is being given subcutaneously (SQ) or intramuscularly (IM). IM is the most dangerous method and should be avoided if possible. The risk of hemorrhage or hematoma at the site is great. Preferably, therapeutic heparin is given IV by continuous infusion (Nordin, 1980).
   c. Give any other IM injections just prior to giving heparin to decrease the chance of bleeding. All drugs should be given orally if possible as well (see "Implications for Nursing" in Section 2.3.2, as well as Section 3.12). All precautions taken for any patient with a bleeding disorder should be taken with persons receiving heparin.
3. *Related to patients with hemophilia:*
   a. Check any site of bleeding for rebleeding after the first clot has formed. Primary hemostasis is unstable in hemophilia.
   b. Prevention of crippling effects due to bleeding into joint spaces or secondary to pain on movement is a major nursing responsibility.
      (1) In the acute stage, elevate the affected joint and immobilize it, to encourage clotting.
      (2) Assist with factor replacement (factor VIII–Hemofil, Humafac, Factorate; factor IX–Konyne, Proplex*) or administration of cryoprecipitate (AHG–antihemophilia globulin; AHF–antihemophilia factor) in hemophilia A. Use of these materials is the major medical approach to both controlling bleeding and preventing further bleeding, which would prevent crippling by eliminating the cause.
      (3) Institute passive range of motion as soon as bleeding stops and the acute phase is over.

*These commercial preparations are rarely used. Most frequently used is cryoprecipitate.

(4) Minor pain control should be maintained with acetaminophen (Tylenol) rather than aspirin to prevent further bleeding effects, yet provide for maximum activity.
(5) Provide pain medication prior to activity.
(6) Consult with physician and physical therapy department in setting up activity programs. Get input from patient and family as to preferred activities and work them into the program to increase compliance.
(7) Teach patient/family/home caretaker when appropriate about the long-range effects of joint involvement to increase compliance with activity regime.

c. Assist patient/family/home caretaker in developing maximum independence. Refer to a home care program if available. If none available, consult with the health care team to set up the most appropriate teaching system possible.
(1) Delay any teaching until the major bleeding emergency is over. Teaching should also be delayed until the process of adjustment to a new diagnosis of hemophilia has occurred for both patient and family/home caretaker. Content areas and some general guidelines on which to base a teaching plan are given below.
(a) Bleeding control: direct pressure; immobilization, elevation; packing with Gelfoam or fibrin foam; application of topical hemostatic preparations such as thrombin; application of cold; and compression with Ace bandages.
(b) Self-administration of scheduled or emergency infusion of factor replacements with emphasis on prevention of further trauma (e.g., use of small-gauge needle, IV technique, minimal venous obstruction with venipuncture).
(c) Signs and symptoms of transfusion reaction (e.g., chills, temperature spike, dyspnea, rash, back pain, edema). (Reactions occur due to presence of anti-A or B isohemaglutinins in solution. Cryoprecipitate must be cross-matched with recipient's blood type.)
(d) Care of stored factor. Cryoprecipitate is stored frozen.
(e) Use of over-the-counter drugs (e.g., no aspirin); teach to read labels.
(f) Need to advise others of diagnosis (e.g., dentist); use of ID card/bracelet/tag with name, doctor's name, and diagnosis.
(2) Refer to National Hemophilia Foundation for literature, films, counseling, special children's camps, and newsletter.

d. All precautions and teaching areas listed for other bleeding problems apply to the individual with hemophilia (see "Implications for Nursing" in Section 2.3.2, and Section 3.12).

4. *Monitor related laboratory findings* with bleeding problems of the intrinsic pathway.
   a. Whole blood clotting time is usually prolonged.
   b. Prothrombin consumption time is usually decreased.
   c. Bleeding time is usually normal (there is no platelet deficiency in hemophilia A and B, but there is with Von Willebrand's disease).
   d. Prothrombin time is usually normal.

3.6 PLASMA FIBRINOGEN

Synonym: Claus fibrinogen

Normal Ranges

Adult	160–300 mg/dL
Senior adult	470–485 mg/dL
Pediatric	
Newborn	150–300 mg/dL
Thereafter	200–400 mg/dL

The plasma fibrinogen test is similar to the thrombin time test in that both measure conversion of fibrinogen to fibrin by thrombin. They differ only in the method of procedure. The fibrinogen test does minimize the effects of any inhibitors of coagulation (antithrombin, heparin), while the thrombin test is sensitive to the presence of inhibitors. The fibrinogen test is helpful in differentiation between liver disease and bleeding due to disseminated intravascular coagulation, since its level is rarely decreased below 100 mg/dL in liver disease but can be much lower in DIC (Wheelis, 1979).

There are several different methods of measuring fibrinogen. Methods such as used for this test, which involve some form of clottable protein determination, are done rapidly; thus they make good screening tests. A chemical assay of fibrin is the most accurate method, but is more time consuming.

Physiology. Fibrinogen (factor I) is one of the major plasma proteins (see Section 1.8) making up about 5% of those proteins. Once clotting has occurred, virtually all of the fibrinogen will have been removed from the plasma. Fibrinogen is produced in the liver by what must be an extremely efficient process since it is uncommon to see decreases except in the most severe forms of liver disease, and decreases that do occur are rarely below 100 mg/dL (Ravel, 1973). This soluble plasma protein is converted by the action of thrombin, in the presence of calcium and factor XIII (fibrin stabilizing factor), to the insoluble protein molecule, fibrin (see Fig. 3.1).

The peptides (A and B) that are split from the fibrinogen molecule in this process are acute-phase reactants which respond to inflammation, making fibrinogen's role in the body a dual one—that of clotting and inflammatory repair (Groer and Shekleton, 1979). The fibrin molecule then forms long fibrin threads that interweave and form the clot, trapping blood cells. The normal presence of heparin and antithrombin in the plasma inhibits the formation and action of thrombin, thus preventing spontaneous activation of fibrinogen and generation of the fibrin clot, assuming relatively small amounts of thrombin being formed. However, in the face of increased tissue or platelet destruction, greater concentrations of thrombin occur and clotting takes place. Blood clotting at an inflamed site helps wall off the area and potentiate other chemical responses to speed repair.

Pathology. Deficiencies of fibrinogen can be congenital or acquired and can result in (1) afibrinogenemia—no measurable fibrinogen; (2) hypofibrinogenemia—fibrinogen present but in amounts less than 100 mg/dL; and (3) dysfibrinogenemia—fibrinogen decreased in function (as measured in its reaction to thrombin) but present in normal amounts (measured immunologically). Acquired deficiencies occur due to liver disorders, active fibrinolysis, or intravascular clotting disorders.

Clinical signs and symptoms of patients deficient in fibrinogen only, and with normal procoagulants otherwise, are less severe than the symptoms of patients with deficiencies of one of the other procoagulants. Therefore, the bleeding that occurs with many congenital forms of fibrinogen deficiencies is not usually life threatening, as the congenital form is usually an isolated fibrinogen deficiency. However, isolated fibrinogen deficiencies are uncommon in acquired bleeding disorders (Davidsohn and Henry, 1969).

FIBRINOGEN INCREASED IN:

1. *The elderly*—a physiologic response, the purpose of which is not clear.
2. *Response to nonspecific stimuli* (e.g., trauma, infections, neoplasm, hemorrhage).

FIBRINOGEN DECREASED IN:

1. *Intravascular clotting disorders* with consumption in excess of production, most commonly disseminated intravascular coagulation (DIC), which occurs secondary to complications of pregnancy, such as:
   a. Missed abortion (long-standing intrauterine death of the fetus).
   b. Premature separation of the placenta.
   c. Amniotic fluid embolism following administration of oxytocin. (All felt to be due to the release of thromboplastin-like substances from the placenta and amniotic fluid into the circulation.)
2. *DIC secondary to other conditions,* such as (these occur more commonly than pregnancy-related DIC):
   a. Prostatic cancer with metastasis, believed to produce a fibrolysin (plasminogen) activator (see Fig. 3.2 in Section 3.9).
   b. Septicemia.
   c. Surgical and postoperative shock.
   d. Postcardiac bypass surgery.
   e. Massive thrombosis.
3. *Liver disease* (cirrhosis, hepatitis) due to decreased production, not usually clinically evident unless accompanied by other factor deficiencies which may cause clinical signs and symptoms.
4. *Conditions causing increased levels of fibrinolysins* (enzymes which destroy fibrinogen) and active fibrinolysis, such as:
   a. Cancer of the prostate with metastasis.
   b. Post thoracic surgery.
5. *Congenital deficiencies,* all other coagulation factors being normal.

FIBRINOGEN NORMAL IN QUANTITY BUT ABNORMAL IN FUNCTION IN:

1. *Congenital dysfibrinogenemia.*
2. *Multiple myeloma,* due to the presence of paraproteins that act as inhibitors of fibrin strand and clot activity.

IMPLICATIONS FOR NURSING

1. *No special patient preparation* is necessary. The fibrinogen test must be performed within 24 hr of blood sample collection. If the nurse obtains the blood sample, the laboratory request slip

should be clearly labeled as to time the specimen was taken and it should arrive in the laboratory as soon as possible.

2. *For persons with congenital fibrinogen deficiencies:*
   a. Treatment is the administration of fibrinogen by plasma transfusions. Since this factor is lost from the body by normal decay in 12 to 21 days when not utilized for clot formation, replacement is done routinely every 10 to 14 days. The nurse should monitor fibrinogen levels for this person when under nursing care between infusions. Fibrinogen levels should be maintained at 50 mg/dL or higher.
   b. True fibrinogen levels for diagnostic purposes can be determined only when there is no active bleeding and there has been no recent (3 to 4 weeks) transfusion of blood or plasma.

3. *A fibrinogen level below 100 mg/dL* is rare in liver disease and can therefore be helpful in ruling that condition out as the cause of low fibrinogen concentrations. Since the alternative possibilities of cause are somewhat limited, a careful nursing history (see "Implications for Nursing" in Section 2.3.2, and Section 3.12) can assist the physician in targeting the problem area.

4. *The test should not be drawn* within 6 hr of a heparin dose, as heparin interferes with thrombin, hence fibrin, generation.

3.7 WHOLE BLOOD CLOT RETRACTION

Synonyms: none

Normal Ranges

Adult	Complete retraction within 24 hr
Senior adult	As for adult
Pediatric	Retraction may be complete within 4 hr but normals generally as for adult

Clot retraction is done as a part of the test for clotting time. Because it is nonspecific and unreliable, it is not used a great deal now. Test tubes filled with blood are placed in a warm bath (37°C) to be observed for clot retraction every 30 to 60 min. The test is open to error because of the differences in the size of the clot formed. Approximately one-half of the total blood volume in the tube should be made up of clot, the other half made up of serum for a "normal"-sized clot.

Clot retraction is a rough indicator of platelet adequacy but is reliable only when packed red cell volume (hematocrit) and fibrinogen concentrations are within normal limits.

Physiology and Pathophysiology. When the coagulation cascade, or process, is complete, a clot has been formed. The fibrin of that clot is acted upon by factor XIII, causing the strands to shrink. The clot's ability to shrink is dependent upon an adequate number of platelets being present and on the action of thrombin. It is thought that platelets may provide the necessary energy (ATP) for the shortening process. The fibrin strands of the clot attach to the edges of the injured blood vessel. The process of shrinking serves to pull the edges closer together, helping to decrease blood loss and begin repair. The retraction process is therefore essential to the process of hemostasis (Watson, 1979).

The clot usually decreases to half of its original size in 1 hr, the fibrinogen free serum being extruded and a definite margin being visible between clot, serum, and test tube wall. The resulting clot, if normal, is much firmer than the original.

The absence of fibrinogen, an increase in fibrinolytic activity, or an increase in packed cell volume will cause red blood cells to be released from the clot into the serum. Smaller clots than normal occur with decreased packed cell volumes or fibrinogen concentrations (Davidsohn and Henry, 1969).

POOR WHOLE BLOOD CLOT RETRACTION OCCURS IN:

1. *Thrombocytopenia.*
2. *Thrombasthenia.*
3. *Fibrinogenopenia.* Because of the small clot size, clot retraction is inadequate, although it may be misinterpreted as normal.

WHOLE BLOOD CLOT DISSOLUTION OCCURS IN:

Conditions with increased fibrinolytic activity (see Section 3.6).

IMPLICATIONS FOR NURSING

The time span necessary for initial retraction to half-size (1 hr) and total clot retraction (24 hr) provides a rationale for the need to immediately immobilize a bleeding part and then to restrict vigorous activity of the part for 24 hr. Immobility promotes clot formation; decreased activity enhances clot stability.

3.8 WHOLE BLOOD CLOTTING TIME, ACTIVATED

Synonyms: activated coagulation time; ACT*

Normal Range: 75–105 sec

Therapeutic Ranges:

150–210 sec (general heparin therapy) (Nordin, 1980)
300–600 sec (extracorporeal heparin therapy) (Widman, 1979)

*Another similar test used to monitor heparin therapy besides the ACT and the APTT, the test of choice in hospital use at present, is the BART (blood activated recalcification time—or recal time). The therapeutic range of the BART test is 1.5 to 2.0 times the normal clotting time (i.e., with the whole blood clotting time, activated, normal range given previously, the BART therapeutic normal would be 113 to 210 sec.

This test measures the overall activity of the intrinsic clotting mechanism, the time it takes whole blood to clot firmly. The predecessor test, nonactivated whole blood clotting test, widely known as the Lee-White clotting test, was the least accurate of coagulation tests, and time consuming. Blood takes 4 to 8 min to clot firmly, and heparinized blood, the kind most often being tested, extends that time to about 20 min. The activated test speeds up that process and can be reproduced more accurately.

Physiology and Pathophysiology. See "Physiology and Pathophysiology" in Sections 3.4 and 3.5.

ACT PROLONGED IN:

As that given with the PTT test (Section 3.5).

ACT DECREASED IN:

As that given with the PTT test (Section 3.5).

3.9 FIBRINOLYSIN

Synonyms: whole blood clot lysis: clot lysis

Normal Range

Adult	Negative (no lysis of clot) in 48 hr
	No available data for indication of any difference from adult normals for other age groups

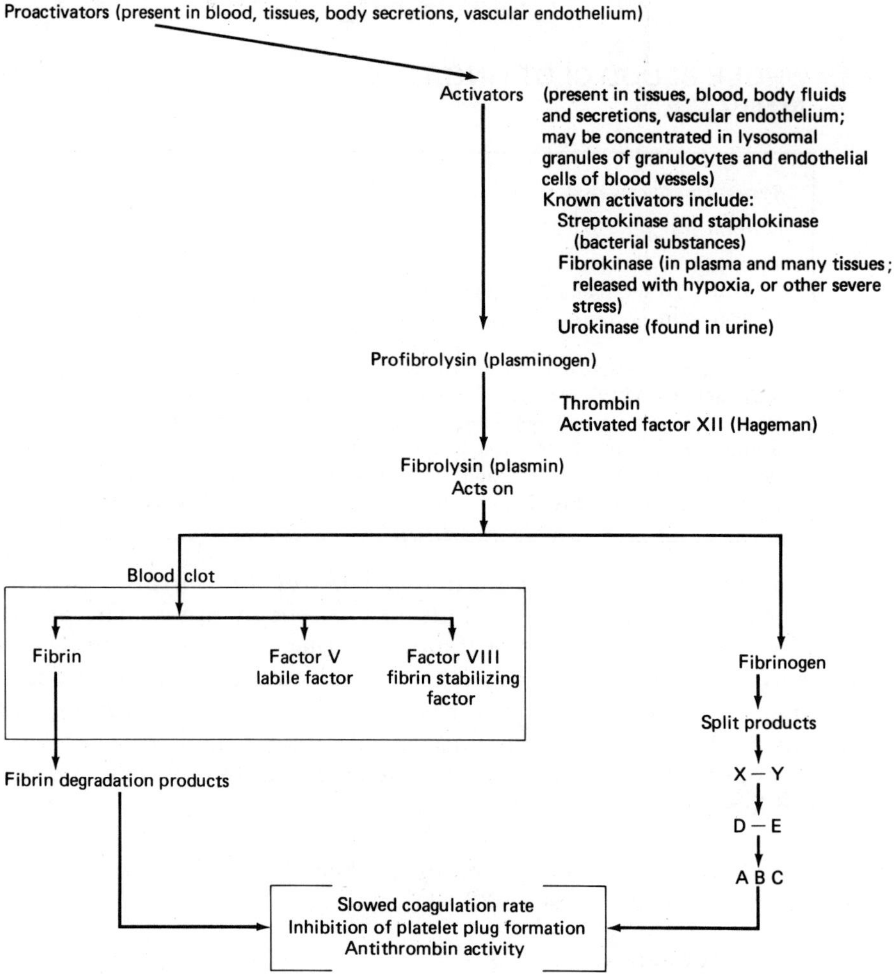

Proactivators (present in blood, tissues, body secretions, vascular endothelium)

Activators (present in tissues, blood, body fluids and secretions, vascular endothelium; may be concentrated in lysosomal granules of granulocytes and endothelial cells of blood vessels)

Known activators include:
- Streptokinase and staphlokinase (bacterial substances)
- Fibrokinase (in plasma and many tissues; released with hypoxia, or other severe stress)
- Urokinase (found in urine)

Profibrolysin (plasminogen)

Thrombin
Activated factor XII (Hageman)

Fibrolysin (plasmin)
Acts on

Blood clot

Fibrin

Factor V
labile factor

Factor VIII
fibrin stabilizing
factor

Fibrin degradation products

Fibrinogen

Split products

X – Y

D – E

A B C

Slowed coagulation rate
Inhibition of platelet plug formation
Antithrombin activity

FIGURE 3.2 Fibrinolysis. (Source: Caprini, 1973; Davidsohn and Henry, 1969; Frolich, 1976; Ganong, 1973; Harper, 1971; and MacBryde and Blacklow, 1970.)

The principle underlying this test is that an increased activity of fibrolysins (plasmins) in the blood will cause a clot, formed from whole blood, to dissolve over a specified period of time—from 1 to 24 hr. A normal clot will remain intact for at least 48 hr. This type of evaluation of the fibrinolytic system is the more common approach used in screening tests or in emergency conditions. Other tests look at the activity of components for fibrinolysis, which components rapidly disappear from the circulation and are, therefore, of limited usefulness in emergency conditions (Caprini, 1973).

Physiology. (See Fig. 3.2 for diagrammatic representation of the fibrinolytic system.) The fibrinolytic system is by intent a protective mechanism to rid the body of clots that are no longer needed and exists in addition to the clotting inhibitors, such as heparin and antithrombin. Preactivators circulate in the blood until activated themselves by the presence of certain tissue enzymes, to profibrolysin (plasminogen), and then converted through further enzyme activation (fibrokinases) to fibrolysin (plasmin). Fibrolysin acts on the blood clot and on fibrinogen as well, breaking them down into products that inhibit the coagulation process (Price and Wilson, 1978). This fibrinolytic sequence is a slow process as opposed to coagulation; it is as complex as the coagulation process; and it is even less well understood than is the coagulation process.

Pathophysiology. At this point in research, it is difficult to determine at what level fibrinolytic activity will result in hemorrhage. Some experts feel the fibrinolytic mechanism is of major significance and others feel there is little clinical significance in its role as a cause of bleeding (Davidsohn and Henry, 1969).

3.10 THROMBIN TIME

Synonyms: None

Normal Ranges

Within 3 sec of control (control usually approximately 10 to 15 sec)
No data available for indication of variation from the above norm in other age groups

As noted with the plasma fibrinogen test, the thrombin time and fibrinogen test evaluate the thrombin-fibrinogen reaction. The thrombin time detects defects in the rate of fibrin formation. The test is done by adding thrombin to plasma and timing the resulting formation of a fibrin clot. This is then compared to a control (or normal). A result ± 3 sec of that control indicates the presence of adequate and functional thrombin. The test is sensitive to the presence of inhibitors of thrombin formation and is more sensitive in detecting heparin inhibition than is any other test.

Physiology. Thrombin formation, already discussed in the general physiology of coagulation, is the central process of blood coagulation and can be generated by both the intrinsic and extrinsic systems. Its presence is essential to the function of platelets and also seems to be a factor in activation of the fibrinolytic system (Mountcastle, 1974; see also Fig. 3.2). It is formed through the action of calcium and factors V, VIII, and X, and functions as an enzyme, stimulating fibrinogen, in the presence of calcium, to form fibrin (see Fig. 3.1). Prothrombin circulating in the blood is not converted to thrombin at any appreciable rate, if at all. Thrombin generation is stimulated by, and appears quickly after, any bleeding. The rate at which it is produced sets the rate of the speed of clotting. Very quickly after maximum thrombin production has been reached, antithrombin progressively inactivates it and it is continuously removed from the system. Were it not removed, it has a half-life of only 3 days. The action of antithrombin and endogenous heparin prevent continuation of the clotting process beyond need.

Thrombin appears to be formed mostly in the arteries, in response to roughened endothelium or collagen exposure.

Pathophysiology. One of the major pathologies directly related to thrombin generation is that of thrombosis. Clots formed in blood vessels are called thrombi (thrombus–singular), which distinguishes them from extravascular clots. The careful balance maintained by the body between blood fluidity and necessary clotting is not yet well understood. Study in the area of intravascular clotting or thrombosis is hampered by the fact that humans are the only animals known to form venous thrombosis (Groer and Shekleton, 1979).

Although thrombin is produced primarily in the arterial circulation, the production of venous thrombus appears to be the result of venous stasis, causing venous *concentration* of thrombin produced at injury sites in the arteries. Venous intimal endothelium of a thrombosed vein is usually found to be normal. Because much activated thrombin is held back (sequestered) in slowed venous circulation, it cannot be adequately destroyed by the liver; thus thrombosis occurs, spreads, and may lead to embolization. Thrombosis can occur in the arterial circulation at the site of injury or at sites of slowed circulation, such as atherosclerotic narrowing of coronary arteries. The elderly are a population at risk for atherosclerosis and consequently thrombophlebitis.

A second major area of pathology is a decrease in thrombin activity due to an increase in fibrinolysis, producing anticoagulant split products, low fibrinogen levels, or the presence of endogenous circulating anticoagulants often seen as an effect of many chronic diseases (Caprini, 1973).

THROMBIN TIME PROLONGED IN:

1. *Persons with plasma fibrinogen levels* less than 100 mg/dL.

2. *Persons with systemic disease,* causing increased production of coagulation inhibitors, such as:
   a. Systemic lupus erythematosis.
   b. Uremia.
   c. Hyperbilirubinemia.
3. *Impaired fibrinogen function* (abnormal fibrinogen).
4. *Inhibitors of thrombin-induced clot formation,* such as:
   a. Exogenous administration of heparin as therapy.
   b. Abnormal globulin.
   c. *Intravascular clotting disorders,* producing increased amounts of fibrinogen split end products (see Fig. 3.2 and Section 3.6 "Fibrinogen decreased in," items 1 and 2).
5. *Most cases of polycythemia vera,* due to a relative depletion of plasma clotting factors, particularly fibrinogen and prothrombin, and due to inadequate platelet function.

THROMBIN TIME DECREASED IN:

Not found clinically significant. Systemic levels are not necessarily altered when either arterial or vascular thrombosis occurs. The thrombin increase is local and quickly eliminated (see "Pathophysiology" above).

IMPLICATIONS FOR NURSING

1. *No special patient preparation* is necessary.
2. *The elderly are at particular risk,* especially when ill and hospitalized, for thrombosis formation. In consequence, their risk of developing disseminated intravascular clotting (DIC) is increased, since massive thrombosis is one etiology for DIC. The nurse then should take a meticulous history and do a thorough, continuing physical appraisal of the elderly patient. Particular attention should be paid to even-higher-risk persons within the elderly as a group. These include females taking replacement hormones; and persons with varicose veins, history of congestive heart disease, and with conditions tending to increase immobility (to include loss of visual or hearing acuity, which can tend to immobilize the elderly due to fear or social embarrassment). A con-

tinuing appraisal for indicators of thrombosis or bleeding should be carried out.

3. *The individual with polycythemia vera* (a fairly rare disorder) is also at dual risk of thrombosis and bleeding from the increased viscosity of the blood and potential heart failure, and from decreased fibrinogen, prothrombin, and ineffective platelet function.
   a. Increased blood viscosity should *not* be treated by provision of increased fluids in this case because of the presence of hypervolemia. Phlebotomy (venesection) removing about 500 ml of blood every 2 or 3 days and the use of marrow suppressants are the medical approach to decrease blood viscosity.
   b. Observe particularly for bleeding from peptic ulcer (hemocult or guiac test for all stools or vomitus), since this is a common problem with this diagnosis (Harvey et al., 1976).
4. *Other pertinent tests to monitor* with prolonged thrombin time include PTT and one-stage PT. Hypofibrinogenemia will be indicated by prolonged values in one or all of these. No clotting will occur in afibrinogenemia; therefore, the prolongation of the tests will be indefinite.
5. *If a repeat thrombin time* is reported as "corrected at 50/50" (or 90/10) control/patient mixture, a coagulation factor or element deficiency is present. If uncorrected, anticoagulant (heparin, fibrin split products) activity is indicated (Caprini, 1973).

3.11 PLATELET COUNT

Synonym: thrombocyte count

Normal Ranges

Adult	250,000–500,000/mm^3
Senior adult	
Age 50*	
Female	255,000–1,392,000/mm^3
Male	330,000–1,430,000/mm^3
Age 94*	100–300,000/mm^3
Pediatric	140–300,000/mm^3
Premature	150–390,000/mm^3
Newborn	200–473,000/mm^3
Neonatal	150–450,000/mm^3
Infant Thereafter	70,266–175,000/mm^3

*Dameshek method.

The platelet count is most consistently accurate when done on an automated counter. Platelets are difficult to count because of the speed and ease with which they disintegrate. In a blood sample drawn for analysis platelets are stable *only* at *room* temperature, not refrigerated, and stable for only 24 hr. Thus there are virtually no functional platelets in stored blood. Bank blood frequently will have the platelets removed immediately for use in platelet transfusion.

Use of venous rather than capillary blood is recommended for this test. The results from venous blood tend to be more reproducible. Capillary sticks tend to lower counts because of the loss of platelets adhering to the wound.

Physiology. Platelets are formed from megakaryocytes in the bone marrow (see Fig. 2.1). They are not true cells as they have no nuclei, but are highly active metabolically when stimulated. They are stimulated by any foreign substance with a negatively charged surface, including glass, which explains blood clots forming in a test tube.

Platelet function is primarily that of hemostasis ("thrombo" means clot and "cyte" means cell, hence a clot cell), actively engaging in the formation of the platelet plug to maintain blood vessel integrity (see Section 3.1.1). They are one of two sources of thromboplastin (or factor III), the other being injured tissue; they are an essential element in the process of coagulation (see Fig. 3.1). They produce serotonin to stimulate blood vessel contraction at the site of injury. Further, they are essential to clot retraction (see Section 3.7).

Platelet regulation is not too well understood. After acute blood loss, production increases; larger platelets appear in peripheral circulation; the platelet count rises. The body produces platelets at a constant rate (from 50,000 to 100,000 per mm^3 per day), maintaining the normal level. Their life span is from 4 to 11 days. There is believed to be a circulating substance called thrombopoietin, as yet not isolated or characterized, that stimulates increased formation and development of platelets (Ganong, 1973). Approximately one-tenth of the circulating platelets are used to maintain the blood vessels endothelial integrity, and about one-third are sequestered in the spleen in the normal person (Davidsohn and Henry, 1969).

Pathophysiology. An increase in platelets can occur. When it does there is a tendency to thrombosis and, less frequently, a tendency to hemorrhage as well. An extremely high count apparently has an anticoagulant effect, which may be that of inhibition of thromboplastin (factor III) generation. Increases can occur secondary to increased production or increased release. Decreases, felt to be of more clinical importance, can occur secondary to a decrease in production, an increase in pooling (sequestration) in the spleen, or increased destruction. Platelets can also be adequate in numbers but ineffective in function.

PLATELET COUNT INCREASED IN:*

1. *For physiologic causes* of changes in platelet levels with platelet estimation, see "Implications for Nursing" in Section 2.3.2.
2. *Myeloproliferative syndrome,* including initial response in polycythemia vera, causing a thrombocythemia. Platelets are abnormal and lead to thrombosis.
3. *Response to acute stress* (e.g., injury, surgery), with an increase in production rather than release from bone marrow. A similar increase occurs when adrenal corticol steroid hormones are used therapeutically.
4. *The period following a splenectomy.* Increases are greater if a preexisting anemia is not corrected by the surgery, and always higher than the levels reached following other surgeries.
5. *The period following hemorrhage* (usually a physiologic response).
6. *Metastatic cancer,* particularly that of the lung and other epithelial cancers.
7. *Acute infections.* Possibly related to the stress response.

PLATELET COUNT DECREASED IN (THROMBOCYTOPENIA):

1. *Conditions causing decreased production,* such as:
   a. Bone marrow failure secondary to administration of drugs, chemotherapeutic agents, or irradiation.
   b. Bone marrow replacement by primary bone marrow malignancies or metastatic malignancies.
   c. Idiopathic thrombocytopenia purpura (ITP), cause unknown. Occurs secondarily to many things. May have an autoimmune mechanism; autoantibodies (IgG) to platelets' protein are often present. Known to occur secondarily to viral infections (especially in children), administration of quinine and quinidine, pernicious anemia, and paroxysmal nocturnal hemoglobinuria.

---

*Two terms are used, frequently interchangeably, to describe platelet increase: thrombocythemia and thrombocytosis. Thrombocytosis seems to refer to an absolute increase in circulating platelets above 500,000 per microliter. Thrombocythemia is used to describe conditions that involve an increase in the number of megakaryocytes in the bone marrow and an increase in circulating platelets over 1,000,000 per microliter (Frohlich, 1976).

2. *Conditions causing increased destruction,* such as:
   a. Immune thrombocytopenia.
   b. Disseminated intravascular clotting (DIC).
3. *Conditions causing increased pooling* (e.g., splenomegaly).

PLATELET COUNT NORMAL IN NUMBER BUT ABNORMAL IN FUNCTION IN:

1. *Von Willebrand's disease.* Platelets lack ability to aggregate.
2. *Persons with high triglyceride levels.* Platelets have decreased ability to aggregate. High cholesterol levels have no effect on platelets.
3. *Persons on a high dosage of aspirin,* causing inhibition of platelet aggregation, due to decreased ADP release. [0.5 millimolar (m*M*) concentration of aspirin in the blood can be achieved by as little as four 5-g aspirin tablets and can cause a bleeding tendency (Groer and Shekleton, 1979).]
4. *Nitroglycerin and prostaglandin* E_1 also inhibit platelet aggregation.

IMPLICATIONS FOR NURSING

1. *See* "Implications for Nursing" in Section 2.3.2, and Section 3.12.
2. *If the nurse takes the blood sample* for a platelet count, the laboratory request slip should have the time of sample collection clearly indicated, and the tube should be kept at room temperature until turned over to the laboratory, which should be done as soon as possible.
3. *Unless absolutely necessary, peripheral blood* (finger stick) should not be used for the test. If peripheral blood must be used, indicate this on the request slip.
4. *Check pertinent laboratory tests* other than platelet count. Severe thrombocytopenia should be accompanied by an increased bleeding time and poor clot retraction–both tests of platelet function.
5. *Identify risk populations for thrombosis.*
   a. Persons with metastatic malignancies, especially of the lung.
   b. Persons over 60 with sedentary life-styles.
   c. Persons at bedrest or otherwise immobilized.

d. Those with increased platelet counts.
e. Those with atherosclerosis.

6. *Implement nursing measures* to help prevent thrombus formation. Measures to decrease venous stasis include:

   a. Use of properly fitted, properly worn elastic hose, removed at least once daily, left off at night. The legs should be visually examined each time the hose are removed for evidence of venous stasis (e.g., cool extremeties, varicose veins, capillary dilitation). Hose should be reapplied with the leg elevated at least to the level of the rest of the body.
   b. Frequent change of position, independent or assisted.
   c. Sequential elevation of dependent parts of the body.
   d. Elimination of any pressure in the popliteal area—no knee pillows.
   e. Whenever possible, body weight should be evenly distributed over the largest body area possible. No crossed legs; lying better than sitting and sitting better than standing.
   f. No massage of leg muscles.
   g. Bed exercises should be passively instituted, then taught and actively practiced by the patient when possible. Examples of bed exercises include flexion and extension of knees alternating legs; foot lifted from mattress with back of knee pressed to mattress; flexion, extension rotation of ankle with heel off bed; gluteal muscle setting (buttocks tightly contracted, then relaxed).
      (1) Exercises should be done independently by the patient, if possible. Set up mutually agreed on environmental clues to remind the person of the exercises, such as doing a set of exercises each time a nurse enters a room, or if that seems to predict too little exercise, each time a commercial comes on television.
      (2) Passive ROM is still indicated in a patient at risk for thrombosis, even if that person is up walking. Not all muscles are used equally in ambulation, and some not at all.
   h. Encourage swimming or wading in water as a recreational pursuit, or if a pool is available in the physical therapy department, consult with appropriate members of the health team to allow this activity while the person is hospitalized. Water exerts equal pressure about the leg, and when wading, the water pressure is exerted most strongly in the area with most need of venous support. Muscular activity requires less effort when swimming with an equal increase in muscle pumping of blood.

3.12 GENERAL IMPLICATIONS FOR NURSING RELATED TO PROBLEMS IN COAGULATION

1. *Observe persons with undiagnosed bleeding problems* carefully for origin of bleeding. Although the specific diagnosis is ultimately made by the physician based primarily on laboratory data, data collected by the nurse based on the following generalizations can also be helpful. Bleeding into deep tissue spaces or joints usually indicates a coagulation disorder, whereas superficial bleeding is more often due to a vascular or platelet disorder (Caprini, 1973).

2. *Principles that are helpful* in understanding how diagnoses of coagulation defects are made include:
   a. Factors I, II, V, VII, IX, and X are synthesized in the liver; therefore, liver disease may affect their production.
   b. Liver-synthesized factors II, VII, IX, and X are dependent on vitamin K; therefore, any process that interferes with vitamin K intake, absorption, or utilization may affect their production.
   c. Only factors I, II, V, VIII, and XIII and platelets are consumed in the process of blood clotting. Other factors act as true enzymes. Therefore, in conditions of rapid and/or prolonged clotting (e.g., DIC), the listed factors may be depleted.
   d. Banked blood, as well as platelets, will be deficient in factors V and VIII, since they are unstable on storage. Replacements are possible only with fresh blood or plasma.
   e. Platelets, which must be used immediately, and cryoprecipitate, which can be frozen and is rich in factors I and VIII, are commonly removed from banked blood for individual administration (see Table 14.4).

3. *Certain requirements should be met in obtaining blood samples* for coagulation tests. Although this activity is not always the responsibility of the nurse, seeing that the requirements are met may well be in order to assure valid test results.
   a. Select a vein of adequate caliber; use of the veins on the back of the hand is not recommended.
   b. Use at least a 19-guage, thin-wall needle to help prevent hemolysis.
   c. A clean venipuncture (no residual bruising) will give the most accurate results.
   d. Before use, the first few milliliters of blood collected should be discarded to remove tissue thromboplastin generated by the tissue trauma of venipuncture.

e. The tourniquet should not be left in place for over 1 min, as stasis facilitates blood clotting and changes the normal distribution of blood cells.
f. Use only a very light pressure to immobilize the vein without compressing it. This avoids mobilizing vessel-wall enzymes that can falsely elevate fibrinolytic levels (Caprini, 1973).
g. Usually, blood should not be taken from a patient having been given heparin within 6 hr prior to the time of sample taking, and blood is best taken from the arm without a heparin lock.

4. *Complete and accurate history taking and physical appraisal* are of great importance in the determination of cause, and thus treatment, of bleeding disorders. In addition to those observations suggested with the nursing implications for platelet estimation (Section 2.3.2) and those given with individual tests in this chapter, the nurse can assist the physician in the assessment process by observation or inquiry into the following areas:

   a. Duration of bleeding tendency—lifelong or of only recent origin?
   b. Presence of chronic disease, originating before or concurrent with the bleeding problem, especially hepatic or renal disease?
   c. Diet history, with special emphasis on deficiencies in protein, fat, and vitamins K or C intake?
   d. In the newborn, note bleeding from the umbilicus that is prolonged or occurring after normal clotting time (24 to 48 hr). This may indicate a defect of the extrinsic pathway or a fibrin defect. Inquire into family history of bleeding, or consanguious union (such bleeding is a hallmark of a rare autosomal recessive trait).

5. *Active observation* should be done for bleeding or thrombosis in all risk populations [e.g., at the time of delivery (bleeding), the elderly (thrombophlebitis), patients with medical history of bleeding problems in themselves or their families]. With these persons it would be sensible to guaiac or hemoccult all urine, stools, or vomitus.

6. *Institute nursing actions to reduce trauma and prevent bleeding.* Review "Implications for Nursing" in Section 2.3.2. In addition:

   a. Teach and help the person to practice good dental hygiene to prevent extractions and probable severe hemorrhage.
   b. Avoid rectal temperatures with the possibility of damage to fragile mucous membrane, particularly if the platelet count is less than 20,000 per mm^3.

c. The person taking oral anticoagulants may be advised by their physicians to carry vitamin K at all times. This individual requires instruction as to the purpose and effect of vitamin K and how to use it in self-treatment of spontaneous hemorrhage.

7. *Despite the need for calcium* in almost all the steps of the coagulation process, a low serum calcium is not considered a cause of abnormal bleeding. Deficiency of calcium low enough to cause bleeding is incompatible with life (Sodeman and Sodeman, 1974).

Urinalysis Screen: Urinalysis Routine

chapter 4

The routine urinalysis is one of the first tests used in identification of pathology of the urinary tract and is an indispensable part of clinical pathology. It can provide an estimate of renal function, give information as to possible causes for dysfunction, and can even indicate systemic disease. The urinalysis is a careful, systematic study of the physical, chemical, and microscopic properties of urine. Data thus obtained help provide only a tentative diagnosis at times, but at the same time guide the selection of more specific tests for more definitive diagnosis.

Tests commonly included in a routine urinalysis are gross examination, specific gravity, pH, glucose, protein, ketone bodies, occult blood, bilirubin, and a microscopic examination of the urinary sediment if indicated or ordered. To understand the implications of abnormalities in these tests, it is necessary to understand how urine is formed.

4.1 PHYSIOLOGY OF URINE PRODUCTION

All blood circulating through the body eventually passes through the kidney. The blood enters the nephron(s) of the kidney at the glomerulus, where it leaves most of its protein content in the capillaries, since the

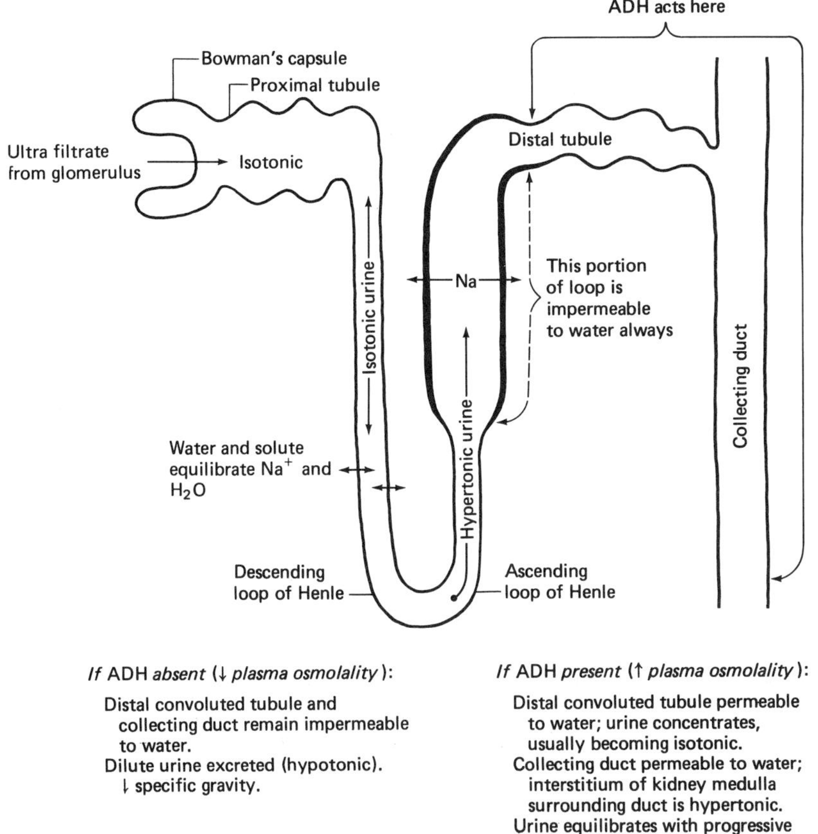

If ADH *absent* (↓ *plasma osmolality*):

Distal convoluted tubule and collecting duct remain impermeable to water.
Dilute urine excreted (hypotonic).
↓ specific gravity.

If ADH *present* (↑ *plasma osmolality*):

Distal convoluted tubule permeable to water; urine concentrates, usually becoming isotonic.
Collecting duct permeable to water; interstitium of kidney medulla surrounding duct is hypertonic.
Urine equilibrates with progressive concentration.
Hypertonic urine.
↑ specific gravity.

FIGURE 4.1 Dilution and concentration of urine. [Adapted by Tami Bruce and printed with permission from A. McGehee Harvey, Richard Johns, Albert Owens, and Richard Ross, ***The Principles and Practice of Medicine,*** 19th ed. (New York: Appleton-Century-Crofts, a Publishing Division of Prentice-Hall, Inc., 1968), p. 141.]

healthy glomerulus is relatively impermeable to the larger molecules. The resulting plasma, which contains most of the organic and inorganic chemicals of the blood (e.g., glucose, amino acids, urea, uric acid, sodium, potassium, chloride, and bicarbonate), in much the same concentrations as that of whole blood (specific gravity of 1.010, the same as protein-free plasma), goes into the tubule system of the nephron (see Fig. 4-1). The tubules selectively secrete waste products not useful to the body and reabsorb those needed by the body (see Table 4-1). The waste products, together with at least enough water to keep them in solution, are excreted into the kidney pelvis, ureter, and bladder, to be removed from the body when sufficient amounts of this waste solution, now called urine, stretch and stimulate the bladder muscles to contract.

TABLE 4-1 *Segmenta functions of the renal tubules*

Segment	Functions
Proximal tubule	Reabsorption 70% filtered H_2O and NaCl Glucose Urea Uric acid Amino acids K^+, Mg^+, Ca^{2+}, HPO Secretion Organic acids and bases H^+ and NH_3
Henle's loop	Reabsorption via countercurrent multiplier NaCl in excess of H_2O
Distal tubule	Reabsorption Filtered H_2O and NaCl (small fraction only) Secretion H^+, NH_3, K^+
Collecting ducts	Reabsorption NaCl H_2O (depends on ADH concentration) Urea K^+ (depends on aldosterone concentration) Secretion H^+, NH_3 (pH of urine may be reduced to 4.5–5.0) K^+ (depends on aldosterone concentration)

Source: Reprinted with permission from Maureen E. Groer and Maureen E. Shekleton, *Basic Pathophysiology: A Conceptual Approach* (St. Louis, Mo.: The C. V. Mosby Company, 1979), p. 291.

Some 180 L of fluid is filtered daily in the healthy adult. The filtrate forms approximately 1 to 1½ L of urine. About 25,000 mEq of sodium and 25 g of urea, the major inorganic and organic solutes, are processed with the water and, of that amount, about 150 mEq of sodium and 15 g of urea are excreted.

In short, urine is formed by the filtering of plasma through the glomeruli, the selective reabsorption and secretion activity of the tubules, and the excretion of the formed urine by the urinary tract (Collins, 1975).

There are some age-related physiologic changes in kidney function. Urine osmolality decreases slowly from a high at age 30, to a low at age 80, and other slight tubular function changes occur due to a loss of tubular cell mass with age progression. In infancy all renal functions are less efficient, due to immaturity. However, these changes are not felt to be clinically important in the healthy infant or older person. They do pose a threat in illness, or imbalance of fluid, electrolytes, or acid-base levels, because of their influence on the body's ability to adapt.

4.2 PATHOPHYSIOLOGY OF URINE PRODUCTION

Dysfunction of urine formation and excretion has profound effect on the body's homeostasis. The kidney is primarily a volume organ. Although one of its major functions is to excrete waste, that process is dependent on an adequate circulatory volume that is composed of a specific balance of certain chemicals and water. Should fluid volume decrease, more waste will be retained; if there is a proportional increase of solute to water, additional water is required to remove additional solute. The kidney strives to maintain the body's extracellular fluid (ECF) osmolality at a norm, usually 285 milliosmols (mOsm). The person with renal insufficiency loses this flexibility. The lack of, or a decrease in the functional ability of either ADH or aldosterone can alter the kidney's flexibility as well, since kidney function is controlled mostly by these hormones.

Alterations in the glomerular filtration rate (GFR) will also impair kidney function. Such alterations can occur with changes in arterial blood pressure for any reason, an increase or decrease in oncontic pressure (pressure of plasma proteins), an increase in glomerular permeability (e.g., nephrotic syndrome), or a decrease in the filtration area of the glomeruli. Any alteration in GFR will alter urine production.

The next priority for kidney function, after volume, is that of acid-base balance. The kidney works to excrete fixed acids in the free state, as well as in combination as a titrable acid and as ammonium, and to reabsorb bicarbonate (HCO_3) as needed. However, when the extracellular volume (ECV) is threatened, that threat takes precedence, and the kidney is stimulated to increase sodium reabsorption in exchange for hydrogen ion (H^+) or potassium ion (K^+) via the distal tubule's cation pump, in order to maintain ECV, this despite its effect on the acid-base balance. This is the basis for persistent metabolic alkalosis due to K^+ or chloride (Cl^-) deficit (Stroot et al., 1977).

4.3 RISK POPULATIONS

Senior adults, especially females, are more prone to urinary tract infections, due in part to decreased immunological response, a delayed and prolonged kidney response in acid-base regulation, and decreased tubular cell mass. Glucose reabsorption is also decreased, which can enhance nutritional problems (Carnevali and Patrick, 1979).

Newborns have a less efficient buffer system, both in the blood and in the kidney, and are more likely to develop acidosis. The kidney's ability to adapt to changes in serum Na^+ levels is reduced, leading to fluid volume problems, and, as in the elderly, the infant's kidney reabsorbs glucose less efficiently (Whaley and Wong, 1979).

Pregnancy also predisposes to urinary tract infection (UTI) because of the occurrence of dilatation of the urethra, and urinary stasis (Harper, 1971).

4.4 GROSS EXAMINATION OF URINE

Synonym: visual examination of urine

Normal Ranges

Color	Pale to dark yellow
Transparency	Clear or slightly cloudy
Odor	Mild, faintly pungent or aromatic

The appearance and odor of a urine specimen are often reported only when they are abnormal. Newborns and the aged tend to have less ability to concentrate urine; therefore, the urine is more likely to be pale when normal. When less precise laboratory measurements were available, much unwarranted importance was given to the gross characteristics of urine. Presently, such examination does not, perhaps, receive enough attention. Active awareness of changes in the characteristics of a patient's urine is highly recommended as an independent nursing action of no small value (see Table 4.2).

TABLE 4.2 *Changes in urine and corresponding nursing action*

Change in urine	Cause	Related nursing
Color and Transparency		
Colorless	Very dilute due to inability to concentrate (infant, diabetes insipidus, some diuretics); increased fluid intake	Check history; keep input and output (temporary increased output = diuresis; prolonged = polyuria); observe for change

TABLE 4.2 *Changes in urine and corresponding nursing action (cont.)*

Change in urine	Cause	Related nursing
Color and Transparency (*cont.*)		
Cloudy	Most often due to phosphate precipitation in alkaline urine	Report; manipulate diet to provide acid ash foods, restrict alkaline ash
	Presence of phosphates, carbonates, urates; uric acid (precipitate in acid urine)	Report; manipulate diet to provide alkaline ash foods, restrict acid ash (see "Implications for Nursing," Section 1.7)
	Presence of leukocytes, bacteria, yeasts, clumps of pus, calculi, gravel	Depends on how specimen obtained; may be normal; observe urine and patient for signs/symptoms of UTI
Smoky	Minimal red cells, prostatic fluid; spermatozoa; mucin; mucous threads	Usually normal, possible menses; normal
Milky	Many PMN (pyuria)	Obtain culture; institute infection control measures (see Section 4.13)
	Chyluria (filiarasis)	Check for lymph enlargement, especially of lower extremities
Opalescent	Fat due to nephrosis; crush injuries, especially of long bones	Check for concentrated urine, signs and symptoms of renal insufficiency; monitor for potential fat embolism
	Bacteria	Check for characteristic unpleasant ammonia odor, obtain culture
Bright yellow	Many drugs [e.g., acriflavine, mepacrine (Atabrine), nitrofurantoin (Furadantin), riboflavin—large doses]	Instruct patient/family that this color change is an expected effect; instruction best if done before medication started
Yellow-orange	Concentrated urine due to increased metabolic rate (fever, thyroid increase): lack of water intake or excessive losses (dehydration)	Increase water intake if appropriate place on input and output; determine cause of losses and correct if possible, or refer
	Urobilin in excess due to liver or gallbladder disorders (colorless until exposed to light)	Will cause a white or colorless persistent foam when shaken
	Bilirubinuria due to liver or gallbladder disorder	Will cause a yellow persistent foam when shaken Both indicate a bilirubin disorder (see "Implications for Nursing," Section 1.10)
	Pyridium (urinary disinfectant)	Instruct patient/family that this is an expected effect
Yellow-green	Bilirubin—biliverdin due to bilirubin dysfunction, possible hemolysis; some drugs: senna, cascara; some foods: rhubarb	Causes a yellow persistent foam when shaken (see "Implications for Nursing," Section 1.10); assess bowel management; assess diet

TABLE 4.2 *Changes in urine and corresponding nursing action (cont.)*

Change in urine	Cause	Related nursing
Color and Transparency (*cont.*)		
Red	Hemoglobin (bright red when fresh) due to intravascular hemolysis greater than haptoglobin can bind	Seek source, report (possible transfusion reaction); check RBC count, Hgb, and Hct (see "Implications for Nursing," items e and f, Section 2.3.2)
	Red blood cells due to trauma of urinary tract/kidney or may be menstrual contamination	Seek source; if not menstrual, blood in urine always significant; report and follow up with repeat urine specimens
	Myoglobin	Look for muscle damage; report
	Porphyrin due to genetic disease (colorless until exposed to light)	Check medical history; report
	Phenindione (anticoagulant similar to coumarin)	Causes benign color change in alkaline urine, inform patient family to expect this; the drug can also cause urinary bleeding with similar color changes which can be differentiated by acidifying urine; benign color change will disappear
	Some foods: beets, candy, and some other foods containing fuscin dye	Response to beets is genetic; check diet history for possibly dyed foods
	Menses	Look for accompanying clots and mucus
Red-pink	Phenophthalein (found in many laxatives, e.g., Ex-lax, Feen-a-mint); senna, cascara, rhubarb	Usually occurs in response to the drugs and/or food listed when urine is alkaline; check medications being taken and inform patient/family of cause-and-effect relationship when found
	Sulfobromephthalein and phenolsulfonphthalein used in certain gallbladder tests	Inform patient of possible color change of urine following test and that it is temporary
Red-purple	Phenolphthalein	As above
	Porphyrin	As above
Red-brown	Red blood cells, older cells	As above
	Hemoglobin on standing;	As above
	Methemoglobin (an abnormal hemoglobin associated with excessive smoking or heavy-metal poisoning)	Assess smoking history and record; check CBC for report of basophilic stipling of WBCs (lead intoxication); record findings; report if positive
	Myoglobin	As above
Brown-black	Methemoglobin	As above
	Hemogentisic acid due to a rare genetic disorder–alkaptonuria	Color change occurs in alkaline urine on standing
	Phenols;	As above
	Melanin due to Addison's disease, but a rare occurrence	
Blue-green	Dyes used in diagnostic tests and/or in medications (e.g., Evans Blue, methylene	Inform patient/family about to have such tests, or who is to receive medication containing dyes, of

TABLE 4.2 *Changes in urine and corresponding nursing action (cont.)*

Change in urine	Cause	Related nursing
Color and Transparency (*cont.*)		
Blue/Green (*cont.*)	blue, indigo carmine, indicans)	the probability of urine color change
	Pseudomonas infection	Check for characteristic odor (rather pleasant, fruity, but somewhat cloying); obtain culture if necessary to establish diagnosis; requires antibiotic susceptibility test before treatment due to resistance to many antibiotics[a]
Odor—Physiologic Changes		
Strong, sharp, penicillin-like	Vitamin B Multivitamin ingestion	If client or family is upset by urine odor, it is sometimes helpful to explain the cause
Pungent, grass-like	Asparagus	Foods can be avoided
Penetrating, ammoniacal	Decomposing urine	Urine should be disposed of as soon as possible
Odor—Pathologic Changes		
Sweet, heavy, thick (at times described as pleasant/fruity)	*Pseudomonas* infection	See "Blue-green" above
Stale urine, ammoniacal	Uremic acidosis	See "Implications for Nursing," Section 1.5
Acetone odor, heavy, sickening, sweet	Ketonuria with diabetic acidosis; lighter or no odor, usually with appearance of ketones in urine in starvation	Ketonuria associated with glucosuria places the patient at special risk for infection and overgrowth of monilial infection, especially in women; frequent and meticulous perineal care needed
Sharp, acrid, "fishy," unpleasant even when fresh; as it becomes older, more markedly ammoniacal	Urinary tract infection—bacterial	Culture and sensitivity tests should be run and followed up with treatment; depending on medication used, the urine pH may need manipulation, so frequent pH checks should be made; maintain urine at most advantageous pH; increase fluid intake when appropriate
"Mousy," "horsey," musty odor—in infant	Phenylketonuria	Report notice of odor; routine testing usually done for this condition on newborns (see Section 1.14.1)
Asparagus odor	Hepatic failure	Less noticeable odor in urine than in other body secretions such as breath vapor
Fecal odor	Usually due to a rectal fistula	Report; institute infection control measures (see Section 4.13)

[a]This section compiled from the following resources: Beck, 1971; Davidsohn and Henry, 1969; Govoni and Hayes, 1978; Harrington and Brener, 1973; Price and Wilson, 1978; Ravel, 1973; and Watson, 1979.

Source: Compiled from Sorensen and Luckmann, 1979; Whaley and Wong, 1979; Beck, 1971.

4.5 pH OF URINE

Synonyms: none

Normal Ranges

Adult	5 – 7 pH units*
Senior adult	No age specific difference
Pediatric	
Newborn/Neonatal	5 – 7
Thereafter	4.5–8

*This normal range is for a group of hospitalized persons, which group might be expected to run a more alkaline urine than the general population due to the combination of the effects of immobility and posttraumatic tendency to extracellular alkalosis (Sabiston, 1977).

The urine pH is a fairly simple test to perform. It reflects the kidneys' ability to maintain the hydrogen ion (H^+) concentration of the body's plasma and extracellular fluid.

Physiology. Ultimately it is the kidneys' function to correct acid-base disturbance. Their action is more thorough and selective than that of body buffers and respiratory control. The urine can sustain H^+ concentration 1000 times greater than that of the blood. Maximum urine acidity is pH 4.5; that of blood is 7.35. The kidneys can eliminate hydrogen in three ways: (1) formation of ammonia (NH_3) in the distal tubular cells—60 to 75% of all H^+ is excreted from the body by this mechanism; (2) excretion as a titratable acid (e.g., sulfuric, phosphoric, hydrochloric, pyruvic, lactic, citric) and some ketones from the glomerulus and the proximal tubule—25 to 40% of all H^+ is excreted by this method; and (3) excretion as free H^+ in exchange for Na^+, which usually returns a bicarbonate ion with it. The process has the net result of conserving sodium and bicarbonate, and excreting the acid products of metabolism. More acid than alkali is formed by the body in its metabolic process, yet the normal ratio of bicarbonate to acid is 20:1 in the body. This results in an acid urine in health.

Physiologic Alterations of Urine pH

1. *Alkaline urine occurs in* (increased pH):
   a. Infancy. Hydrogen excretion is reduced—less acid is secreted—in the first year of life. In the first few days of life the infant has a diminished capacity to produce ammonium ions as well.

b. Urine that has been left standing due to loss of carbon dioxide and/or the action of some bacteria on urine.
c. Individuals on a primarily vegetarian diet.

2. *Urine pH increases* following a meal, due to the increased secretion of HC1 into the stomach for digestion (alkaline tide).

3. *Urine pH decreases* (increased acidity) in:

a. Early morning urine samples, or after any fairly prolonged period of sleep, due to the mild respiratory acidosis occurring with sleep and the renal compensation to that acidosis.
b. Individuals on a diet high in meat protein and some fruits [e.g., cranberries (acid ash)].

Pathophysiologic Alterations in Urine pH

1. *Alkaline urine occurs in* (increased pH):

a. Renal disease, such as:
   (1) Chronic glomerulonephritis due to decreased glomerular filtration, which causes a diminished excretion of phosphate, sulfate, and other acids.
   (2) Renal tubular acidosis due to impaired distal tubular function, which causes a decreased ability to exchange H^+ (secretion) and a decreased formation of ammonia (Cameron et al., 1976).
b. Metabolic or respiratory alkalosis from any cause due to the kidneys' compensatory action in retaining H^+ and eliminating excess base. Ammonia production is also decreased.
c. Hypoaldosteronism (Addison's disease) at times, due to H^+ retention secondary to sodium loss. Potassium often is retained, even preferentially, which allows H^+ to be excreted. In that case urine pH would be within normal limits (Thorn, 1971).
d. The presence of some bacterial infections (e.g., *Pseudomonas, Proteus*).
e. Individuals who are immobilized.

2. *Increases in urine acidity occur in* (decreased pH):

a. Metabolic acidosis and respiratory acidosis from any cause, as a compensatory response to retain bicarbonate and eliminate excess acid. Titratable acid production is increased, as in ammonia production.
b. Hypokalemic, hypochloremic alkalosis (such as occurs in hyperaldosteronism or with prolonged vomiting). This is a

paradoxical aciduria which occurs despite the presence of metabolic alkalosis. Both K^+ and H^+ are excreted in response to the elevated aldosterone levels, which obligates Na^+ reabsorption. In the absence of chloride, bicarbonate is reabsorbed with the Na^+, prolonging the alkalotic state and increasing urine acidity (Biglieri and Stockigt, 1971).

Pharmacologic Alteration in Urine pH. Although alkalinity may occur only as a side effect of the administraton of drugs, drugs can be given specifically for that purpose. Usually this is done to facilitate action of other drugs that are most effective in an alkaline media (e.g., neomycin, kanamycin, streptomycin, sulfadiazine, and sulfamerazine).

Acidic urine suppresses the growth of both gram-negative and gram-positive organisms, including *Escherica coli, Staphylococcus Aureus, Staphylococcus albus,* and some streptococci. Gram-negative organisms are one of the most frequent urinary tract contaminants. *Escherica coli* accounts for roughly 80% of cultured infections (Kunin, 1972).

1. *Alkaline urine occurs with the administration of:*
   a. Excess amounts of sodium bicarbonate and other antacids that are absorbable [e.g., calcium carbonate (Tums), magnesium hydroxide].
   b. Potassium citrate, sometimes used as a expectorant with other drugs or as potassium replacement, as in K-Lyte (Mowad, 1979).
   c. Acetozolamide (Diamox) or other carbonic anhydrase inhibitors [e.g., methazolamide (Neptazane)].
   d. Chlorothiazide (Diuril), a diuretic that promotes K^+ loss and bicarbonate excretion.

2. *Acidic urine occurs with the administration of:*
   a. Ammonium chloride, sometimes used as a mild expectorant, a diuretic, or systemic acidifier. It is only effective in creating acidic urine for short periods of 1 to 2 days because of the renal compensatory mechanisms it stimulates (Kunin, 1972).
   b. Methenamine madelate (Mandelamine). However, the use of this drug or other methenamine compounds, such as methenamine hippurate (Hippox), contributes to urine acidification only when the urine pH is at 5.5 or less at the time of administration (Govoni and Hayes, 1978).
   c. Methionine, which is useful over prolonged periods.
   d. Ascorbic acid.

IMPLICATIONS FOR NURSING

See Section 4.13.

4.6 SPECIFIC GRAVITY OF URINE

Synonyms: None

Normal Ranges

Adult	1.003–1.030
Senior adult	1.016–1.022
Pediatric	
Newborn	1.001–1.020
Thereafter	1.001–1.030

The urine specific gravity test can be defined as the weight of urine compared to the weight of an equal volume of distilled water. It can also be defined as a measurement of density, which depends not only on weight, but also on the number of solute particles in solution. This definition is probably a more accurate reflection of the kidney function being measured. The kidneys' capacity to concentrate is related to the concentration of particles in a solution (osmolality), not to their weight. The correlation between specific gravity and osmolality is close enough to use specific gravity as a clinical guide to urine osmolality, even though methods for measuring specific gravity are not as precise as the measurement of osmolality.

It is a relatively simple, inexpensive, and convenient method for evaluation of the kidneys' ability to dilute and concentrate urine. The test gives some information about renal tubular function.

Physiology. The cells of the kidney tubules in each nephron function to modify the glomerular filtrate presented to them by removing some of the substance from the filtrate (tubular reabsorption) or by adding more of a substance to the filtrate (tubular secretion). Most of the reabsorption occurs in the proximal tubule. In a healthy kidney, with "normal" filtrate, about 98% of the filtrate is reabsorbed. It is through this process of tubular absorption and secretion that the final composition of urine is determined. Part of the process is the ability of the tubules to respond to the osmolality of the filtrate, keeping it constant. This serves to either concentrate or dilute the urine. Figure 4-1 describes the fairly specific process of tubular function by nephron segments.

The function of concentration of urine is directly under the control of antidiuretic hormone (ADH). Na^+ and water diffuse passively in or out of the descending limb of Henle's loop, as the interstitial and intravascular fluids equilibrate with the glomerular filtrate. However, in the ascending loop, the membrane is impermeable to water, and Na^+ must be actively transported out of that section of the loop. Beyond this point, at the beginning of the distal convoluted tubule, ADH, if present, acts on the membrane, allowing water to flow out. If ADH is absent, the entire distal tubule is impermeable to water and the hypotonic urine produced in the ascending portion of Henle's loop is excreted unchanged. The collecting ducts, under the influence of ADH, progressively concentrate the urine (see Fig. 4-1) (Harvey et al., 1976).

Pathophysiology. In renal disease, and in many conditions causing renal dysfunction, the mechanism most commonly lost is the ability to concentrate urine, which can threaten, or cause, severe water loss. A specific example of this occurrence is found in pyelonephritis. The kidney can no longer respond to the presence of ADH. The actual loss of the hormone, as in diabetes insipidus, will obviously cause the inability to concentrate urine. Yet there is otherwise a relatively normal tubular function.

Concentration of urine depends in part upon the amount of water available for excretion, assuming adequate ADH secretion and the kidneys' ability to respond to it. The amount of water available for excretion, then, in turn, depends upon the amount of water taken in, the amount lost through the lungs or skin, and on the amount of blood perfusing the kidney. In conditions of reduced blood perfusion of the kidney, renin is secreted, and angiotension and aldosterone are produced, all of which enhance the production of a highly concentrated urine, almost without sodium (Cameron et al., 1976).

Although there is a general, moderate decrease in specific gravity with aging, the decrease is not thought to influence findings in any clinically important way, being a reflection of the loss of cell mass rather than of function of the existing tubules.

During the neonatal period the infants glomerular filtration rate (GFR) is very low, remaining low for several months. Coupled with this, the infant's ability to concentrate urine is very limited. The infant then has the potential for difficulty in both concentration and dilution of his urine.

SPECIFIC GRAVITY INCREASED IN:

1. *Inaccurate reading due to the use of too small an amount of urine* for testing, or too narrow a vessel in proportion to the size of the urinometer.
2. *Inaccurate reading due to the use of refrigerated urine,* or urine that is colder or warmer than room temperature (20°C). A correction by adding 0.001 for each 3°C the sample is above or by subtracting 0.001 for each 3°C the sample is below 20°C should be made (Davidsohn and Henry, 1969). Normal room temperature may be calculated differently in different places. Check the local laboratory for the proper calculation.
3. *Individuals who have had an IV pyelogram,* for a day or two after the injection of the dye.
4. *States of dehydration or water deprivation,* due to lack of available water to be excreted. Can occur in many situations and conditions (e.g., diarrhea, vomiting, excessive sweating, inability to respond to thirst, as with decreased levels of consciousness).
5. *Excessive ingestion of sodium chloride,* causing true hypernatremia.
6. *Urine with glucose or protein in excessive amounts* (e.g., uncontrolled diabetes mellitus, nephrotic syndrome).
7. *States causing decreased glomerular filtration rate* (GFR), such as shock or heart failure.

SPECIFIC GRAVITY DECREASED IN:

1. *Conditions that increase the GFR,* such as severe hyperthyroidism or fever.
2. *Conditions causing decreased tubular absorption,* such as:
   a. Diabetes insipidus, due to loss of hormonal influence of ADH.
   b. Early pyelonephritis.
   c. Occasionally in sickle cell anemia.
   d. Acute renal failure. The specific gravity is fixed at 1.010 to 1.012 (Metheny and Snively, 1979).
3. *Individuals on diets severely restricted in salt or protein* due to inadequate intake of solute.
4. *Individuals on potent diuretics* that decrease tubular reabsorption of salt and water.

5. *Individuals having a marked increase in water intake.* This can occur due to oral intake or parenteral administration of electrolyte free solutions, such as 5% glucose in water.
6. *Severe K^+ deficiency or calcium excess,* due to possible inhibition of tubular reabsorption.
7. *Inaccurately measured samples,* due to use of warm urine. Urine measured when it is at 35°C will measure 0.005 too low (see correction formula given in "Specific Gravity Increased in" on page 223).
8. *Urine containing large amounts of urea.*

IMPLICATIONS FOR NURSING

The nurse can perform specific gravity tests totally independently, and without increasing the patient's cost for care. Since the procedure can be so helpful in determining the state of hydration of a patient, and can also indicate acute renal failure, the nurse should not only become adept at the technique, but also should become as knowledgeable as possible about the implications of the changes in specific gravity values.

1. *Test procedure:*
   a. The urine sample should be fresh and at room temperature. It should also be well mixed, that is, a representative sampling of the urine. Urine taken from the bottom of a catheter bag, for example, would not yield accurate results.
   b. Check that the urinometer to be used is the correct size for the container. There are varying sizes available and the urinometer from one set, used with the container of another, will produce inaccurate readings.
   c. Test the urinometer if unsure of container size or accuracy of calibration, by filling the container at least three-fourths full of distilled water. (In many areas tap water contains many solutes and should not be used.) Insert urinometer (process given below). The reading should be 1.000. If the reading is incorrect, be sure to correct your urine sample reading by the same variation. Have the urinometer recalibrated as soon as possible.
   d. Dry the urinometer thoroughly before using for the test.

e. Fill container with urine—three-fourths at least, or to marked level. There must be sufficient fluid to "float" the urinometer.
f. Insert urinometer gently without allowing it to touch the sides or bottom of the container. Before releasing the urinometer, twist it between finger and thumb to cause it to spin. It should then float freely without touching the sides or bottom of the container.
g. Read with meniscus of fluid at eye level.
h. The urinometer is calibrated with lines similar to a thermometer. The denser the solution, the higher the meter will float in it. Therefore, the greater numbers are toward the base, the smaller ones toward the top. The numbers usually range from 1.060 to 1.000.

2. *Correlation with other tests:*
   a. Specific gravity should correlate fairly closely with osmolality. A minimum specific gravity of urine is 1.001, which corresponds with about 40 milliosmoles (mOsm). Maximum specific gravity of urine is about 1.040 or 41.6 mOsm (1 unit of specific gravity = 40 mOsm).
   b. Specific gravity can be expected to be increased in the presence of glucosuria or proteinuria. It will be decreased in the presence of increased urea excretion.
   c. Specific gravity exerts effects on other tests. The patient demonstrating proteinuria will appear to have a greater amount of protein in the urine in the face of an increased specific gravity. The amount of protein excreted remains the same, but its concentration in solution changes, depending on whether the urine is dilute, normal, or concentrated.

3. *General guidelines for evaluating specific gravity findings:*
   a. The specific gravity of an individual kept NPO overnight should be at least 1.022 to be considered normal (Davidsohn and Henry, 1969).
   b. If urine does not concentrate overnight, this may be an early sign of renal disease.
   c. Expect decreased urine specific gravity in persons on diets severely restricted in sodium or protein due to the decrease of available solute.
   d. A first morning urine specimen tested for specific gravity might be considered adequate if it reaches 1.016, given that it is negative for glucose or protein (Metheny and Snively, 1979).
   e. The oliguria of acute renal failure can be differentiated from that of water deficit by the presence of a fixed specific gravity of 1.010 to 1.012 in acute renal failure.

4. *Special concerns in caring for infants* (Cameron et al., 1976):
   a. Because of their limited ability to concentrate urine, infants require feedings rich in protein, which help increase the urine concentration.
   b. Urea excretion is hampered in the infant because of the difficulty in urine concentration. To assure excretion of urea, the protein-rich feedings must contain adequate amounts of water—an excellent rationale for breast feeding.
   c. At times it is difficult to acquire enough urine (approximately 15 mL with small urinometer sets) for a specific gravity test for the infant. There are available on the market so-called "specific gravity beads," supplied in a series of different weights, that will sink in urine of equal or matching specific gravity. The weight is inscribed on the bead. However, even this method requires 10 mL of urine.

Refractometers may be available on some pediatric units for this test. They have the advantage of requiring only a few drops of urine, are highly accurate, and are simple to use. However, they are relatively expensive, thus not often found.

4.7 URINE GLUCOSE

Synonym: urine fractional*

Normal Range: negative for all age groups

*Urine fractional is actually a misnomer, as it is not a precise synonym for the urine glucose test. It is, however, often used interchangeably, particularly when urine is being checked routinely on the hospital unit to help determine insulin dosage. Urine fractionals are, in fact, the testing of a certain *group* of urine voidings, excreted in a given time frame. This provides information as to when the most sugar is excreted in the urine and dosage of insulin can be planned accordingly.

An example of the timing and procedure are: All urine voided is collected from just before breakfast to just before lunch (7 to 12 A.M.), mixed and tested for glucose and usually for acetone as well. Another collection is made of all voiding from the last voiding for the first collection until just before dinner; then from dinner to bedtime; then bedtime to early morning—6 A.M. approximately. Each collection is mixed and tested as a group (Phipps et al., 1979).

The urine glucose test is a qualitative test for the presence of glucose in urine, done as part of a routine urinalysis. It is a relatively simple and accurate test. Attempts to quantify the results (see "Implications for Nursing", this section, item 3) are as accurate as the person performing the comparison is accurate in technique. Similar methods of testing are used by nurses on the clinical unit. The procedure is done with a dipstick, or test strip, impregnated with glucose oxidase. This substance is very sensitive to the presence of glucose and will change in color when exposed to very low concentrations in the urine (0.1 g/dL). In pediatric testing, or after a positive response in adult testing, a Clinitest may be done to confirm clinically significant concentrations of sugar, usually present as glucose, or to indicate the presence of any other reducing sugars (e.g., lactose, xylose, fructose or galactose, as well as homogentistic acid). Use of Clinitest expands the procedure to screen for genetic carbohydrate metabolism dysfunction (SHMC, 1978).

Routine urinalysis, and thus the urinary glucose test, is most often done on random voidings, or on the more concentrated first voiding of the morning. The urine should be collected as a midstream, clean-catch sample (see Section 4.13). In doing "fractionals," single-specimen urinary glucose testing, on the hospital unit for the purpose of regulating insulin administration, a double-voided specimen is often required (see "Implications for Nursing" in Section 1.4). Catheterized specimens are rarely necessary and should be avoided if possible because of the high risk of infection, which risk is even greater in the presence of glucosuria.

Physiology. When blood sugar, specifically glucose, rises, the glomerular filtrate may contain more glucose than can be reabsorbed. Tubular reabsorption of glucose is limited by the concentration of an enzyme necessary to the process in the tubule cell. The rate limit is approximately 350 mg/min. When this rate is exceeded, the excess glucose is excreted into the urine. The result is glucosuria. The blood level at which this spillover occurs is approximately 170 mg/dL and is called the *renal threshold* for glucose. The concentration thus spilled into the urine is sufficient to be detected by the usual screening methods.

Pathophysiology. The most frequent cause of glucosuria, at least in the adult, is diabetes mellitus, in which the lack of insulin, or presence of ineffective insulin, causes increased blood glucose levels. However, nine other precipitants of increased glucose levels, and subsequent glucosuria, have been listed previously (see "Serum Glucose Increased in" in Section 1.4).

Glucosuria can occur without increased blood glucose levels, although it occurs much less frequently. Renal diabetes, also known as renal glucosuria, or nondiabetic glucosuria, is so named because of the source of the defect, a renal tubular deficiency in the reabsorption of glucose. This defect, coupled with two other renal defects [vitamin D-resistant rickets in children, or idiopathic osetomalacia (milkman's syndrome) in adults; and excessive excretion of amino acids] is usually referred to as Fanconi syndrome, or more recently de Toni-Fanconi syndrome.

Another glucosuria occurring without increased blood levels of glucose has been found in a small percentage of pregnant women. Their renal threshold becomes lower and they spill glucose. The condition is usually temporary and the cause has not been defined.

POSITIVE URINE GLUCOSE TESTS OCCUR IN:

1. *Conditions causing increased blood glucose concentration* beyond renal threshold maximums (see "Serum Glucose Increased in" in Section 1.4).
2. *Renal tubular defects* due to genetic inheritance.
3. *Rare instances during pregnancy.*
4. *Conditions causing false-positive reactions,* such as:
   a. Individual tested with Clinitest and taking drugs excreted as conjugated glucournides [e.g., salicylates, PABA, chloral hydrate, paraldehyde, cephalsporin (Keflex, Keflin) [Danovitch et al., 1971).
   b. Individuals tested soon after ingestion of large amount of carbohydrate.
   c. Postgastrectomy in some persons.

FALSE-NEGATIVE URINE GLUCOSE RESULTS OCCUR IN:

1. *Some older diabetic patients with arteriosclerosis,* due to an increased renal threshold.
2. *Persons taking large quantities of ascorbic acid (vitamin C)* with dipstick tests.

IMPLICATIONS FOR NURSING

1. *See* "Implications for Nursing" in Section 1.4.
2. *Since the accuracy of the test* depends on the technique of the person doing the test, the nurse should learn and practice meticulous technique:
   a. There are a number of different types of dipstick or test strip materials available for use, (e.g., Combistix, Tes-tape, Clinistix,

Diastix). They vary in color response, the time required for the reagent to be exposed to the urine, and the number of urine tests that can be done on the same strip or stick. For these reasons, as well as acceptance of the concept as a sound one in almost any case, the nurse is cautioned to read directions with care, and to carry them out precisely.

b. Some generalizations concerning urine tests done with glucose oxidase reagent strips or sticks include:
   (1) Protect the materials from moisture or excessive heat. Reagents tend to lose sensitivity when so exposed. Store in cool dry area, but not a refrigerator.
   (2) If strip or stick is brownish in color, do not use. Such color indicates a significant loss of sensitivity.
   (3) Do not take more out of the container than will be immediately used. Recover the container immediately.
   (4) Do not touch test areas, or allow them to touch other areas. Lay the stick or strip on a clean piece of paper if it must be put down.
   (5) Be sure that the urine to be tested is well mixed.
   (6) Completely wet the reagent area so as to completely cover it.
   (7) Avoid prolonged dipping, which can leach reagent from the strip.
   (8) Read at the time indicated, exactly. Time with a second-hand.
   (9) Hold the strip immediately by appropriate color chart to compare color. Do not use one company's chart for another company's product, even if the colors seem identical.
   (10) Reading is best done in direct daylight. In any case, lighting conditions should be the best possible.

c. If the test material used does not include testing area for ketones (acetone), the test should usually be done in addition to the glucose test. The presence of ketone bodies indicates the seriousness of the diabetic's condition. The absence of a positive ketone test in the presence of a 3+ or 4+ urine glucose also demands prompt attention. In an older (50 or above) known diabetic, in a state of dehydration and with a decreased level of consciousness, the possibility of nonketotic, hyperosmolar, hyperglycemic coma should be suspected and checked out.

3. *Many laboratories report rough quantitative results* of urinary glucose testing as a series of pluses, from 1+ to 4+, depending on the amount of glucose present as indicated by the color change. As mentioned previously, the lowest concentration of glucose in

urine that will cause a positive reaction in this type of testing is 0.1 g/dL. However, that concentration does not equate with a "trace" as given on the numerical scale. The following table may serve as a rough guide in determining just how great the urinary spill of glucose is. This is a Clinitest scale.

Concentration (g/dL)	Numerical scale
0.25	Trace
0.5	1+
0.79	2+
1.0	3+
2.0	4+

4. *If there is no glucose found* in a 2-hr postprandial [after meals, or p.p.; also sometimes called p.c. (postcibum, after eating)] urinary glucose test, it is unlikely that untreated diabetes mellitus is present.
5. *Related tests:*
   a. Elevated 2-hr p.p. blood glucose (greater than 160 mg/dL) in repeated tests, with or without positive urinary glucose, confirms diagnosis of diabetes mellitus (Davidsohn and Henry, 1969).
   b. Glucose tolerance test (GTT). Done when the above finding is doubtful.
   c. 24-hr urine specimen for glucose determination when above finding is doubtful, or done instead of a GTT.
   d. Serum sodium (Na^+). To determine possible fluid loss with osmotic diuresis secondary to glucosuria.
   e. Serum potassium (K^+). Done in cases of possible, or diagnosed, ketoacidosis, to determine need for replacement.

4.8 URINE PROTEIN

Synonyms: none

Normal Range: negative for all age groups*

*Newborns have higher levels of protein in the urine the first few days of life, but no specific value alterations are available (Davidsohn and Henry, 1969).

Measurement of urinary protein is an important evaluation of glomerular function. As with the screening test for urinary glucose, the screening test for urinary protein is most frequently that which utilizes a reagent-impregnated strip or stick—a qualitative test. Also, as in the urinary glucose test, the quantity of protein present can be roughly estimated, based on a scale of increasing concentration. The scale can be roughly quantified as follows (SHMC, 1978):

Protein concentration (mg/dL)	Numerical scale
Less than 5	Negative
5–10	Trace
10–30	1+
40–100	2+
200–500	3+
500 or more	4+

The reagent test (dipstick test, such as Albustix, Combistix, or a strip test such as Albutest) is most sensitive for albumin and least sensitive, if sensitive at all, for globulin. It does have the advantage of avoiding many of the false positives that plague globulin-sensitive proteinuria tests. It is important, then, to confirm a positive reaction to the reagent test with another qualitative or quantitative test, particularly if there is any question as to the significance of the proteinuria. To do this, frequently a 24-hr urine sample will be analyzed for confirmation; the method for this provides a fairly accurate evaluation of urine protein concentration. It also avoids the problems of variation in dilution or concentration found in random sample testing.

Physiology. Not all urine protein is pathologic, and not all pathologic proteinuria is persistent (Ravel, 1973). But measurable, significant, persistent proteinuria almost always indicates renal disease (Price and Wilson, 1978).

The healthy glomerular membrane prevents most of the protein constituents of blood from entering the tubular ultrafiltrate (see Fig. 4-1). The small amount of the smaller molecular proteins that do get through may be reabsorbed by the tubules. Less than 0.1 g/24 hr is normally excreted. This amount usually cannot be detected by routine screening tests but may be detected in 24-hr samples. An increase in the glomerular filtration rate (GFR) can increase normal protein excretion slightly.

Pathophysiology. According to Price and Wilson (1978), "the direct cause of proteinuria is always an increase in glomerular permeability." As with most generalizations, that is not quite true. Protein can appear in the urine due to postrenal problems, in which case the glomerular permeability is not a factor.

Proteinuria can be classified in two ways:

1. *Extent* (Davidsohn and Henry, 1969):

Heavy proteinuria	More than 4 g/day	Nephrotic syndrome
Moderate proteinuria	0.5–4 g/day	Most renal diseases in some phase, and most systemic diseases with nephropathy (e.g., diabetes mellitus, multiple myeloma, preeclampsia
Minimal proteinuria	Less than 0.5–1.0 g/day	Chronic glomerulonephritis, postural proteinurias

2. *Relationship of proteinuria's etiology to the kidney* and the mechanism involved (Ravel, 1973):
   a. Functional. Not obviously associated with pathology, renal or systemic.
   b. Organic. Associated with pathology, renal and/or systemic.
      (1) Prerenal—not due to kidney disease primarily.
      (2) Renal—due to primary kidney disease.
      (3) Postrenal—due to release of protein into urine at a point below the kidney parenchyma (e.g., renal pelvis, ureters, bladder, urethra, or contamination from vaginal, prostatic, or seminal secretions).

POSITIVE REACTION IN URINARY PROTEIN SCREENING TESTS FOUND IN:

1. *False positives* due to the presence of hemoglobin, or contamination of urine with chemicals such as the ammonium compounds.

2. *Functional conditions* such as:
   a. Severe muscular exertion. Proteinuria is seen quite frequently in pregnant women at the time of labor.
   b. Severe dehydration, due to increased concentration of solute in solution.

c. Orthostatic proteinuria, which occurs only when the person is standing erect, and may be due to renal congestion/ischemia secondary to an exaggerated lordotic position.
d. In response to temperature change (e.g., internal temperature: fever; external temperature: exposure to cold).
e. Severe emotional stress.
f. Contamination with vaginal secretions.

3. *Prerenal pathology,* such as:
   a. Conditions leading to a hypoxic renal state (e.g., shock, severe acidosis, acute cardiac decompensation, severe anemia, preeclampsia of pregnancy).
   b. Multiple myeloma (Bence Jones protein–primarily globulin excreted, so a false negative is possible).
   c. Hypertension.
4. *Renal pathology,* such as:
   a. Glomerulonephritis, poststreptococcal infection; less commonly, postcollagen disease, or very rarely following sickle-cell disease. It can also be idiopathic.
   b. Nephrotic syndrome.
   c. De Toni-Fanconi syndrome, or renal tubular acidosis.
   d. Tumors or infarcts causing destruction of the parenchyma of the kidney.
5. *Postrenal conditions,* such as:
   a. Infection of kidney, pelvis, or ureter.
   b. Cystitis.
   c. Urethritis or prostatitis.

FALSE-NEGATIVE RESPONSES TO URINARY PROTEIN SCREENING TESTS OCCUR IN:

1. *See* item 3 in "Positive Reaction" above.
2. *Dilute, random urine samples,* or the reaction may be falsely low.
3. *Highly buffered alkaline urine.*

IMPLICATIONS FOR NURSING

1. *Some renal disease can be prevented,* or its severity modified, by consistent preventative measures. Nursing measures to help pre-

vent infection are given at the end of this chapter. Awareness of these measures will help the nurse to include appropriate prevention in the care of *all* patients.

2. *Encourage culturing all sore throats,* especially in school-age children, a high-risk group. Although costly, the cost is considerably less than that incurred in the treatment of glomerular nephritis, even when treatment of the sore throat, should it be indicated, is included in the cost.

3. *In taking a history of a patient with proteinuria,* inquire into recent acute infections, even those seemingly far removed from the present problem some 10 days or 2 weeks previously.

   a. Check voiding history for changes. Decreased or increased volume? Increased frequency? Change in color? Change in odor?
   b. Check for presence of edema (periorbital in morning?) or undue fatigue.

4. *Assess related laboratory tests:*

   a. Urine. The presence of pyuria (pus cells found in the urine) in the absence of proteinuria tentatively indicates a postrenal infection. Pursue questions concerning pain or discomfort related to urination with occurrence of pyuria.
   b. Urine: specific gravity. Will increase in uremia; will increase markedly in the nephrotic syndrome until the late stages.
   c. Blood: RBC count, Hct, Hbg. Anemia accompanies almost all renal disease, and is roughly proportional to the severity of the uremia. BUN increases in uremia. RBC life span reduced to about one-half normal when BUN exceeds 200 mg/dL.
      (1) Serum sodium—markedly increased in nephrotic syndrome.
      (2) Serum potassium—may decrease due to urinary washout. May increase with urinary obstruction.
      (3) Serum total protein—albumin: decreased with severe to moderate prolonged proteinuria.

5. *Teach patient/family home caretaker* the purpose of any medications given or dietary restrictions made.

   a. Severe anemia secondary to renal disease may be treated with androgens, which act directly on the bone marrow to increase renal secretion of erythropoietin. One happy side effect for males may be the return of libido, which kidney disease can suppress. Side effects for women are masculinizing changes, for which they should be prepared. The changes are reversible, but not immediately on cessation of the drug. (Children may be given corticosteroids.)

b. Transfusions are rarely used because of the depressive effect on erythropoietin and bone marrow.
c. Increased blood pressure may not be treated medically. Explain rationale to patient/family if lack of therapy is questioned. Decreased blood pressure causes decreased GFR, decreased renal perfusion, and further renal damage. When there is reason to believe that treatment of the original pathology will effectively decrease the blood pressure, given time, the risk of prematurely decreasing it is not taken.
d. Edema due to decreased protein in the circulating volume (decreased serum protein = decreased oncotic pressure intravascularly = movement of fluid out of the capillaries) is treated frequently with sodium restriction and diuretics, to remove excess sodium (e.g., nephrotic syndrome). Plasma expanders can be used when the circulating volume is very low, particularly when potent diuretics are given. Most, however, contain sodium. A high-protein, high-carbohydrate diet is usually prescribed to attempt replacement of renal losses of protein and to provide a ready form of energy (Harrington and Brener, 1973). Antibiotics are frequently given due to the renal patient's increased susceptibility to infection as well as to treat renal disease due to infection. The nurse should see that he or she is personally informed as to the expected effects, desired effects, side effects, and untoward effects; the dosage and how it should be adapted to this patient's renal condition; and the desired outcomes of its use.

6. *For nutritional needs,* see "Implications for Nursing," items 4b, 5b and 6 to 8, in Section 1.8.

7. *For nursing measures related to anemia,* see Section 2.1.6, item 1f.

8. *For nursing care in renal disease,* see "Implications for Nursing," items 1 to 8, 12 and 13, in Section 1.5.

9. *For nursing care in azotemia,* see "Implications for Nursing," items 2, 3, and 9, in Section 1.6.

4.9 URINE BILIRUBIN

Synonym: urine bile

Normal Range: negative for all age groups

Bilirubin is normally not found in the urine. When present it is an indicator of an increase in the serum levels of conjugated (direct-reacting, water-soluble) bilirubin, which may be due to liver disease or biliary obstruction. When present in great amounts in urine, the color changes to very dark amber or a deep yellow orange and produces a persistent yellow foam when agitated (see Section 4.4).

Physiology. See "Physiology" in Section 1.10.

Pathophysiology. (See also "Pathophysiology" in Section 1.10.) Bilirubin, conjugated by the liver, may be unable to be excreted into the bile, due to obstruction of bile canaliculi from many causes. With the blockage of its normal excretory route, the conjugated bilirubin is ultimately excreted into the urine (see Fig. 1.1). Its appearance in the urine can even precede the appearance of jaundice.

Indirect-reacting, or unconjugated bilirubin, apparently cannot pass the glomerular filter and does not appear in the urine. Increased serum levels of this substance will ultimately cause an increased production of direct-reacting conjugated bilirubin, which eventually enters the urine.

At the same time that urinary bilirubin excretion increases, the production of urobilinogen is increased with increased excretion of that substance into the urine. Thus when a serum bilirubin indicates an increase in the unconjugated, indirect-reacting bilirubin concentration, one would expect to see a rise in urine urobilinogen, and later, frequently urine bilirubin (Sodeman and Sodeman, 1974).

When increased red cell destruction alone causes serum bilirubin to rise, only the unconjugated (indirect-reacting) fraction is increased and, consequently, bilirubinuria will not occur.

Despite a physiologic jaundice, little or no conjugated bilirubin is found in the neonates serum or urine during the first few days of life (1 to 4) due to the immaturity of the liver, which cannot form conjugated bilirubin.

POSITIVE REACTIONS TO URINE BILIRUBIN FOUND IN:

1. *Liver disease* due to:
   a. Obstructive jaundice, due to gallstones or other mechanical obstruction, such as cancer of the head of the pancreas.
   b. Inflammation, due to infectious processes in the liver, such as hepatitis.
   c. Fibrosis of the biliary canaliculi in conditions such as cirrhosis.
   d. Exposure to toxins, or ingestion of certain drugs that are hepatotoxic.

2. *See also* "Total Serum Bilirubin Increased in," items 2 and 3, in Section 1.12.

NEGATIVE REACTIONS TO URINE BILIRUBIN:

Not clinically significant.

IMPLICATIONS FOR NURSING

See "Implications for Nursing," item 2, in Section 1.12.

4.10 URINARY HEMOGLOBIN

Synonym: occult blood

Normal Range: negative for all age groups

The test for urinary hemoglobin, or occult blood, indicates the presence of microscopic (occult–hidden) blood, macroscopic blood (visible indications of blood due to change in urine color), intact red blood cells, or lysed cells with free hemoglobin present. An abnormal number of red blood cells in urine is called "hematuria." The presence of free hemoglobin in the urine is called "hemoglobinuria." Normal urine may contain about 1000 RBC/mL. Some 66,000 RBC/mL are usually required to be clearly detected in a microscopic examination of urine (Davidsohn and Henry, 1969).

The test can be done with a reagent strip, a tablet, or as a wet chemical test. The reactive substance is usually orthotolidine, which is sensitive to a hemoglobin level equivalent to 10 million red blood cells per liter (10,000 RBC/mL) of urine, and reacts positively to myoglobin and the intermediate hemoglobin chemical derivatives, as well as to hemoglobin. It is more sensitive to hemoglobin than to RBCs, but free hemoglobin occurs in at least 90% of all urine specimens containing red blood cells.

Physiology. Ordinarily, proteins of large molecular structure, such as the red blood cell, do not pass the glomerular membrane in any significant number. (Significant is defined by Ravel as over six red blood cells per high-power field on microscopic examination.)

Pathophysiology. In hemolytic anemias, or other types of intravascular lysis of red blood cells, free hemoglobin is produced in excess of the available haptoglobin for binding. The excess is excreted by the kidney (see "Compensatory Mechanism: Physiologic" in Section 2.1.2). Free hemoglobin also occurs in the urine in response to severe, unaccustomed exercise; in deficiency of glucose-6-phosphate dehydrogenase due to ingestion of certain drugs or fava beans; in autoimmune hemolytic anemias; and in several abnormal hemoglobinopathies (Davidsohn and Henry, 1969).

Hematuria occurs with damage to the endothelial lining of the small glomerular arterioles. This damage can occur secondary to a number of different precipitants (e.g., trauma, hypertension, systemic disease). Hematuria also occurs secondary to problems of the lower urinary tract (e.g., infections, tumors, or mechanical trauma due to renal stones).

Causes of hematuria or hemoglobinuria can be organized as (Harvey et al., 1976):

1. *Local disorders* of the kidney and genitourinary tract:
   a. May have slight (rarely more than a few hundred milligrams/day) proteinuria.
   b. Often associated with some discomfort or pain (e.g., suprapubic discomfort, dysuria, renal colic).
   c. Blood may appear only at the beginning or end of micturation.
   d. No casts are seen.
2. *Diffuse renal disease:*
   a. Usually associated with proteinuria.
   b. Usually painless hematuria or hemoglobinuria.
   c. Distribution of RBCs or hemoglobin is uniform in the urine.
   d. RBC casts are a characteristic feature, unmistakably identifying the nephron as the source of bleeding.

POSITIVE URINARY HEMOGLOBIN TEST RESPONSES OCCUR:

1. *As a false-positive reaction* in urine contaminated with a high bacterial content due to the presence of bacterial peroxidases.
2. *In some physiologic conditions,* such as:
   a. After vigorous exercise undergone immediately before the test, which produces a microscopic hematuria.
   b. Benign recurrent hematuria, found in children. Frequently precipitated by a viral respiratory infection or other mild febrile illness. There is no loss of renal function (Whaley and Wong, 1979).

3. *Consistently after renal trauma.* The severity of the bleeding into the urine is not a reliable indicator of the seriousness of the injury.

4. *In infections of the lower urinary tract,* particularly in acute cystitis.

5. *In genitourinary tumors.* Hematuria is the most frequent sign of urinary tract cancer, and often may be the only sign. Tumors are unlikely to occur in children (Ravel, 1973).

6. *In the presence of renal calculi.* It may also be an isolated finding with this diagnosis, in the absence of pain.

7. *In inherited disorders* such as:

   a. Hemoglobinopathies: Hemoglobinuria is usually grossly visible without other signs or symptoms.
   b. Polycystic kidney disease: Rapidly fatal in infants but may be consistent with a normal life span in adults.

8. *In thrombocytopenia purpura.* In small children, ages 6 months to 3 years, a similar condition occurs known as hemolytic uremia syndrome. It is an uncommon disease, but of importance in that it is one of the most frequent causes of acute renal failure in children.

9. *In diffuse renal lesions* due to glomerulonephritis (acute and chronic); autoimmune hemolytic anemia seen with systemic lupus erthematosis, lymphomas, polyarteritis, viral pneumonias, Goodpasture's syndrome (lung purpura with nephritis), allergic nephropathies (Henock-Schönlein syndrome); malignant hypertension (severe); or focal embolic glomerulitis (usually secondary to bacterial endocarditis).

10. *Due to drug ingestion* such as sulfonamides, phenacetin, quinine, arsenic, carbon tetrachloride, or those that inhibit glucose-6-phosphate dehydrogenase activity, such as primaquin, nitrofuantoin, and pheothiazine.

11. *Due to systemic infections,* such as blackwater fever (*Plasmodium falciparum*) or clostridium.

12. *Secondary to incompatible blood transfusions* causing intravascular lysis, an immunohemolytic process. RBCs or hemoglobin can occur in the urine both as a result of direct hemolysis, and secondary to renal damage occurring because of the hemoglobin obstruction of the renal tubules.

13. *Paroxysmal nocturnal hemoglobinuria.*

FALSE-NEGATIVE URINARY HEMOGLOBIN REACTIONS OCCUR IN:

1. *The presence of large amounts of ascorbic acid* in the urine. Large amounts of ascorbic acid are present in many parenteral antibiotics as a preservative (e.g., tetracycline).

IMPLICATIONS FOR NURSING

1. *In risk populations:*
   a. Check the microscopic examination of the urine for the presence of red cells as well as the positive reaction to blood. If the specimen examined was not fresh, total hemolysis may have occurred. Conversely, the absence of a positive reaction for blood does not necessarily rule out the presence of red blood cells in the sediment.
   b. If urinalysis is positive for hemoglobin, but urinary sediment is normal, suggest that a fresh urine specimen be examined. The presence of both RBCs and hemoglobin is expected; absence of RBCs suggests urine that has been standing.
   c. Check each voiding for change in color. Smoky color indicates small amounts of blood; red or brown indicates gross hematuria.
   d. Get a complete voiding history: changes in amount of urine, change in color, pattern of occurrence with color change [e.g., only after unusual exercise, just at the start and completion of the urinary stream (may indicate the urethra or bladder as the source of bleeding)].
2. *With the presence of massive hemoglobin* in the urine and the absence of other indicators of kidney disease:
   a. Observe for bleeding tendencies.
   b. Check coagulation screening tests if available. Request such tests if evidence of bleeding tendencies is found.
   c. Look for report of RBC casts. Presence indicates kidney disease; absence a disorder of the lower urinary tract.
3. *Hematuria accompanying a urinary tract infection* usually disappears as the acute infection subsides. If this does not occur, the possibility of relapse, or reinfection with another organism, should be explored. Consult with physician regarding the need for further cultures (Turck, 1980).

4. *Hematuria or hemoglobinuria accompanying, or following transfusions:*
   a. Reactions usually appear during the infusion, but hematuria or hemoglobinuria may not be evident for several hours, even after all other signs have been allayed.
   b. Specially diligent monitoring should be instituted with those individuals who are felt to be at risk for transfusion reaction (e.g., known history of previous transfusion or prior pregnancy).
   c. Prior to administration of blood:
      (1) Check for completion of type and cross-match tests and compatibility between patient and donor blood.
      (2) Check blood to be given, validating with another nurse or a physician; see that the label is correct in *all* details. *Any* discrepancy on the label means that the blood is not to be given.
   d. Start infusion slowly, not to exceed 20 drops (gtts) per minute, and run at that rate for the first 50 mL. The usual rate in the adult, depending on the person's condition, is 30 gtts/min, or 500 mL run in over 4 hr. If the person should receive more than 100 mL of incompatible blood, irreversible shock, total renal shutdown, and death can occur.
   e. Check vital signs every 15 min to ½ hr, depending on the general condition of the person getting the blood. Particularly close surveillance is suggested if the individual's mobility or awareness is impaired.
   f. Observe for, or inquire after, any sign or symptom of reaction (e.g., chills, fever, low back pain). Occasionally, early signs may be urticaria or flushing, a sense of uneasiness, and/or mild air hunger. Should a person receiving blood complain about "feeling funny," this vague complaint should be given much attention. A *minimal* response on the part of the nurse is to decrease the rate of blood flow and report the complaint. Stay with the person and watch carefully for any other untoward sign.
   g. With any confirmed sign of reaction:
      (1) Discontinue the blood.
      (2) Change the IV tubing and maintain the vascular access with normal saline or one-quarter normal saline. It is best not to use glucose in water immediately after giving blood. The absence of electrolytes can precipitate hemolysis and/or clotting in the needle, or in the tubing if it has not been changed.
      (3) Notify the physician. Epinephrine HCl 1:1000 and sodium lactate (1/6 *M*) may be given to reduce the precipitation of hemoglobin in the kidney (Phipps et al., 1979).

(4) Evaluate renal function. Monitor input and output. If the reaction is severe, a catheter may be required. Frequent urine specimens may be examined for hemolysis. Retain urine until it is known whether it will need to be examined. Maintain hydration via IV, but check for any evidence of overload. Check for bleeding (hemolysis may be severe enough to cause consumptive coagulopathy with massive platelet loss, and defibrination; see also "Types of Transfusion Reactions," page 469).

4.11 URINE KETONES

Synonym: ketone bodies

Normal Range: negative for all age groups

Testing for ketone bodies in the urine is another fairly simple, straightforward test. Ketonuria of sufficient concentration to produce a positive response in testing reflects an alteration of carbohydrate metabolism with secondary disturbance in lipid metabolism.

Diabetes mellitus is the only disease in which ketonuria has a true diagnostic importance. Ketonuria in slight to moderate amounts is fairly common. But in most cases it is only incidental to the variety of conditions in which it can occur. The presence of ketonuria in diabetes mellitus is a major indicator of impending or established ketoacidosis. Its absence, or a less than strong testing response, does not rule out diabetes mellitus, however, if other signs or symptoms of the condition are present.

With the advent of laboratory use of reagent strips, especially the combined strips, testing for urine ketones has become a more frequent part of a routine urinalysis. In the past it was often routinely done only on young children. The reagent strip is the simplest form of testing. There is also a tablet form of the same testing material (nitroprusside and alkali) which is similar in sensitivity. The strip test is most sensitive to acetoacetic acid (also referred to at times as diacetic acid) and less sensitive to acetone. It does not react at all with the third ketone body—β-hydroxybutyric acid. It is felt, however, that there is little need to distinguish between acetone and acetoacetic acid, as both have essentially the same significance.

Davidsohn and Henry (1969) provide the scale given in Table 4.3 for comparison of testing responses and to provide a rough quantification of the urine ketone tests.

TABLE 4.3 *Urine ketone testing*

Sodium nitroprusside tests		Approximate level of ketone bodies (mg/dL)	
Reagent strip scale	**Tablet test scale**	**Concentration of acetoacetic acid**	**Concentration of acetone**
–	Trace	5	20–40
Small	1+	10	100
Moderate	2+	20–100	250–500
Large	4+	100–300	800–4,000

Physiology. (See also "Physiology" in Section 1.4.1). When fat is used as a body fuel, as in dieting for weight loss, one of the first steps in processing it for use involves lipolysis, that is hydrolysis of triglycerides to glycerol and free fatty acids (FFA). Thus FFA formation is increased. The glycerol fraction is broken down for glucose by the liver as it reverts from glucose utilization to glucose production. The remainder of the fat molecule, approximately 90%, becomes waste products, such as ketone bodies, and must be eliminated. Usually the body metabolizes all ketones produced, but, in the face of markedly increased ketone production, not all ketones can be metabolized and the excess must be excreted in the urine (ketonuria). For the dieter this process is a compensatory one, at least for a while (Howard and Herbold, 1978; Frolich, 1976; Tietz, 1970).

Pathophysiology. When ketone bodies are produced in excess, as occurs when fat is mobilized for fuel, their levels may rise from 1 mEq/dL to as high as 30 mEq/dL. They circulate in the blood stream (ketonemia) and are subsequently excreted in the urine. The body is in a state of ketosis. In the absence of glucose (e.g., starvation), or the inability of the body to utilize it due to lack of insulin (e.g., diabetes mellitus), the body can to some extent utilize ketones in lieu of glucose. However, in diabetes mellitus with the absence of insulin to transport the liver-produced glucose into the cells, the body soon reaches a state of cellular starvation. The unused ketones are excreted rapidly due to a low renal threshold. Ketone bodies are organic acids, but few of them can be excreted as acid. Instead, they require sodium for their excretion, causing sodium loss. They are also fairly large molecules and tend to add to the osmotic diuresis, rapidly depleting the extracellular volume (Blevins, 1974).

Because ketone bodies are organic acids, they produce excessive amounts of free hydrogen, causing metabolic acidosis. Slight to moderate degrees of ketonuria are fairly common conditions, secondary to a number of causes. Ketoacidosis is not as frequent an occurrence as ketonuria, but it can, and does, occur in uncontrolled diabetes mellitus. The amount of ketones present in the urine in such states is in fact a good indication of the severity of the ketoacidosis and may provide warning of impending coma.

POSITIVE URINE KETONE TEST RESPONSES OCCUR IN:

1. *Physiologic conditions, treatments, or other illnesses causing nondiabetic positives:*
   a. Individuals ingesting high-fat, low-carbohydrate diets for weight loss, or for control of certain types of seizure activity.
   b. Persons receiving *L*-dopa (Parkinson's disease), or medications containing phthalein compounds (bromsulfalein) may have low-grade false positives.
   c. Infants with untreated phenylketonuria, although high enough levels are seldom present in the disease state to cause positive reactions to general screening tests for ketonuria.
   d. Occasionally seen following exposure to cold or severe exercise.
2. *Pathologic conditions* such as:
   a. Diabetes mellitus, in which the presence of ketones is an indicator of metabolic acidosis.
   b. The first trimester of pregnancy in latent, or otherwise controlled, diabetic women. The stress of fetal growth can cause a hypoglycemic state which, when coupled with nausea and vomiting and decreased food intake, actually produces a starvation ketosis with ketonuria and decreased serum glucose. This state can have an effect on the fetus's mental development (Metheny and Snively, 1979). Ketoacidosis is more common in the second half of pregnancy of diabetic women due to an increase of placental hormones, which are antagonistic to insulin. Ketoacidosis can be fatal to the fetus, particularly during the second trimester (Howard and Herbold, 1978).
   c. Starvation, due to lack of available food or an inability to digest and/or absorb food adequately, or due to an increased and excessive body demand for nutrients (e.g., cancer, thyrotoxicosis, and increased tissue catabolism). A type of starvation occurs in postanesthesia patients. Because of tissue destruction during the surgery, the stress response increasing tissue catabolism and the lack of nutritional intake, perhaps before, and certainly after the surgery, they are prime candidates for nondiabetic ketonuria.

d. Febrile diseases and toxic states, usually or especially in children, accompanied by vomiting or diarrhea.
e. Glyocogen storage disease (e.g., Gierke's), in which ketonuria is accompanied by hypoglycemia.

IMPLICATIONS FOR NURSING

1. *Daily routine testing* for ketonuria for diabetic patients is not always necessary. After the initial learning period when the process should be practiced several times daily, the diabetic with a stable blood sugar, and who has never evidenced hypoglycemia or ketonuria during his or her stabilization period on a treatment regime, usually may test for acetone only when glycouria is increased beyond his or her "norm." Many diabetics routinely run a trace or more of sugar.

2. *The diabetic person* must become capable of examining his or her own urine for ketones, or a family member or home caretaker must have this skill if the patient is to live outside a hospital setting. Since the process varies slightly, or greatly, depending on the product used, the process per se will not be discussed here. Generally, the dipstick or reagent strip is more convenient for home use. Care of these products and general instructions in the use of testing material are given with nursing implications for urine glucose. The procedure to be followed at home should be the same as that taught in the hospitals, and any adaptation to the home environment should be worked out before discharge.

   One of the more important points to clarify in the teaching process is the knowledge and understanding of the patient/family/home caretaker as to what to do should he or she get a positive result. There are several options available: repeat the test, increase insulin dosage, note any accompanying signs or symptoms of ketoacidosis, assess for possible precipitants of ketoacidosis, increase frequency of testing, call the doctor, and/or inform a clinic or visiting nurse. Usually, the doctor likes to be notified *whenever* ketonuria occurs, but this needs to be validated with the doctor as well as other steps to be taken.

3. *The use of the combined Keto-Diastix* (acetone/glucose) has the disadvantage of giving a false low glucose reading when there are moderate or large amounts of ketones present. The patient/family/home caretaker needs to be aware of this possibility if using this

product. Further, he or she needs to know how to retest the urine with Clinitest tablets and to understand the rationale.

4. *Further subjects to be covered in preparing the diabetic patient to go home* include understanding the need for and the process of evaluating the testing material for deterioration. (Measures to prevent deterioration are included under urine glucose, this chapter.) Any strips produced by the Ames Company can be tested for effective acetone reagent by placing the strip in a solution made up of ¼ teaspoon of *freshly opened* Cutex or Revlon nail polish remover (or any remover that is known to contain primarily acetone), mixed with 2/3 cup of water. Any result showing less than "small," or one that produces a color response that does not match those of the color chart, indicates deterioration and the testing material should be discarded (Blevins, 1979).

5. *Identification of risk groups* for ketonuria in a hospital population, or in any situation in which patients contact nurses, is of importance for provision of complete preventative care. Risk populations include:
   a. Any pregnant women but particularly those with a history of diabetes in the family, or "prediabetes" themselves, and certainly those diagnosed as diabetic.
      (1) Check urine for ketonuria on each visit, whether glucosuria is or is not present.
      (2) Teach the procedure and rationale to the women and set up a regime for preventative testing.
      (3) Be especially alert during the first two trimesters. The women should be impressed with the need for daily testing during that time.
   b. Postoperative patients:
      (1) Particularly those who had extensive periods without food prior to surgery.
      (2) Those who face prolonged periods on parenteral nutrition only (not to include those on hyperalimentation).
      (3) Those who had extensive preparation of the gut prior to surgery (gut sterilization):
         (a) If possible, check the urine daily for ketones.
         (b) If (a) is not possible, monitor any routine urinalyses that are done for the presence of ketones.
         (c) If at all appropriate to the case at hand, discuss with the physician the possibility of increased nutritional intake for the patient as soon postoperatively as possible. Elemental diets via nasogastric tubes have

been given immediately postoperatively in at least one study with totally beneficial, rather than detrimental, results (Moss, 1977, pp. 73-82). The better the nutritional state, the more rapid the recovery, and a person demonstrating ketonuria is also demonstrating starvation.

6. *For related nursing implications,* see also "Implications for Nursing" in Sections 1.4 and 4.7.

4.12 MICROSCOPIC EXAMINATION OF THE URINE

Synonyms: none

Normal Ranges

Cell count
- RBC 2–3
- WBC 4–5/hpf (per high power field)

Casts
- Occasional (occ.) hyaline

No age variation in the healthy infant, child, or senior adult

Examination of urinary sediment can indicate, or confirm, evidence of renal disease. It provides information about the kidneys and/or urinary tract not found elsewhere, when correlated with the clinical status of the patient. Since there is no widely accepted standardized procedure for this examination, and urinary sediment is concentrated by centrifuging to greater or lesser degrees, depending on many variables, strict interpretation of quantitative reports is difficult.

The urinary sediment is routinely examined for cells, casts, crystals, and oval fat bodies. The cells and casts are often called *formed elements* and are usually of the most importance. Any other materials found in the urine are reported and commented on. Further testing is done as indicated to confirm the findings (e.g., urine culture for a finding of urinary bacteria) (Davidsohn and Henry, 1969).

As in all tests included in the routine urinalysis, proper collection and handling of the urine is vital in obtaining valid results. For example, white blood cells in the urine sediment will lyse rapidly. Some 50% of the WBCs present can be lost in 2 to 3 hr at room temperature. Therefore, examination of urinary sediment should be prompt.

Physiology

Cells. Cells are normally found in urine and come from either normal desquamation of the lining of the urinary tract (epithelial cells), or from the blood (white and red blood cells). Epithelial cells appear in very small numbers as a result of normal cell aging and sloughing. Certain epithelial cells cannot be easily identified as to source and at times may not be distinguished from white blood cells. In some counting procedures (Addis counts) white blood cells and epithelial cells are counted together. An increased number of epithelial cells will be found after prostatic massage in males.

Just how white blood and red blood cells enter the urine when there is no pathology present is not known, but in proportion there are a greater number of WBCs to RBCs in the urine than in the blood. The excretion rate of WBCs by way of the urine varies from hour to hour in the same individual. Excretion rates also increase with strenuous exercise or fever. Females tend to have a greater concentration of white blood cells than do men.

Casts. Normally, the number of cells present in urine is too small to form casts, so very few casts are seen in normal urine. An occasional hyaline cast may be seen, often after exercise or in the person having postural proteinuria (see Section 4.8), since cast formation is closely tied to the presence of renal protein, and hyaline casts are almost entirely protein. Hyaline casts are hard to see on microscopic examination, and when they are seen, if they are the only type of casts present, they have little significance (Ravel, 1973).

Crystals. The importance of crystal formation in urine is questionable. Except when an unusually large number of one type are seen, or the crystals are abnormal, they are not routinely reported. They may have been somewhat overemphasized in the past. Crystals can, however, contain clues to calculus (stone) formation, or certain metabolic disease. Crystal formation is pH-dependent. Crystals that normally appear in acid urine include calcium oxalate, uric acid, and urate. Alkaline urine produces phosphate and carbonate crystals. Neutral urine can also produce crystals, such as calcium oxalate and calcium phosphate. A generalization can be made. If urine is alkaline, phosphates crystalize; if urine is acid, urates crystalize (Davidsohn and Henry, 1969).

Pathophysiology

Cells. Epithelial cells increase in number in relationship to the amount of tissue deterioration present. Fatty degeneration of the epithelial cells occurs in some conditions. The epithelial cell includes fatty droplets with inflammatory changes in the tubule cells. In the presence of marked proteinuria, the cell degrades to the point of becoming only a fatty droplet, found floating free in the urine. This is called an *oval fat body* and occurs in conditions such as the nephrotic syndrome. The source of the fat is thought to be the lipoproteins that can pass the damaged glomerulus in this condition. Oval fat bodies are also found in many other diseases [e.g., lupus erythematosus, subacute glomerulonephritis, the nephrotic stage of glomerulonephritis, with certain tubular poisons (mercury), and in rare hypersensitive states]. Active degeneration of the tubules with increased epithelial cell excretion occurs in acute tubular necrosis or necrotizing papillitis (Ravel, 1973).

Red blood cells. A significant increase in microscopic hematuria occurs in substantially the same disorders given previously in this chapter for urinary occult blood, or hemoglobinuria. Some conditions related to only occasional gross bleeding in the urine, but with significant microscopic hematuria include: bleeding and clotting disorders (e.g., purpura, effects of anticoagulants); blood dyscrasias (e.g., sickle cell anemia, leukemia); renal infarction; malignant hypertension; subacute bacterial endocarditis; collagen disorders (e.g., lupus erythematosus, periarteritis nodosa); and various bladder, urethral, or prostatic conditions. Extrarenal sources can also contribute to microscopic hematuria (e.g., acute appendicitis; salpingitis; diverticulitis; tumors of the colon, rectum, and pelvis) (Davidsohn and Henry, 1969).

White blood cells. Increased numbers of leukocytes, particularly neutrophils, are seen in almost *all* renal disease or disease of the urinary tract. They can come from any point in the urinary tract and are generally accompanied by significant proteinuria, if from renal origin. Bacteriuria usually accompanies lower urinary tract infection with only slight proteinuria (Ravel, 1973).

Casts. Casts are formed protein gel conglomerations, outlining the shape of the renal tubules in which they are formed. They are produced in two ways: (1) the precipitation and gelling of protein from a high solute concentration of tubular fluid; or (2) by the clumping of the cells in the tubules in a matrix of protein (Davidsohn and Henry, 1969); see Fig. 4-2.

Some factors that influence the formation of casts include:

1. *pH.* Protein casts tend to dissolve in alkaline medium, so an acid pH favors formation.
2. *Casts tend to dissolve* in a very dilute medium; thus concentrated, high-solute solutions favor their formation.

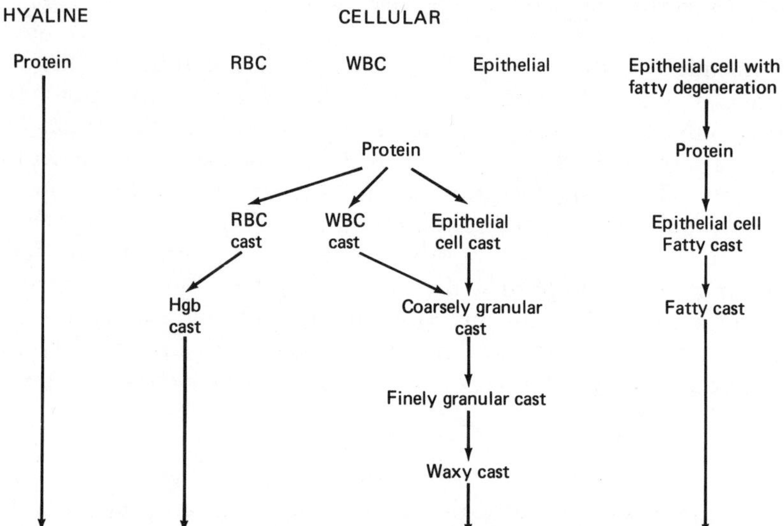

FIGURE 4.2 Formation of casts. (Reproduced with permission from R. Ravel, *Clinical Laboratory Medicine: Clinical Application of Laboratory Data,* 3rd ed.; copyright © 1978 by Year Book Medical Publishers, Inc., Chicago.)

3. *Protein is the basic matrix* for cast formation; therefore, proteinuria from a renal or prerenal source is a necessity for cast formation.
4. *Stasis.* To provide the time for protein precipitation in the tubules, a slowing of the urine flow through the tubules is necessary. This usually occurs with a protein obstruction intratubularly. Ordinarily, the distal, or collecting tubules, are where casts are formed. This may be due to the fact that urine acidification takes place there, as well as to the fact that urine concentration is the greatest at this point.

There are three main types of casts formed (see Fig. 4-2). The cellular cast may be made up of one, or all, of the cells present in the urine. As the cellular cast is excreted, disintegration may take place, leaving only coarse or fine granules. Or the full cast may be expelled. *Broad casts,* which are casts of the larger collecting tubules where large ducts drain several small ones, indicate a more widespread and severe stasis, and are often found in kidneys close to total renal shutdown; hence another name for broad casts is "renal failure casts" (Ravel, 1973).

An increase in the number of casts appearing in the urine is called *cylinduria,* and an increased number is diagnostic of renal rather than lower urinary tract disease, since they are formed in the nephron (Davidsohn and Henry, 1969).

IMPLICATIONS FOR NURSING

Microscopic findings	Cause and/or significance	Assessment and nursing care
CASTS		
RBC	Localizes source of bleeding as the kidney; presence of any casts indicate presence of proteinuria, increased urine concentration, and renal stasis	1. Any urine specimens must arrive at lab stat. 2. Mark any urine sample with time of collection 3. Report presence of increased numbers of casts; bring to attention of physician
WBC	Localizes source of infection as in the kidney	4. Increase fluid intake if appropriate—especially important in the aged
Fatty	Indicates renal tubular damage; frequently due to nephrotic syndrome	5. Manipulate diet for alkaline ash if appropriate (see Section 4.5); again of particular importance in caring for the aged 6. See "Implications for Nursing," Section 4.8
Broad	Indicates severe stasis, potential renal shutdown	Report immediately to physician
Hyaline	If persistent and increasing in face of therapy, can suggest serious intrarenal problem; further diagnostic work-up indicated Individual occurrence, or only occasionally found, usually benign but does indicate that conditions necessary for formation were present	Bring persistency to attention of physician; assess for change in urinary output
CRYSTALS		
Cystine, tyrosine leucine, sulfonamide	All abnormal in urine; indicate loss of amino acids through urine; may be due to an inherited metabolic disease	Report; usually a recheck will be done; presence and identity confirmed; cystinuria in itself benign, easily overlooked; can cause massive renal calculi
CELLS		
WBC in clumps	Strongly indicates renal infection, but not conclusive	Urine specimen should go to lab stat, or be kept cool; WBCs lyse on standing and in alkaline urine
With WBC or mixed epithelial and WBC casts	Definitely shows kidney origin of infection	
Many	Usually with acute infection	Obtain a culture; with repeated sterile cultures and continued WBCs may indicate Tbc or a lupus nephritis

Implications for Nursing (*cont.*)

Microscopic findings	Cause and/or significance	Assessment and nursing care
Gross amount	May indicate rupture of renal or urinary tract abcess	Look for changes in vital signs (decreasing temp. for example) or complaint of pain
Slight increase	Usually indicates urethral calculi, renal calculi, or acute or chronic cystitis, urethritis, prostatitis	To determine presence of urethritis over renal or bladder infection, a two-container specimen may be ordered: initial voiding in container 1, rest in container 2; in urethritis, most leukocytes will be in container 1
Epithelial clumps	Seen in acute tubular necrosis	
RBC	Poorly preserved in dilute or alkaline urine; sp. gr. 1.006–1.010	If RBCs expected and not reported by lab, consult with physician for second order; might be well to check sp. gr. before requesting second order Report should have been positive for hemoglobin or occult blood due to hemolysis; if not, no RBCs present, hemolyzed or intact Prevent contamination of urine specimen, especially in females; bacteria from vagina or rectum may be cause of alkalinity of urine
BACTERIA	Could be due to urinary tract infection or due to contamination of specimen	Prevent contamination by proper technique (see Section 4.13); suspect contamination when numerous bacteria and squamous epithelial cells are reported
Trichomonas	Almost always a contaminant	Report; may indicate need for WBC

Source: Data from Davidsohn and Henry, 1969; Harper, 1971; and Saxon and Etten, 1978.

4.13 GENERAL IMPLICATIONS FOR NURSING

1. *Identify risk groups* for urinary tract infections (UTI) (e.g., females—due to the short urethra—extremes in age, the debilitated in health, adult diabetics).
   a. Assess risk groups for signs and symptoms of UTI. They may be easily missed because the signs or symptoms are often

vague. A high index of suspicion should be applied in general assessment of any member of a risk group.

(1) Check for UTI any time an elderly person presents signs or symptoms of an altered state of health.

(2) Check for lethargy, change in mental status, as possible symptoms of uremia.

(3) Anorexia, vomiting, and restlessness can also relate to a UTI.

(4) Any change in voiding habits (nocturia, dribbling, incontinence), as well as the more specific signs of UTI (e.g., frequency and dysuria), should be noted and followed up.

b. Keep careful intake and output records on all risk patients, particularly when urinary problems are suspected. Such records kept routinely on all risk individuals are of great value. Such a record is *the* most effective nursing assessment tool.

c. Urinary dipstick or strip screening can be utilized independently by nursing personnel to help determine increased UTI risks (e.g., alkaline urine).

d. Individuals with a history of bacteriuria should have:

(1) Careful inquiry into the history of the frequency of occurrences, and possible causes in the past.

(2) History of the type(s) of treatment used in the past and their response to the treatment(s).

(3) History taken of the type of follow-up care done in the past to help prevent further occurrences and its effectiveness.

(4) A flow sheet kept that documents daily voiding patterns, general health status, intake and output, and dipstick findings (if done).

(5) Instruction in maintaining the individual's own flow sheet when discharged to pick up on early signs/symptoms of UTI, and to be shared with the physician should another infection occur.

e. Preventative measures should be instituted for *all* patients, but such measures are imperative for the groups at risk.

(1) Fluid intake should be increased with any signs or symptoms of UTI unless contraindicated by other disorder(s).

(2) Teach and assist the individual to carry out measures to prevent urinary stasis and/or infections, such as:

(a) Providing easy and safe access to bathroom, day and night (night light, bedside commode).

(b) Preplanned waking to toilet during night if sleep patterns not unduly disturbed.

(c) Maximizing physicial mobility during day.

(d) Appropriate positioning to urinate: females seated upright, no slouching or crouching; bending forward to help empty bladder; males standing with back in alignment, bending forward at hips to help empty bladder.

(e) Preventing contamination of urinary tract due to poor hygiene by the following means. First, provide for, or remind the individual to change underwear, keeping it clean and dry. Second, if diapers used at night, change them as soon as possible after they have been wet. Third, discourage elderly women from using a sanitary napkin throughout the day, or make sure that it is changed as soon as it becomes wet. A wet napkin provides a good environment for bacterial growth and will tend to irritate and inflame the perineal area. Fourth, provide and teach the need for excellent perineal care daily. Show women the technqiue of cleansing with a cloth by stroking *toward* the rectum only, never from the rectum forward. Same technique to be practiced with the use of toilet paper, after voiding. Finally, in hospital settings; use disposable bedpans or urinals, or establish routines of *thorough* cleansing and routine disinfection and culturing of nondisposable items; and provide cleansing, disinfection and culturing of bathtubs.

(f) Providing sexually active older women with special instruction as needed (e.g., voiding immediately after intercourse to flush the urethra; bathing just before or after intercourse; change of position for the sexual act if male superior position usual, as it can cause extraurethral stress and irritation).

(3) When a UTI does not respond to the administration of an antimicrobial agent (cultures remain positive; signs and symptoms remain active):

(a) Request a Gram stain, culture, and sensitivity test.

(b) Consult with physician for a change in treatment.

(4) At times dietary manipulation to foster acid urine is indicated [e.g., in the presence of a proteus infection or in the care of a sedentary person with urinalysis findings of phosphate crystals (which tend to precipitate in alkaline urine and may form calculi)].

(a) Provide acid ash foods (cranberries, plums, prunes, eggs, meat, fish).

(b) Consider need to restrict use of alkaline ash foods (whole milk, nuts, other fruits*).

2. *With systemic diseases* that predispose to acid-base imbalances, the individuals at extremes in age must be closely monitored and protected against such imbalances, as they have little reserve for adapting in acid-base disorders.
   a. Testing urine for pH is one way to monitor acid-base balance.
      (1) Only fresh urine should be used.
      (2) The testing strip, or stick, should be left in the urine for just a few seconds; excessive fluid can wash away the reactive chemicals.
      (3) Observe for change in color in a good light, using the proper scale for the test agent being used.
      (4) When accuracy is imperative, use a fresh urine sample taken between meals, and when the patient has been awake for several hours. (Recall, sleep causes a slight respiratory acidosis, which leads to a more alkaline urine, and food intake will alter the acid-base response, depending on what has been eaten and on the "alkaline tide" following meals due to hydrochloric acid utilization.)
   b. Individuals on intensive, or prolonged, antacid therapy, particularly those among the elderly with diminished renal adaptation to correct acid-base disorders, should be taught to:
      (1) Observe themselves, or have a family member assess, for symptoms of milk-alkali syndrome (nausea, vomiting, confusion, polydypsia, polyuria, and a profound distaste for milk). The potential for this problem is greatest in those taking readily absorbed base products, such as Tums.
      (2) In caring for the hospitalized patient on antacid treatment, the nurse should monitor laboratory values for urinary pH and venous CO_2, which are indicators of the base content of blood.

3. *Proper urine collection* is absolutely essential in getting accurate test results in cases of pyuria (presence of WBC in urine) and is important in almost all tests on urine. Contamination from the

---

*A rather thorough study was done on the effect of cranberry juice in decreasing urinary pH. It was found that in young subjects only, given 450 to 720 ml of 80% of cranberry juice/day (not a commercially available preparation), there was a significant decrease in urinary pH. Little or no effect was noted in other age groups, or at lower amounts of concentrations of cranberry juice. There were also side effects of frequency of voiding–increased body weight and diarrhea in the successful group (Kinney and Blount, 1979).

periurethral area and the vagina is a significant factor in causing inaccurate visualization of WBCs in the urinary sediment

a. Procedure (Female; clean catch, or midstream):
   (1) Wash hands and rinse well. If patient is collecting own specimen, this must be stressed.
   (2) Spread the labia.
      (a) Using three separate cleansing wipes [prepackaged wipes, soft clean cloths saturated with cleansing detergent or Betadine, or (last choice) cotton balls, also saturated], wash downward from just above the inner labia on one side, stopping before reaching the rectum. Discard wipe.
      (b) Repeat on opposite side.
      (c) With third wipe, cleanse between the inner labia.
   (3) Rinse well with water pouring from front to back.
   (4) Continuing to hold the labia apart, when rinse water has dripped off, the individual should begin voiding.
   (5) As soon as some urine has cleansed the urethral opening, place the collecting container in position with your free hand, not touching the inner surface or edge about the opening with fingers or the body.
   (6) When the specimen is in the container, cap it as soon as possible to prevent bacterial contamination from the air. Do not touch the inner surface of the cap. Container and cap preferably sterile; *must* be clean. The fuller the specimen container, the less the chance of bacterial contamination.
   (7) Take immediately to the laboratory, or if it *must* wait more than an hour, refrigerate the specimen.
   (8) If the individual has been having difficulty with either concentration or dilution of the urine, for whatever reason, that fact should be indicated on the laboratory request slip or on the specimen label.

b. Procedure (male; clean catch, or midstream):
   (1) Retract the foreskin if uncircumsized.
   (2) Cleanse the glans using a circular motion from tip of penis to foreskin, and discard wipe. Do not retrace with same cleansing wipe. Repeat with remaining wipes. Often, two are sufficient.
   (3) Follow steps (5) through (8) above. The tip of the penis should not touch any part of the collecting container at any time (Mowad, 1979).

Diagnosis of Infectious Disease

PART 2

Introduction to Infectious Disease

chapter 5

5.1 DEFINITION OF TERMS

There is a difference between infection and infectious disease. Many terms used to describe infection tend to be used interchangeably and are confusing for that reason. The following defines frequently used terms for the purpose of this book.

Colonization. The presence in the body of a bacterium, virus, yeast, fungus, protozoa, or rickettsia organism which may or may not be capable of producing disease. The interactions between bacteria and humans are more often than not equally beneficial (mutualism). The presence of such an organism in the body is most commonly trivial and unapparent, or helpful (e.g., normal flora of the intestinal tract digest protein for absorption by the body). The person is indeed colonized, but he or she is *not sick.*

For an insight into the microorganisms normally present (normal flora), the common contaminating microorganisms, and the unusual—or abnormal—microorganisms most likely to cause an infectious process in a given body site, see Appendix F.

Infectious process. The state occurring when the invasion of organisms, or their toxins, is in sufficient numbers and virulency to stimulate an inflammatory response in the part of the body overwhelmed so that notable signs and symptoms occur [e.g., fever (local or systemic), redness, pain, discomfort].

Infectious disease. A condition occurring in much the same manner as an infectious process, but is capable of being transmitted from one person to another by transfer of the organism. The term "infectious disease" is used interchangeably with "communicable disease." An infectious disease *is* an infectious process, but an infectious process is localized and not considered a disease in the truest sense of the word. As a person can be colonized and not "sick," so may a person have an infectious process but not be considered "diseased."

Local infection. An infectious process confined to one area of the body (e.g., an abcess, a furuncle).

Focal infection. A local infectious process with systemic symptoms (e.g., increase in body temperature with a postoperative wound infection).

Systemic or generalized infection. Organisms spread throughout the body, may be a septicemia or pyemia (see below).

Opportunistic infection. Infectious process caused by organisms of low pathogenicity, often endogenous to the host, because some factor, or set of factors, has compromised the intrinsic defense mechanisms of the host, or has in some way altered the ecology of the normal resident microbes (see Section 5.2).

Secondary, or superimposed infection. An opportunistic infection which occurs during the course of another infection, the *primary infection.*

Nosocomial infection. The term applied to hospital-acquired infections as opposed to community-acquired infections. They are usually, but not necessarily, opportunistic in type.

Acute infection. An infectious process characterized by a rapid onset, usually severe symptoms, and a fairly rapid course.

Chronic infection. An infectious process characterized by a slow, probably insidious onset, although it can be a residual state following an acute infection. Symptoms are insiduous and often nonspecific. The course is protracted. Chronic disease may have periods of remission and exacerbation.

Bacteremia. Presence of bacteria in the blood; may be transient or constant; may be a sign of an infectious process or a momentary happening prior to bacterial destruction.

Septicemia. Presence of bacteria or their toxins in the blood. Usually associated with a severe infectious process and involves active multiplication of the microorganism in the bloodstream and/or production of toxin. Known in lay terms as "blood poisoning."

Pyemia. A type of septicemia with the presence of pyogenic (pus-forming) microorganisms in the bloodstream (e.g., streptococci, staphylococci). Secondary abcesses can form wherever the microorganisms lodge. Organisms causing pyemia kill the neutrophils that phagocytize them. The resulting cellular debris is called pus [Nonpyogenic organisms (e.g., *Salmonella, Brucella, Mycobacterium*) persist within the macrophages that attack them, rather than killing them, causing chronic, low-grade infections.]

Toxemia. A term used to imply a concentration of bacterial toxins in the blood.

5.2 GENERAL INFORMATION ABOUT INFECTIOUS DISEASE AND ITS CONTROL

It is no longer possible to classify microorganisms as pathogens and nonpathogens in humans. Many organisms, supposedly part of the "normal flora," are now found to cause disease. There are multiple causes for this change. Drugs have been discovered to eliminate certain pathogenic organisms. In their absence the usual ecological balance is upset, allowing a previous nonpathogenic organism to emerge and grow out of all proportion, causing a disease state. Further, some therapies developed over the last two decades depress the normal immune mechanism.

Most interactions between humans and bacteria are unaccompanied by disease. Many body parts are always "colonized" with normal flora, and most infectious diseases in humans are mild (see Appendix F). The acute, fulminating, and highly contagious bacterial diseases of the past are less frequently seen, due to environmental sanitation and preventative medicine. When they do occur such acute infectious diseases are relatively simple to diagnose and there are specific and effective therapy for most. More difficult in the present is the interpretation of a culture to determine the primary infective agent, since the likelihood of secondary contributors to the infectious process is greatly increased.

Control of infectious disease is a great deal broader than are the identification and treatment of a given infectious disease. The diagnosis is only a beginning of the control process and that process is most frequently contained in the scope of nursing practice. Control consists of prevention based on known methods of microorganism transmission, and identification of the population at risk; surveillance through identification of outbreaks, extensive data collection, organization, and reporting; and preparation, implementation, and updating of infection control techniques specific to the locale.

5.3 PHYSIOLOGY

(See also "Physiology" in Sections 1.9.2 and 2.2.1, and Table 2.3.) The body has a great number of natural barriers to infection as well as a variable number of acquired defenses. The natural, or innate, barriers include the intact skin and endothelial linings of body organs; the limited ability of the skin and endothelial linings to decontaminate themselves by the "washing" action of area fluids [e.g., sweat, urine flow, mucus, and through the presence of antibacterial substances on those surfaces (e.g., lysozymes, hydrochloric acid, digestive enzymes, sebaceous secretion)], cilia and ciliary movement in the respiratory passages; phagocytosis; and antibody response. Many microorganisms cannot survive in the environment of a healthy body due to the ambient temperature or the oxygen tension.

Acquired defenses include active immunity secondary to immunization, usually including diphtheria, tetanus, pertussis, poliomyelitis, measles, and at times mumps, rubella, and smallpox; active immunity occurring secondary to certain infectious diseases (e.g., mumps, chickenpox); and passive immunity due to administration of immune serum or gamma globulin.

5.4 PATHOPHYSIOLOGY

Infections occur secondary to invasion and colonization of microorganisms. These microorganisms include:

1. *Bacteria.* Unicellular forms of plant life, classified as to shape and visible only under a microscope.

2. *Viruses.* Chunks of genetic material (DNA, RNA) that are obligate intracellular parasites; that is, they cannot live apart from animal cells, and can insert themselves into host cells. They tend to remain there in a dormant state in many cases. Individual organisms are visible only with electron microscopy.
3. *Fungi.* Multicellular mold-like organisms. These are often "opportunistic" infectors, as they are not usually particularly pathogenic unless they enter an already compromised host. Many forms tend to occur in rather typical geographic distribution (e.g., histoplasmosis in the midwestern and eastern parts of the United States).
4. *Protozoa.* Single-cell animal organisms that are motile and much more structurally complicated than are bacteria.
5. *Rickettsia.* Biochemically resembling bacteria and spread by vermin (e.g., ticks, fleas, and lice) and, like viruses, cannot live apart from animal cells.

Identification of Causative Organisms

chapter 6

6.1 METHODS FOR DIRECT EVIDENCE OF INFECTIOUS ORGANISMS

6.1.1 Examination of Direct Smears

A. Gram stain

Synonyms: none

Reported Results

Negative	Expected result from a specimen taken from a normally sterile site; indicates no visualization of microorganisms
Presence of mixed flora	Indicates the identification of expected resident flora (normal flora) from the site
Positive for shape and Gram result	Indicates the identification of probable causative organism by virtue of the number seen, or its presence in a normally sterile site
Presence of an increased number of polymorphonuclear neutrophils (PMN)	Increases the index of suspicion for infection

In most laboratories the examination of specimens received involves examination of direct smears, unstained and stained, and culture on appropriate media. There are many staining procedures, the most common and useful being the Gram stain. It is the one most likely to provide valuable information about the greatest number of organisms and is, therefore, usually indicated whenever staining is indicated. It is routinely used to examine cultures to identify organisms and determine purity of the colonies (i.e., single microorganism's growth).

The Gram stain provides a method of distinguishing between the many bacteria that have similar morphology. It artificially groups bacteria into gram-positive (stain purple) and gram-negative (stain red) categories as well as making the bacteria more visible on the slide so that form, size, and other structural details can be identified. There is correlation between the Gram stain and many other morphologic properties of related forms. The microbiologist can accurately predict by expert reading of the Gram stain some forms of anaerobic infection, resulting in early specific chemotherapy.

Portions of gram-negative bacteria cell walls possess endotoxins (toxins retained in the bacteria) which can produce lethal shock states, yet some gram-negative bacteria form part of the normal flora of the intestinal tract of man and animals. Their endotoxins are not released into the host in the disease-free state.

Certain gram-positive rods are spore formers, tending to contaminate soil [e.g., anthrax, *Clostridium*]. Many gram-positive cocci product exotoxins (toxin released from the body of the organism) [e.g., staphylococci, streptococci], and/or enterotoxins (toxins specific for the cells of the intestinal mucosa) which cause food poisoning.

When a smear is stained and examined, the presence and type of inflammatory cells are noted as well as the staining characteristics of the microorganisms present. If there are no accompanying inflammatory cells, it may indicate the presence of colonies of the organisms unable to elicit inflammatory response, although they can cause an invasive infection—the infected but *not* sick individual discussed in the definition of terms previously, or may indicate an immunodeficient host.

IMPLICATIONS FOR NURSING

See Chapter 7.

B. Acid–fast stain

Synonyms: Ziehl-Neelsen method; acid-fast bacilli stain; AFB; *Myocobacterium;* tubercle bacilli; Kinyoun carbolfuchsin acid-fast stain

Reported Results: no AFB (acid-fast bacilli); negative; positive for acid-fast bacilli [false positives possible with occurrence of saprophytic (nonpathogenic contaminants) acid-fast bacilli; differentiation made by correlation with the clinical picture]

Acid-fast organisms cannot be stained readily by Gram stain. Therefore, in cases of a suspected acid-fast bacterial infection (e.g., tuberculosis or leprosy—the most common conditions caused by acid-fast bacilli), special staining methods must be used. (Leprosy is caused by *Mycobacterium leprae.*) *Mycobacterium tuberculosis, Mycobacterium kanasii,* and *Mycobacterium bovis* (almost never isolated in humans) cause most tuberculosis in humans, but a tuberculosis-like disease is caused by other *Mycobacterium* organisms, known as atypical, or Group III, or Battey strains of *Mycobacterium.* There are still other forms (e.g., Group II) that cause cutaneous lesions and lymph node infections, seen more frequently in children. It is important that atypical strains be identified, as treatment will differ. Atypical strains tend to be resistant to currently available drugs.

The term "acid-fast" is derived from the staining characteristics of the bacteria. The organisms have such an affinity for certain stains (e.g., carbolfuchsin) that they retain the dye when washed with strong acids, a procedure that decolorizes most other types of bacteria. They are also quite resistant to strong alkaline solutions; thus both acid and alkaline solutions can be used to cut down on the presence of other organisms in the specimen. Such decontamination is necessary to culture the acid-fast organism because it is much slower growing than most bacteria—it needs 2 to 6 weeks for culture growth. Left with other organisms in the specimen, the culture would soon be overgrown.

Because the culture takes so long to yield results, treatment for disease caused by acid-fast bacilli is usually begun on the strength of the smear/stain identification. In suspected tuberculosis, sputum for smear evaluation is usually done in a series of not less than three first-morning-cough specimens collected on three separate days, in order to catch the sporadic discharge of the bacilli from the tubercle.

SPECIFIC IMPLICATIONS FOR NURSING

1. *The acid-fast stain* can be done on any body fluid or exudate.
2. *Gastric washing* may be done for AFB that have been coughed up and swallowed. The specimen must be taken to the lab immediately (properly labeled), before the concentrated stomach acid can kill the bacteria.

6.1.2 Specimen Culture

Synonyms: none

Reported results

No growth	Expected in cultures from normally sterile sites
Mixed flora	Reported with the identification of expected resident microorganisms from the site; any organisms found that are not normally present in the area, or "normal" organisms that are present in increased numbers, are specifically noted by the microbiologist and an antibiotic sensitivity test is often done and reported as soon as possible thereafter

A culture involves the collection of suspect material in an aseptic manner, or sterile collection from normally sterile body sites if possible, and introduction of that material to an environment in which the organisms present can grow—an appropriate culture media, gel, broth, or living cells. The cultures are then incubated and observed for growth for a specified length of time under specific conditions of ambient temperature and presence or absence of certain gases (e.g., CO_2). Different types of nutrients can be added to an agar or broth culture to be inoculated to meet specific microorganism's needs; and growth, or lack of it, on the different media helps to identify the organism.

Specimens for culture can be collected from blood, sputum, urine, feces, the discharge or scrapings from wounds, spinal fluid, and throat secretions. Droplets can be collected on a "cough plate" as well for detection of pertussis, although it is not often done at present.

The process of culturing an organism is done for three purposes:

1. Isolation of an organism—accomplished by streaking on an agar plate to ensure the appearance of isolated, and hopefully pure, colonies when incubated.
2. Identification of the organisms present by the characteristics of colony growth, such as color and morphology of the colony; growth requirements (e.g., specific nutrient media, anaerobic conditions); effect on media nutrients (e.g., fermentation of carbohydrates); and response patterns to the addition of certain antimicrobials or serological tests.
3. Maintenance, or preservation, of the live organism for further study. Staining kills the bacteria.

Identification of organisms from culture characteristics is validated by use of a direct smear/stain evaluation.

The decision as to whether to interpret the laboratory findings as normal, as an infection, an infectious process, or as an infectious disease is made by the physician and/or the pathologist based on symptoms, clinical history, clinical findings, antimicrobial findings, and any other relevant data.

IMPLICATIONS FOR NURSING RELATED TO SPECIMEN COLLECTION: REQUIREMENTS AND PRECAUTIONS

1. Usually, the laboratory does not collect culture specimens, except perhaps blood cultures. Most are collected by the nurse or other unit personnel. Some *general requirements and precautions* related to collection of any specimens include:
   a. The quantity of the specimen collected should be as large as necessary for laboratory processing: 5 to 10 mL of sputum for routine AFB or fungus culture; 2 to 3 mL of urine for routine urine; for AFB culture, 100 to 200 mL of urine is needed of first morning voiding. Check with lab personnel.
   b. All specimens should be collected as early in the disease as possible, preferably before antibiotic therapy or chemotherapy have begun.

c. Note time of collection on test request form and/or specimen label. The lab usually records the time the specimen is received and inoculated, but needs to know the collection time to assure adequate recovery of all significant organisms. Immediate processing must be done to recover certain ones (cocci such as gonococci, meningicocci, pneumonococci) and knowledge of the collection time will provide information as to the possibility of recovery.

d. Labels/request forms should include the following information:
   (1) Give *complete* information as to type and source of the specimen (e.g., "Throat swab from posterior pharynx through mouth"), which helps identify contaminant organisms.
   (2) If a full routine culture is not necessary (e.g., the physician wants only to rule out the presence of a specific organism), order the culture accordingly: "For beta strep. only."
   (3) Note any antimicrobial therapy being administered prior to the specimen collection and specify it by name and dosage, so that proper techniques can be used to identify or grow the organism.

e. Deliver culture specimens, particularly those collected on swabs, as soon as possible to the lab to prevent drying of the organisms. (Check with the lab regarding the availability and use of "transport media.")

f. Specimens should be collected where the suspected organism is most likely to be found with as little external contamination as possible (e.g., well within a draining wound rather than from the surrounding skin).

g. If possible, collect specimens at a stage of the disease when the organisms are present in greatest numbers (e.g., the diarrheal stage of intestinal infections, the first 3 to 5 days of viral infections).

h. If the patient is to be involved in the collection of a specimen, he or she will need precise and full instructions in the process, as well as the reasons for the requirements. Further, he or she will need to be encouraged in the process by reminders, and positive reinforcement.

i. The container for the specimen must be sterile for collection from a sterile site. Clean, disposable plastic containers with tightly fitted lids (preferably screw caps) may be used for such specimens as expectorated sputum, clean voided urine, and the like. The specimen should be introduced into the container so that the outer surfaces are not contaminated. This will prevent contamination of the specimen with outside organisms and contamination of health care personnel handling the container.

j. Frequently, advance notice to the lab about the type of organism to be cultured is necessary so that special media or handling can be prepared. Check with the lab servicing the facility in which you work for a list of such organisms. Organisms such as *Chlamydra,* viruses, Legionnaires' disease bacillus or botulism bacillus, for example, require materials or transport media that may not be available in the ward.

2. *Specific requirements and precautions* for specimen collection include:

   a. Abscesses, wounds, exudates (to include genital area—vagina, urethra, Bartholin's cyst, Skene's glands, etc.):
      (1) Specimen should be collected via sterile swab (many labs have special swabs that do not shed lint), or aspirated with a sterile needle and syringe from the most moist area. Bacteria from the absolute center may be nonviable. Therefore, the near periphery should be cultured, where organisms are most viable and active.
      (2) Expel air from syringe after collection. Cap and send stat to lab, properly labeled.
      (3) Genital area cultures (cervical, urethral, vaginal) should be clearly marked as to origin, as they are usually cultured for gonococci as well as other pathogens.

   b. Catheter tips (intravascular):*
      (1) Cut tip with *sterile* scissors 4 to 5 in. from the skin, holding it directly over a sterile specimen cup or wide-mouth bottle. (The cup is best, since it allows the broadest opening for collecting the tip and also allows the tip to be cultured in the lab without removing it from the container.)
      (2) Sterile technique is *essential,* since catheter infections are usually due to common skin organisms, which will also be the contaminating organisms if a sterile technique is not used.
      (3) Deliver as soon as possible to prevent drying of the organisms.

   c. Catheter sites:
      (1) Culture at the time of catheter removal or at the puncture site if culturing a venous catheter.

*Culture of urinary catheter tips is not advised, as they tend to grow a plethora of bacteria whose significance is not well determined in disease (Harris, 1980).

(2) Vein may be carefully "milked," or pressure placed on nearby tissue to express fluid.
(3) Send to lab with catheter tip, both property labeled.

d. Nasopharyngeal and throat:
(1) Nares: Insert swab to culture as far back as possible without bending the swab. Rotate the swab gently but using some pressure against the side.
(2) Pharyngeal: Use swab through mouth, exploring any obvious lesions or visible crypts. Rotate swab, getting it below the surface. In the absence of lesions, vigorously rotate swab over tonsillar or any inflamed area. Avoid touching the tongue or teeth, since many contaminating microorganisms from these areas can overgrow pathogens from the posterior pharynx.
(3) Nasopharyngeal: Use a swab attached to a narrow flexible wire. Clear nares and insert swab taking a mucus sample from above and behind the uvula. If only a small quantity of the specimen is available for collection, some labs suggest moistening the swab with sterile saline beforehand.
(4) Throat: Swab posterior wall of throat below level of the uvula. Depress tongue with tongue blade and do not touch tongue with the swab.

e. Rectal:
(1) Wearing a clean (not sterile) glove, insert swab approximately 1 in. into rectum, which has been cleared of feces if possible. If swab does enter the stool, discard it and start over, except when culturing *Shigella.* In that case the swab should be totally covered and saturated with stool. This may require deeper insertion of the swab—3 in.—and/or help of the patient in bearing down.
(2) Move swab from side to side to sample crypts. Allow 10 to 30 sec for organisms to be absorbed into the swab.

f. Spinal fluid:
(1) Collected by the physician in most cases.
(2) Keep the fluid warm in the tube during transport. You can use body heat from a warm hand or place the tube in a glass of tepid water. A common pathogen sought from spinal fluid is *Neisseria meningitidis,* which is very sensitive to cold (anything less than 35° C).

g. Sputum:
(1) Have patient rinse his or her mouth well with water without swallowing before trying to raise material by

coughing. This decreases the amount of saliva present. Do *not* use mouthwash, as this will kill the bacteria.

(2) Demonstrate technique of effective coughing for patient and assist him or her in learning the process (e.g., need for several deep breaths to help mobilize secretion, hands on diaphragm coordinating expulsion of air with upward hand pressure, preparation by intake of adequate fluids to thin secretions if needed). Explain the need for sputum and not saliva and the difference between them.

(3) If sputum is difficult to raise, have the patient lie with head and shoulders below chest level for a few minutes, if not contradicted by his or her condition.

(4) If specimen does not contain mucoid, or mucopurulent material, consult with the physician if necessary for alternate procedures (e.g., induced sputum, or nasotrachial aspiration).

(5) Early morning is often the best time for sputum collection, as it takes advantage of the overnight collection of pooled bronchial secretions.

(6) With nonproductive coughs, the use of cold steam or nebulized vapor may help raise sputum. Use of propylene glycol in the nebulizer should be avoided if the specimen is to be tested for *Mycobacterium tuberculi,* as it will inhibit growth or could even kill the bacteria.

(7) If the sputum cup is left with the patient, he or she will need careful instruction in its use—the need to keep the inner surfaces untouched and to keep it closed when not in use.

h. Stool:

(1) Stool specimens must be delivered to the lab while still warm, usually within 30 min or less. If allowed to stand longer, normal resident organisms may overgrow the less adaptive pathogens.

(2) Keep lid and outside of container clear of stool. The container should not be completely filled.

(3) Presence of barium in the stool does not usually interfere with most cultures if adequate feces is obtained. Barium will, however, interfere with parasitic studies.

i. Tissues, biopsies:

(1) Usually obtained by the physician.

(2) Place in a sterile tube or sputum cup with a small volume of sterile *nonbacteriostatic* saline or a sterile moist gauze.

(3) Do *not* place the sample in a preservative solution such as formalin or alcohol.

j. Urine:
   (1) See collection procedure in Section 4.13, item 3.
   (2) Endeavor to see that urine cultures are taken before antimicrobial therapy is started, especially in the case of an elderly patient or a patient recently rehospitalized and suspected of UTI. The pathogen is likely to be more resistant to antimicrobials in these instances.

6.1.3 Living-Tissue Culture

As discussed previously, two forms of microorganisms, virus and rickettsia, are obligate intracellular parasites and require animal cells in order to live. Thus the ordinary means of culture growth is not feasible for these microorganisms. Also, at times all usual means of isolation of a bacterium can fail. Another approach is necessary and living-tissue culture can be used.

A. Animal inoculation

The only available source of living cells in the past was the living, intact, experimental animal. Animals used included mice, hamsters, cotton rats, guinea pigs, rabbits, and monkeys. The animal used depended on the microorganism to be grown. Animals were inoculated intracerebrally, intranasally, or intradermally, again depending on the microorganism. The animal was then observed for a set time, usually a matter of weeks rather than days, sacrificed, and carefully autopsied. If successful, the organism was isolated in the living host and could then be identified by indirect (immunological, biochemical, pathological) methods.

Animal inoculation is still used on rare occasions as an aid in the final identification of acid-fast bacteria or for recovery of fastidious microorganisms when there are doubtful outcomes from stain and/or culture processes. The guinea pig (negative Mantoux reacting) is the animal of choice in human or bovine tuberculosis.

B. Chick embryo

Since its introduction, chick embryo inoculation has been used more frequently than has animal inoculation. The process is less expensive than animal inoculation, better accepted by the general public, and in most cases, equally effective in isolating some microorganisms, such as viruses. Lesions are produced on the membrane of the egg yolk sac and are examined by a number of techniques to identify the organism.

C. Dispersed cells in culture

This is the more recent living-tissue culture method. Microorganisms, especially viruses, grow and multiply when introduced into the culture. As viruses grow in the tissue culture they produce biologic effects on the cells present in the culture, which permits identification of the agent. The presence of the virus is confirmed by use of a type-specific antiserum (see Section 6.2.1). The cell or tissue culture is the most widely used method for isolating viruses from clinical specimens.

6.1.4 Colony Count

A colony is a discrete group of organisms on a culture. At times, such as in urinary tract infection, it is important to count the numbers of discrete colonies of a specific organism found on a given culture; 100,000 colonies per cubic milliliter of urine from a voided specimen; 10,000 colonies per mm^3 from a catheterized specimen is felt to be significant. Lesser counts are usually attributed to contamination with urethral flora, and in the absence of prior therapy largely rule out bacteriuria.

6.1.5 Biopsy

A biopsy is an examination of tissues taken from a living body. At times, a biopsy can be a useful diagnostic aid in infectious disease. For example, in may cases of prolonged fever of unknown origin (FUO), all the routine tests—culture, smear, and so on—fail to isolate and identify the causative organism of the fever. Surgical exploration of the suspect area may be done and a biopsy with histologic examination of the tissue cells may produce the identification of the microorganism and the diagnosis.

In miliary (disseminated) tuberculosis, clinical and culture investigations may fail to confirm the presence of the mycobacterium. Without evidence of the organism the diagnosis is not absolutely certain and biopsy of the bone marrow, or less frequently the liver, may be done, successfully demonstrating the microorganism through culture and acid-fast stain.

Use of biopsy and examination of the biopsied tissue are important in the diagnosis of some types of systemic fungi and for Legionnaires' disease.

6.1.6 Antibiotic Sensitivity

Most organisms are either sensitive (susceptible) or resistant to a specific group of antimicrobials. Although this reaction can help identify microorganisms, that is not the purpose for which a test is usually performed. The decisive factor in the physician's choice of antibiotic in the treatment of infectious disease is the relative susceptibility of the invading microorganism to the antibiotic.

Each antibiotic tested is listed and its effect on bacterial growth is indicated as:

Resistant	bacterial growth not inhibited
Sensitive	bacterial growth inhibited (see discussion of MIC below)
Intermediate	some inhibition (usually considered as resistant)

Antibiotic susceptibility (sensitivity) testing, when available, helps the physician select the most effective agent for treatment of the organism in question. The narrower the spectrum of action of the antimicrobial, the more preferred its use when the specific organism is known. Broad-spectrum antibiotics have value when treating an as-yet-unknown infection.

The Kirby-Bauer Agar Disc Diffusion Test. This test and its modifications are indirect approaches to describing the minimum inhibitory concentration (MIC) of certain antimicrobials. MIC is defined as the "lowest concentration of an antimicrobial at which no bacterial growth occurs for a given bacterial strain" (Henry, 1979). The test is performed after isolation of the suspect bacteria. The bacteria are placed on an agar plate, completely covering it. Specially prepared discs of a variety of antibiotics thought to be effective against the suspected microorganism are then placed at intervals on the agar plate surface. The plate is incubated and examined for clear areas (inhibition of bacterial growth) around the antibiotic impregnated discs. The clear areas are measured and compared to a predetermined norm for minimum inhibitory concentration. Commercially prepared dilution sets are now available as a modification of this method. Automated methods are rapidly replacing the Kirby-Bauer test and will give the MIC directly.

Microbroth Dilution Test. A form of MIC test, this test is a modification of the Kirby-Bauer test and is still in frequent use. Uses a standard suspension of antibiotics and a single concentration of bacteria derived from the patient's infection. If a low dilution does not inhibit growth, the therapy is thought to be ineffective.

The information gained tells the physician the inherent susceptibility of the infecting organism to the antibiotics tested. The most appropriate agent can then be selected for treatment.

Other considerations in the selection of an antibiotic include:

1. *The clinical pharmacologic properties* of the antibiotic: what concentrations will be achieved in the blood at recommended dosage, whether it can reach the site of infection (cross the blood-brain barrier, for example), or the route of administration and excretion (a drug not excreted by the kidney would be of little value in a urinary tract infection).
2. *Previous clinical experience* with the antibiotic and the organism (e.g., difficulty in maintaining a therapeutic blood level without danger of toxicity or ineffective levels—narrow therapeutic antibiotic concentration).
3. *The nature of the underlying pathologic process* (e.g., infectious disease in some body areas, or with some microorganisms, makes it difficult to get adequate blood concentrations to the site, as with multiple abcesses, or the tubercle of tuberculosis).
4. *The immune status of the patient.* Individuals with little or no immunologic defense will require greater concentrations of the antibiotic, and run greater risk of secondary and/or opportunistic infections.

Susceptibility tests are considered unnecessary by some authorities in the treatment of certain organisms that have shown little or no tendency to change in resistance (e.g., *Streptococcus pyogenes, Streptococcus pneumoniae, Neisseria gonorrhoeae*) (Henry, 1979). There is not total agreement on this approach.

Other Tests Related to Sensitivity Testing. *Antimicrobial assay*—determination of the concentration of an antimicrobial present in serum and other body fluid—is used to help predict the likelihood of success in the use of a given antimicrobial and to prevent potential toxicity, of particular concern in the patient with compromised renal or liver function. Types include:

1. *Radioimmunoassay* (RIA)—a direct and absolute measurement.
2. *Bioassay.*
3. *Enzymologic assay.* Both bioassay and enzymologic assay give individualized information about each drug and do not base data on general norms.
4. *Bactericidal assays* ('cidal assays or Schlichter tests) measure effective levels of antibiotics in the blood. They look at the combined effect of an isolated culture of the patient's infected body fluid and the antibiotic he or she is receiving. Bactericidal activity is anticipated at a given dilution. Such an indirect test can also

predict success in the use of the drug, and can also monitor the appropriateness of the treatment.

Susceptibility tests usually reflect inhibition levels; however, certain categories of infections may require knowledge of bactericidal concentrations (e.g., bacterial endocarditis or subacute bacterial endocarditis); MBC = minimum bactericidal concentration.

6.2 METHODS FOR INDIRECT EVIDENCE OF INFECTIOUS DISEASE

6.2.1 Serologic Tests (Immunologic)

Serologic tests are those based on observation of antibody-antigen reactions. They are of diagnostic value only late in the course of an infection. Their use in short-term illnesses is primarily for epidemiologic purposes, that is, identifying a disease in retrospect so as to prevent or treat the disease occurring in others. In some cases, as in very mild infections or those treated with antibiotics prior to specific diagnosis, serology may be the only way a diagnosis can be made.

Serology is used to collect evidence of past infections. Antibodies formed in response to the infection are identified and their concentration (titer) measured at different stages of the disease process. This provides a tool for following the course of an active infection and monitoring therapy. A single test seldom provides adequate information (e.g., whether a disease is active, or whether a negative response rules out a given disease). Usually, at least two tests are necessary, one during the active process and one during convalescent stage. Paired testing such as this provides comparative data. A fourfold or greater rise in titer to a specific microorganism is usually considered diagnostic.

Blood serum is the only body fluid that gives adequately high antibody titers to be useful. No other body fluid is usually tested. The five categories of serologic tests generally used to identify infectious disease are given, defined, and some examples shown in the following sections.

A. Agglutination tests

Agglutination is the process of an antibody attacking an antigen [defined as a protein which may be an organism, tissue cell (leukocytes) or other large protein molecule] which causes clumping of the antibody, antigen, and the microorganism. Agglutinins are specific antibodies developed in response to an antigenic agent (in infectious disease, the infective microorganism). They are protein–gamma globulins–and are part of the immune mechanism of the body. Agglutination tests (Table 6.1) can be done in test tubes, or directly on slides by mixing the patient's serum with a specific antigen.

TABLE 6.1 *Agglutination tests*

Name (synonyms)	Reference range reaction results	Purpose	Comments
Anti-streptolysin-0 (ASO; ASL)	Normal: 12–100 Todd units Significant: 100–2500 Todd units	Diagnosis of acute glomerulonephritis (AGN) and rheumatic fever	Until recently the ASO was felt to be the most helpful of the many antistreptococci antibody measurements
Brucella agglutination test (brucellosis test; undulant fever test)	Normal: 1:40 or less Significant: 1:80 or greater	Diagnosis of brucellosis	Because of many cross-reactions (false positives), results confirm, but do not diagnose brucellosis; history (e.g., drinking raw milk or working with large domestic animals: cattle, pigs, goats) helpful in increasing certainty
Cold agglutinins	Less than 1:32 to 1:65	Diagnosis of primary atypical pneumonia (PAP)	Called "cold" since agglutination occurs only at 37°C or lower; formed in response to a number of diseases other than PAP at lower titers; high titers *in vivo* can cause hemolysis; a Coombs (indirect) test also usually ordered to check for this
Febrile agglutination group (febrile agglutinins; febrile screen)	Can include any, or all, of the following tests: Salmonella-typhoid (paratyphoid, and enteric); rickettsial disease (those included depend to a great extent on which ones are endemic in an area; see Proteus OX19) (see Widal test for typhoid); brucellosis; tularemia; see specific tests for further information		
Heterophile screen (monospot; test for infectious mononucleosis; heterophile glutination)	Normal: negative (no agglutination)	Diagnosis of infectious mononucleosis	Heterophile refers to having an affinity to more than one antibody; there are close similarities between a normally appearing antibody in all human serum (Forsmann) and the specific antibody found 2–3 weeks from onset of infectious mononucleosis
Proteus OX19 (Rocky Mountain spotted fever test; test for RMSF)	Negative: 1:60 or less Significant: 1:80 or greater	Diagnosis of Rocky Mountain spotted fever (RMSF)	A high percentage of people have a normal low titer because *Proteus* are common infective agents not necessarily causing disease; important that more than one titer be done with at least a fourfold rise between acute and convalescent sera for diagnosis

Name (synonyms)	Reference range reaction results	Purpose	Comments
Streptozyme	Negative: less than 1:100 (correlates with less than 166 Todd units)	Diagnosis of AGN and rheumatic fever	Similar to the ASO but thought to be more sensitive, detecting 95% of streptococcal infections (ASO = 80–85%); also thought to be quite specific—90% chance to detect recent strep. infection; good correlation between the tests
Tularemia	Negative: no agglutination Significant: 1:40–1:80 or higher	Diagnosis of tularemia	Titers of 1:80 are diagnostic of actual infection; elevations may persist for years, but at less than 1:80; history of visits in endemic areas or work/leisure activity causing exposure (game warden/hunting)
Widal	Negative: 1:40 or less Significant: 1:80 or greater	Diagnosis of typhoid H and O; paratyphoid A and B	Two serotypes of *Salmonella* organism, somatic (0) and flagelar (H) cause typhoid and paratyphoid fever; other serotypes of *Salmonella* cause a well-known type of food poisoning (salmonellosis); many variables affect results: titers increase in disease course; agglutination not due to disease found in elderly, drug addicts, previous vaccination, and as an effect of antibiotics early in the disease
Venereal Disease Research Laboratory test (VDRL; RPR)	Negative: no agglutination of antigen (reagin), or less than 2+ Positive: more than 2+ agglutination of antigen	Diagnosis of syphilis	The RPR, a modification of the VDRL, is the most commonly used *screening* test for syphilis (reagin)

B. Complement-fixation tests

Serum complement is a globulin and makes up an important serum enzyme system. There are nine major components of the complement system, identified by letter/number designations, C1 through C9. The numbers assigned are not in the order of their sequence in activating the system and are, therefore, confusing. The total system, total complement, is also referred to as C. Most pathologic conditions tend to decrease total complement.

Complement-fixation tests (Table 6.2) are based on the activity of complement in the serum. During an antigen-antibody reaction, all available complement is bound, or "fixed." If complement is activated indicating that an antigen-antibody reaction did *not* take place, complement will hemolyze the red blood cells. Therefore, the presence of hemolysis in a complement-fixation test is interpreted as a negative response; the absence of hemolysis, as a positive reaction.

C. Precipitin tests

Precipitin tests (Table 6.2) are used primarily in identification of antibodies produced in response to certain fungi and bacterial exotoxins. They are also helpful in typing various bacteria and in identifying unknown protein. When properly done, they are very sensitive and highly specific. The tests are done by producing antisera, usually in rabbits, by immunization with a known protein antigen. The antisera taken from the rabbits contain precipitins (antibodies produced by the reaction of soluble antigens with antibodies). These precipitins, when placed in solution with the protein used for immunization, will form a distinct white cloud—a visible precipitate.

D. Neutralization tests

Neutralization tests are used to detect viruses and rickettsiae. They are the most common method used to confirm and serotype viral or rickettsial microorganisms. Neutralization speaks to the process on which the tests are based. The unknown virus (patient's serum) is mixed with a type-specific antisera (an antisera developed against the suspected infective microorganism). At the same time a control with known virus, antigen to the type-specific antisera, and the antisera, is also mixed. After a short incubation both are inoculated into appropriate tissue cultures. The two are compared for neutralization effect on viral growth. (No examples given.)

TABLE 6.2 *Complement-fixation and precipitin tests*

Name (synonyms)	Reference range reaction results	Purpose	Comments
Complement-fixation tests			
Influenza serology (influenza A and B; flu test)	Negative: hemolysis Positive: no hemolysis	Diagnosis of influenza A or B	Titer increase of fourfold or greater indicative of recent infection; confirmed by viral isolation
Rickettsial serology	[Usually a group of rickettsial diseases are done and reported as a group, including rickettsial pox, Q fever, RMSF (New World spotted fever or tick-borne typhus fever); epidemic louse-borne typhus fever]		
	Negative: hemolysis Positive: no hemolysis		A fourfold difference between acute and convalescent titers probably significant for all the above-listed diseases
Serologic test for syphilis (standard test for syphilis; STS; Wasserman)	Negative: hemolysis Positive: no hemolysis	Diagnosis of syphilis	Rarely used now, but of historical interest as the first practical serologic test;antibody produced is not specific to the syphilis causative organism and thus called a "reagin" rather than antibody; the most used test to confirm syphilis at present is FTA-ABS (fluorescent treponemal antibody absorbed) (see E., p. 282)
Precipitin tests			
Beta streptococci	Typing and grouping Lancefield method		—
Schistosomiasis test	As in text above	Identification of infestation by flukes	Rare in the United States; precipitin tests a useful routine test for the infestation

E. Fluorescent-antibody tests

Synonyms: FA; immunofluorescence tests.

Tests of this type (Table 6.3) are meant to identify suspected, specific organisms and cannot be used to identify unknown organisms. Fluorescent testing is based on tagging either a specific antibody or an anti-immunoglobulin (an anti-antibody) with fluorescein labeling. If the specific microorganism is present in the patient's sample, the fluorescent antibody, or anti-antibody, attaches and the organism will be visible under a fluorescent microscope. Two methods are available for the test, the direct and the indirect. The indirect method is simpler and is used more frequently.

6.2.2 Skin Tests

Skin tests (Table 6.4) are generally used to determine hypersensitivity or immunity. Hypersensitivity refers to an alteration in the strength of reactivity of the body to a foreign or harmful agent. Allergy is a form of hypersensitivity. Immunity is the resistance of the body to the effects of harmful agents.

Many agents can, without causing obvious illness (subclinical disease states), trigger cell-mediated immunity. A fairly simple way to test cell-mediated immune function is by doing skin tests with commonly encountered antigens. The absence of any skin reaction to these antigens indicates probable impaired immune function in the person tested.

In infectious disease, hypersensitivity, or "infectious allergy," is demonstrated by a positive, delayed inflammatory response at the site of an intracutaneous (intradermal) injection of the antigenic agent. The positive or inflammatory response indicates two things: (1) the individual being tested has an intact cell-mediated immune function; and (2) it indicates either a present or a past experience with the specific antigen used—evidenced by the "sensitized" response. A negative response indicates two possible causes: (1) no prior exposure to the infective agent; or (2) active infection with temporary loss of reactivity, a state known as *anergy*. A good example of this hypersensitive response to infectious disease is the Mantoux test done to detect tuberculosis.

Anergy, as defined above, occurs not only in the far advanced stages of many infectious diseases, but also accompanies some chronic diseases (e.g., Hodgkin's disease and sarcoidosis). It accompanies some of the exanthema of childhood (e.g., measles) and is found in individuals on immunosuppressant drugs, such as the corticosteroids and anticancer or antithyroid drugs.

TABLE 6.3 *Fluorescent-antibody tests*

Name (synonyms)	Reference range reaction results	Purpose	Comments
Fluorescent treponemal antibody (FTA; treponemal antibody test; syphilis confirmation test)	Negative: nonreactive Positive: 1+ to 4+ (weak to strong reaction)	Confirmatory test for positive or weakly positive VDRL, STS tests	The Venereal Disease Research Laboratory Test (VDRL), a flocculation test, is still in frequent use but has many cross-reactions; the FTA helps confirm a positive diagnosis, but has many cross-reactions as well
Fluorescent treponemal antibody absorption test (FTA-ABS)	As for FTA above	As for FTA above	This test is a modification of the FTA to eliminate many of the cross-reactions; it causes cross-reacting antibodies to be absorbed and increases test specificity
Immunofluorescent study, urine (antibody coating, urine)	As for FTA above but without indication of strength of positive reaction	Differentiation between cystitis and pyelonephritis	If bacteriuria is due to cystitis, the test will be negative; if due to pyelonephritis, it will be positive; false positives occur with autofluorescence of staphylococci and *pseudomonas*
Legionnaires' serology (indirect fluorescent antibody; Legionnaires' indirect antibody test)	Normal is negative or nonreactive; if positive, a titer is reported	Diagnosis of Legionnaires' disease	Several different tests can be done to identify this disease [culture, direct immunofluorescent (IF) stain, tissue stain-Warthin-Starry]; this test was included because it is simple and can be reported rapidly; diagnosis is by fourfold increase in titer, or in an "outbreak," a single positive, plus clinical signs and symptoms; very high titers have been reported in nonaffected individuals
Direct fluorescent antibody tests: FA (fluorescent antibody) for specific microorganisms (Group A beta hemolytic strep; *Neisseria gonnorrheae; Legionnaires' bacillus; Bordetella pertussis*)	Negative: no fluorescence Positive: fluorescent staining of suspected microorganisms	Demonstration of suspected etiologic agents of disease in patient exudate or secretions	The most simple of fluorescent tests; diagnosis of etiologic agents is more rapid than by traditional culture methods (Harris, 1980)

TABLE 6.4 *Delineation of skin tests*

Test name	Disease	Antigen	Reaction time	Criteria for positive reaction/discussion
		Skin tests to determine susceptibility or resistance to infectious disease		
Dick	Scarlet fever	Erythrogenic toxin	18–24 hr	Induration 3–5 mm, very red erythema, marked by swollen sharply raised edges; indicates insufficient circulating antigen and susceptibility to scarlet fever
Maloney	Diphtheria	Plain toxin	12–24 hr	12 mm or greater erythema; used to detect hypersensitivity prior to immunization; with a positive reaction, toxoid may be given only in very small doses and carefully monitored to prevent anaphylaxis
Schick	Diphtheria	Diphtheria toxin	24–48 hr	Induration 25–50 mm in diameter; erythema not measured; fading leaves brownish pigmented area; positive reaction indicates lack of antitoxin and need for immunization
Schick control	–	Heated toxin	12–24 hr	Used to indicate immediate inflammatory response due to an allergic reaction to the protein; control compared to delayed response to eliminate false positives
		Skin tests used primarily to test immune competence[a]		
Candidin	*Candida albicans*	Candidal cell wall	48–72 hr	10 mm or greater induration plus erythema; most persons with active immunocompetence systems will show a positive reaction; negative response, no reaction = anergy of T-lymphocyte response
SKK	Streptococci infections	Varidase streptococci enzymes	48 hr	Induration of 10 mm or greater; used to assess cellular immune response (immunocompetence); also used to evaluate anergy
Trichophyton	Ringworm	Extract of trichophyton	48–72 hr	Induration of 5 mm or more; used to assess cellular immune response; most persons react positively; positive response increases with age
		Diagnostic skin tests		
Brucellin	Brucellosis	Killed bacteria or protein nucleate	24–48 hr	Over 5 mm induration; not well standardized; serologic test may be more helpful
Coccidioidin	Coccidioidomycosis	Culture filtrate of *Coccidioides immitis*	24–72 hr	Over 5 mm induration
Foshay	Tularemia	Killed bacteria	48 hr	Over 5 mm induration

Herpes simplex	Herpes simplex	Killed virus	18–24 hr	Induration of 15 mm or more; positive reaction indicates a primary infection and nonsusceptibility to systemic spread (i.e., encephalitis); local recurrence possible
Histoplasmin	Histoplasmosis (systemic fungal infection)	Killed fungi	48–72 hr	Induration of 5 mm or more; negative reaction = no response, or erythema less than 5 mm; doubtful = induration less than 5 mm; erythema more than 5 mm
Kviem	Sarcoidosis	Sarcoid tissue extract	4–8 weeks	Papule develops, biopsied, and examined histologically for typical sarcoid pattern; positives less likely in chronic states of the disease
Frei	Lymphogranuloma venereum	Killed chlanydral agent	48–72 hr	8–20 mm induration indicates past or present infection with any of the psittacosis group
Mantoux	Tuberculosis	Purified protein derivative (PPD) or old tuberculin (OT)	24–72 hr	Induration of 10 mm or larger; National Tuberculosis Association Criteria on 0 to 4+ scale: Doubtful (+/−1) = erythema, edema 5 mm or less 1+ (+) = erythema, edema 5–10 mm 2+ (++) = erythema, edema 10–20 mm 3+ (+++) = marked erythema, edema exceeds 20 mm 4+ (++++) = erythema, edema, and central necrosis (Davidsohn and Henry, 1969)
Mumps	Mumps	Inactivated vaccine		Erythema of 15 mm or more, with or without induration, indicates some protection against mumps; in a case of active mumps and no previous exposure, the skin test will not become + for several days; + reactions at onset of mumps-like disease may rule out mumps
Schultz-Charlton	Scarlet fever	Antitoxin or convalescent scarlet fever serum	18–24 hr	Injected into area of bright rash suspected to be scarlet fever; + reaction: a blanched area 2–8 mm surrounding needle puncture in cases of scarlet fever; differentiates rash from that of measles, rubella, drug allergies; response increased with allergy to horse serum
Tine	Tuberculosis	PPD or OT	48–72 hr	2 mm or more palpable induration around one or more of the four puncture sites; useful screening test; doubtful reactions should be rechecked with a Mantoux
Trichinin	Trichinosis	Killed larvae	15 min	Wheal and erythematous reaction; delayed reaction occurring after 24 hr is less specific; test remains + for many years, thus possible false positives; many commercial antigens too insensitive, thus causing false negatives

[a]Often done at the same time as other skin tests.

There are three types of biologic or diagnostic skin tests:

1. Tests to determine possible susceptibility or resistance to an infection (see Schick or Dick tests in Table 6.4).
2. Tests for "infectious allergy," described above.
3. Skin tests to determine sensitivity to environmental materials which induce exaggerated reaction in the sensitized host (e.g, hay fever, asthma, food allergies).

The first two categories are discussed in this section (see Table 6.4). The reader is referred to a general medical, surgical nursing test for information about the last category as it is beyond the scope of this section.

In the first two categories no attempt has been made to include all possible skin tests. Instead, a fair sample of the more commonly used tests are presented which should provide an understanding of the process.

IMPLICATIONS FOR NURSING

1. *Skin tests by injection* are done using an intradermal (intracutaneous) approach. Because the reliability of the test response depends in great measure on the process of the injection being faultless, and because these injections are often the nurse's responsibility, the procedure is reviewed briefly here.
   a. Selection of site. The area selected should be free of any edema, chronic skin disease (e.g., eczema), infectious process, scarring, or potential for irritation from clothing or from use of the part. The inner aspect of the forearm is frequently used.
   b. Explanation of the process. Since there are almost always side effects of some kind due to skin tests, the patient and family need to be fully informed as to what to expect; thus the nurse needs to be fully informed prior to beginning the procedure. Patient and family also need reassurance that the benefit of the skin test outweighs the risks involved. The nurse can only undertake such assurance if indeed the benefit *does* outweigh the risk. Therefore, the nurse needs not only to know the expected benefit for *this* individual, but also have at hand, or undertake, a thorough history and physical of the individual so that specific risks peculiar to this one individual

are also known (e.g., history of hypersensitivity of any kind, presence or rash of unknown etiology).

c. Selection of materials:
   (1) Needle: short bevel, 3/8 to 5/8 in. in length, 25 to 27 gauge.
   (2) Syringe: tuberculin or other calibrated in 0.01 mL units, 1 mL capacity.
   (3) Antigen: checked with that ordered; usually kept refrigerated (some exceptions, such as for the Tine test).

d. Check antigen. Measurement of the antigen in the syringe *must* be precise. Overdosage could cause anaphylactic shock. Underdosage would fail to stimulate antibody response, the purpose of the skin test.
   (1) Be sure that the dilution of the antigen is correct. Antigens for skin testing can be provided in many strengths. Most commonly used dilution is 1:100, but not all tests are done with that dilution. Check the physician's order. Usually, the *smallest* concentrations of any given series of dilutions is given first. Use of more concentrated antigens can result in serious side effects in hyperimmune individuals.
   (2) Do not use an air lock in the syringe and needle after drawing up the antigen. (An air lock is 0.2 to 0.3 mL of air in syringe to prevent trailing of an irritating substance intradermally when giving a subcutaneous or intramuscular injection.) The skin test injection is intradermal and is supposed to irritate the tissues.

e. Check the four "R's" of medication administration. Right patient, right medication, right dosage, and right time. Use the recommended skin preparation of the facility. It is most important that *any* substance used to disinfect the skin be allowed to dry thoroughly before injection. Materials on the skin will trail the needle if wet and can cause a false skin reaction.

f. Injection. With the skin held tautly, the needle is inserted bevel up, just under the top layer of skin at about a 10 to 15 degree angle, almost flat with the skin. The needle should be inserted only enough to cover the bevel, the outline of which should be almost visible under the skin. If injected too deeply, a false-negative reaction may occur.

   Inject antigen slowly, making a small bleb, or wheal, under the skin. In some places, and some instances, the wheal is outlined with indelible ink when the needle has been withdrawn to facilitate location of the injection site at the time of reading the reaction.

g. Observe the patient carefully for 20 to 30 min after the injection for any systemic response to the antigen (hypersensitivity). Epinephrine in a *1:1000* solution for parenteral administration should be on hand. At times, standing orders suggest that it be injected directly into the skin at the needle mark of the test site upon appearance of untoward effects.

   Systemic signs and symptoms to observe for include decreased blood pressure; a general feeling of apprehension or doom; weakness; pruritis; signs of perspiration, angioedema, urticaria, dyspnea/shortness of breath (SOB), wheezing, or changes in pulse (fast, irregular, weak, absent); and signs of changes in level of consciousness.

2. *Reading skin test reactions* is frequently a nursing responsibility, or it may be the responsibility of the nurse to instruct the patient and family in the process.
   a. To quantify skin reactions accurately, a metric ruler should be used to measure the diameter of the indurated or erythematous area. Erythema is not usually included in the positive response, but will be in certain select tests such as mumps (see Table 6.4, "diagnostic skin tests").
   b. Reading of reactions should be done in optimum light, preferably daylight.
   c. A rough grading system that does measure erythema, can be made of the +/– approach (Brunner and Suddarth, 1978).

—	No reaction
+	Erythema smaller than a nickel in diameter
++	Erythema larger than a nickel (21 mm)
+++	Erythema and wheal (induration) without pseudopod formation (foot-like protrusions out from the wheal)
++++	Erythema and wheal with pseudopod formation

General Implications for Nursing in Infectious Disease

7

7.1 PREVENTION

One of the major nursing roles in communicable diseases is that of prevention.

7.1.1 Approaches to Prevention

1. *Identification of populations at risk for infectious disease:*
   a. Infants and young adults, particularly for viral and upper respiratory infections, especially in infants of low birthweight, due to ineffective or immature body defense against infection and lack of acquired immunity.
   b. Patients with chronic disease or malignancies, due to decreased resistance.
   c. Persons on immunosuppressive drugs (e.g., organ-transplant patients).
   d. Postoperatively in debilitated and obese patients, due to impaired blood supply to affected tissues, particularly those persons with diabetes mellitus.

2. *Identification of populations at risk for complications* of infectious disease:
   a. The elderly, particularly for progressive viral pneumonia or respiratory failure after an URI.
   b. Persons with chronic obstructive pulmonary disease (COPD) and/or asthma, particularly for lower respiratory infections or respiratory failure.
   c. Persons with diabetes mellitus.
   d. Pregnant women, particularly for lower respiratory tract infection (e.g., influenza, viral pneumonia, and urinary tract infections) due to inadequate expansion with mechanical restriction.
   e. Persons with heart disease due to impaired blood supply, which decreases the available WBCs to fight infection, reduces the body's ability to remove waste and debris from infection, and reduces the ability of the heart to cope with increased metabolic rate, further decreasing perfusion.
   f. Postoperative patients particularly prone to respiratory infection, due to decreased ventilation secondary to pain/immobility and the irritant effect of inhalant anesthesia; also wound infections with potential for septicemia.
3. *Maintaining a high index of suspicion* for manifestations of infectious disease, especially in high-risk populations.

7.1.2 Identification of Infectious Disease

Initial identification is often done by a family member or the patient. The nurse is, however, very frequently the first member of the health team contacted for validation of their conclusions. To screen out innocuous complaints, such as diaper rash, the nurse needs to have acquired a sound knowledge base about the major characteristics of commonly occurring infectious disease in the locality in order to make pertinent assessments. The base should include the order and progression of signs and symptoms in commonly occurring infectious disease (e.g., the type, initial location, and progression of skin rashes); knowledge of which diseases are endemic in the geographical area; and knowledge of the method of transmission of commonly occurring or endemic diseases.

Given this knowledge base, the nurse must then be able to transfer it into clinical action by:

1. *Pertinent questioning* about recent changes in environment—travel in areas where certain diseases are endemic, contact with many household pets, rats in a poor environment, raw animal products,

such as wool, hides, blood—or initiation of drug therapy with an immunosuppressant effect. A nursing history can only be as thorough as the knowledge base of the history taker.

2. *Visual inspection and careful history taking* about progress and changes in signs and symptoms.

7.1.3 Teaching in Prevention of Spread of Infection

The nurse can assist the person with an infectious disease or process in two general ways: direct care and teaching. Teaching should include the patient and any other populations contacted during care.

1. *See* Section 4.13 for nursing implications related to spread of urinary tract infections.
2. *Another common infectious disease* is influenza—a blanket term for a number of different infections. Content to be included in teaching about the prevention of influenza includes:
   a. Use of influenza vaccine. Specific recommendation as to which types and what populations are at risk are made yearly by the Center for Disease Control (CDC) in Atlanta, Georgia. Populations usually included in that report are critical health care workers; police; firefighters; people with COPD, heart disease, diabetes mellitus, or Addison's disease; persons on immunosuppressive drugs or therapy (this group is rarely immunized due to the risk of overwhelming infection from the vaccine); and those over 65. The elderly are usually given full vaccination yearly.
   b. Purpose and effect of amatadine (Symmetrel). The drug is used to decrease the severity of influenzal infections. Since the use of the drug is somewhat controversial, the nurse should understand why it may or may not be used. The drug does decrease the severity of influenza and may shorten its course, but it has disagreeable side effects. When the risk of infection seems negligible, many physicians and patients are unwilling to chance the side effect. Other physicians feel that the side effects are actually infrequent and mild. Mild impairment of intellectual acuteness and decreased motor function have been found to be the most frequent side effects and to impair the elderly particularly. Other side effects include mental depression, nervousness, dizziness, insomnia, and rash.

      The National Institute of Health (NIH) recently issued guidelines that urge use of the drugs with the following risk groups:

      (1) All ages with underlying serious illness.

(2) Individuals in whom shortening of a symptomatic illness by 24 hr is judged important.

(3) Unvaccinated adults performing activities essential to community function (see use of influenza vaccine above).

(4) Unvaccinated individuals in semiclosed environments, especially the elderly. [This last recommendation was modified by the suggestion that the benefit/risk considerations were less clear for this age group (Marks, 1980).]

c. Use of vitamin C to build up resistance to infection or decrease the severity of the disease. This is another hotly debated prophylactic agent. Recent studies have not shown it to be effective in prevention of upper respiratory illness, or influenza. Its use among lay people and some health care workers is rather widespread, however, and evidence of actual damage is not available.

3. *Vaccines* are also available for numerous diseases and should be studied as to use, type of immunity provided (active, passive), and special precautions. Some diseases for which vaccine can be provided include cholera, plague, rabies, Rocky Mountain spotted fever (RMSF), smallpox, typhoid fever, typhus, yellow fever, tuberculosis, and strains of *Streptococcus pneumoniae.*

4. *Immunization program* for normal infants and children:

a. A dramatic decline in the incidence of the "common" childhood infectious diseases has occurred over the last two or three decades due to routine immunization programs. A less desirable outcome has been the decreased importance attached to the need for immunization by some because of lack of experience of widespread infectious disease outbreaks or severe epidemics. The responsibility of the nurse to stress the "whys" of immunization for all infants and children is increased proportionately. A good resource to prepare for such teaching is a pamphlet available from the CDC (Atlanta, Georgia 30333) called "Vaccines and Immunizations."

b. A recommended immunization schedule for infants and young children generally follows the pattern given below (Whaley and Wong, 1979):

2 months	Diphtheria, tetanus toxoid, and pertussis vaccine (DPT), trivalent oral polia virus vaccine (TOPV)
4 months	DPT and TOPV
6 months	DPT, optional TOPV

1 year	Tuberculin test (to precede or coincide with measles vaccine)
15 months	Measles, rubella, mumps vaccine
18 months	DPT, TOPV
4–6 years	DPT, TOPV
14–16 years	Tetanus and diphtheria toxoid (Td), repeated every 10 years

7.2 NURSING MANAGEMENT

7.2.1 Necessary Knowledge Base

Once a specific infectious process is definitely suspected, or diagnosed, the nurse can only provide safe and effective care when in possession of the following knowledge about the suspected or actual microorganism:

1. *The class of infectious agent* (e.g., bacteria, virus). Check lab reports for results of culture and evaluation of smears/stains.
2. *The body parts or secretions* infected with or harboring the infectious microorganisms and thus contagious (e.g., blood, feces, sputum, wound exudate). Assess the patient and review the microbiology of the suspect organism.
3. *The method of transmission* of the microorganism from host to host. Review the microbiology of the suspect organism.
4. *The principal portal of entry* for the microorganism. Review the microbiology.
5. *Unhealthy environments* for the organism; what affects its survival in the host and in the environment. Review the microbiology.
6. *What, if any, immunity* occurs after the infection, and the duration of that immunity (permanent, temporary?). Review the microbiology.
7. *What if any induced immunity* is available (vaccine? toxoid? antisera?) and the duration of that immunity. Review the microbiology. Consult with the physician, infection control officer, or microbiologist.

7.2.2 Application of Knowledge Base

Given the information in Section 7.2.1, nursing care to support the patient's defense against the organism, to prevent spread of the infection to others, and to prevent reinfection or secondary infection of the patient can be planned.

1. *The type of isolation,* if any is predicated primarily on knowledge of items 1 to 5 in Section 7.2.1. Care of items in contact with the patient is also based on that knowledge.
2. *The selection of health care workers* to implement nursing care should be determined primarily from knowledge of items 6 and 7.
3. *Medical treatment* has its premise in knowledge of items 1, 2, 4, and 5. The nurse follows the response of the patient to the treatment prescribed by checking for changes in clinical signs and symptoms of the infection, the appearance of negative lab reports on cultures and slides, and decreasing titers in serologic tests. Collection of specimens for laboratory examination is based on knowledge of items 1, 2, and 5.
4. *Methods of disinfection* require knowledge of items 1 to 3 and 5.

7.2.3 Maintenance of Infection Control Procedures

The scope of this book does not allow coverage of the principles and methods of isolation, or of specific nursing care of particular infectious diseases. The reader is referred to any of a number of medical-surgical or basic nursing texts for that material. It is important, however, to make the point that the effectiveness of infection control is primarily in the hands of the nurse caring for the patient. The nurse, in the role of teacher, has the obligation to help the patient and family understand and cope with the illness, as described previously. However, there exists also the obligation to teach the importance of the control procedures verbally, and, more important, by consistent practice of them. Further, it is the obligation of the nurse to see that *all* other members of the health team practice them as well. This is a difficult task at times. If the measures are judged meaningless by any one health care worker, the patient and/or family will probably follow that lead. It is imperative then that the nurse not only enforce control procedures, but also, by careful study and updating of information, assure that the infection control methods used are indeed based on accurate understanding of the infectious process present *and* are effective in its control if properly followed.

7.2.4 General Approaches to Nursing Management of Acute Infectious Disease Related to Common Patient Problems

1. *Patient problem: actual or potential dehydration* due to fever and/or decreased intake.
   a. Encourage fluids; frequent small amounts up to 2500 to 3000 mL/day minimum unless contraindicated.
   b. In respiratory infections, sipping hot fluids has been found to be of greater value than drinking cold fluids. Sipping hot chicken soup was found to be the most beneficial. It provides fluid, and at the same time increases nasal mucus velocity, which supports the respiratory tract's first line of defense by removing pathogens. Cold fluids have been found to suppress nasal mucus activity.*
2. *Patient problem: fever* due to infectious agent's effect on the body's temperature control center and due to the inflammatory response.
   a. Of particular concern in the elderly or debilitated patient because of the accompanying tachycardia, vasodilatation, and loss of intravascular volume with perspiration.
   b. Aspirin is best given on an around-the-clock basis when possible, every 4 to 6 hr, and started with the first systemic symptom of infection, not necessarily fever. This precaution is especially important in respiratory infections. Its use should be continued even after the temperature returns to normal. Prolonged use will help to eliminate the drenching sweats that occur with rapid fever drops, and will lessen the malaise, arthralgia, myalgias, or sore throat throughout. The use of aspirin is a comfort measure only, but it should be remembered that the presence of body comfort assists in supporting the body defenses. Obviously, aspirin is not to be used when contraindicated by other conditions (e.g., ulcer, bleeding disorders).
   c. Room temperature should depend on the needs of the patient for comfort when possible. Any rapid changes of temperature should be avoided since both shivering and sweating require energy that should be saved.

---

*S. A. Januszkiewics and M. A. Sackner, "Effects of Drinking Hot Water, Cold Water, and Chicken Soup on Nasal Mucus Velocity and Nasal Air-Flow Resistance," *Chest* 74 (1978), 408-410, cited by Scoggin and Sahn (1980, p. 29).

3. *Patient problem: potential reinfection,* or secondary infection, and spread of infection to others. This has been discussed on preceding pages.

4. *Evaluation of nursing plan of care:*
   a. Of necessity, the physician's therapeutic plan of care is also evaluated. As a general rule, expect some improvement in 24 hr after antimicrobials are started. Subjective: verbalized sense of feeling better. Objective: temperature decrease; WBC may begin to return to normal—may have been increased totally (leukocytosis), have a relative increase (e.g., lymphocytosis), or may have been depressed (e.g., neutropenia). A shift to the left may occur in any case (see Section 2.2.3); ESR will decrease.
   b. Check tests of function of specifically involved areas, for example:
      (1) In urinary tract infections. Subjective: verbalized decrease in pain on urination. Objective: urine less cloudy; red cell casts in urine?
      (2) In hepatitis. Check liver enzyme function—SGPT, GTT, SGOT; check platelet dysfunction (i.e., bleeding time), bilirubin—blood direct and indirect, and urine.

5. *In long-term infections* check RBC count and MCV for evidence of anemia.

6. *One of the simplest and most effective,* yet most neglected methods of infection control is the practice of *thorough* hand washing by the nurse *before* and after *any* patient contact.

Laboratory Tests of Specific Body Systems

PART 3

When seemingly unrelated test results from screening procedures are considered together with clinical findings, the body system involved in a disorder may be indicated. Additional tests specific to that system are then in order to lead to a more definitive diagnosis related to that system, or to rule the system out and provide clues to others that may be dysfunctional. The purpose of this section is to indicate the clues from screening tests that can lead to specific system testing, define and describe some of the more frequently used tests of that system, and list procedures necessary to prepare the patient for the test to prevent cross-reactions or false increases or decreases in normal values obtained.

The Endocrine System

chapter **8**

The endocrine and neural systems are the two major integrative, or regulatory systems of the body. They work in close relationship with each other. It is not surprising, then, that endocrine disorders can present themselves as neuropsychiatric disturbances. Because the endocrine system, via its hormones, adjusts and correlates the activities of the various body systems in adaptation to the demands of external and internal environment, it is again not surprising that endocrine disorders are excellent imitators of many other medical disorders.

Because of this ability to look like something other than an endocrine dysfunction, the first, the most critical, and the most difficult clinical problem is to recognize that an endocrine disorder may be present. Endocrine disease often begins insidiously and progresses slowly. The only clue may be a single symptom or physical finding, and that perhaps amid a riot of other symptoms and signs.

Endocrine dysfunction occurs when the levels, or balance of the levels, of hormones produced by the endocrine glands is upset. Endocrine glands may be hyperactive or hypoactive due to a primary glandular problem, or secondary to other factors; for example, the absence of the enzyme renin, elaborated by the kidney, affects the adrenal synthesis of aldosterone. Disorders can occur because the target organ is unable to respond. Disorders can be congenital, infectious, neoplastic, autoimmune, or idiopathic.

Probably the best chance of noting the presence of an endocrine disorder lies in the ability of the health care team to maintain a high index of suspicion for endocrine dysfunction as a possible cause in confusing clinical signs and symptoms.

8.1 THE ADRENAL GLAND

8.1.1 Medullary Hormones

A. Laboratory and clinical indications of adrenal medullary dysfunction

1. Serum glucose: hyperglycemia, due to increased epinephrine levels inhibiting insulin release.
2. Urine glucose: glycosuria, due to hyperglycemia.
3. Increased free fatty acids, due to increased epinephrine release and increased fat metabolism in the absence of insulin.
4. To be compared with the presence of some or all of the following clinical features: Clinical findings are more definitive than the laboratory findings, so must be assessed. Increased epinephrine or norepinephrine, causing intermittent hypertension (may be persistent); signs of increased metabolism such as diaphoresis, hyperactivity, nervousness, heat intolerance, nervous exhaustion; unexplained cardiac arrhythmias; headache; paroxysmal dyspnea; weight loss. Loss of usual sympathetic postural responses, causing orthostatic hypotension. Failure of melanin formation in the skin, causing vitiligo (sharply demarcated, milky white patches of skin with hyperpigmented borders).

B. Tests of medullary function

Vanillylmandelic acid, urine

Synonyms: VMA; 3-methoxy-4-hydroxymandelic acid

Normal Ranges

Adult	0.7–6.8 mg/24 hr
Pediatric	
Newborn	0 –1 mg/24 hr
Neonate	0 –1 mg/24 hr
Infant	0 –2 mg/24 hr
Child	1 –5 mg/24 hr
Adolescent	1 –5 mg/24 hr

Explanation of the Test. The adrenal medulla produces catecholamines (compounds with a sympathomimetic action) [i.e., dopamine (a precursor of the following), epinephrine, and norephinephrine]. 1 to 5% of norepinephrine and epinephrine is excreted unchanged into the urine. The rest undergoes degradation and forms derivatives, metanephrines, and vanillylmandelic acid (VMA). VMA is the principal urinary metabolite. The precursor, dopamine, is degradated to homovanillic acid (see the next test).

The VMA test is a measurement of the amount of VMA found in the urine over a 24-hr period. Assays of plasma catecholamines are available in many hospital laboratories (see test 4 below). However, the 24-hr urine assay is felt to be more reliable since the secretion of VMA is sporadic and diurnal. The VMA test is also technically simpler than the plasma catecholamine assay.

VMA INCREASED IN:

1. *Tumors of the adrenal medulla,* or extrarenal ganglionic tissue, causing increased secretion of epinephrine and norepinephrine, such as (a) pheochromocytoma, and (b) neural crest tumors (e.g., ganglioneuromas). VMA may be normal in these tumors, but the diagnosis should not be ruled out without doing the test.
2. *Other conditions that increase catecholamine production* (e.g., thyrotoxicosis, widespread burns, Cushing's disease and syndrome, myocardial infarct, hemolytic anemia).
3. *Some muscular disorders* due to inability to utilize catecholamines, such as some cases of muscular dystrophy and myasthenia gravis.
4. *Physiologic conditions* in some individuals. Up to a sevenfold increase has been noted when the test was done immediately after *vigorous* exercise.
5. *Many persons with advanced or malignant hypertension.*
6. *False increases,* due to use of several drugs that produce fluorescent urinary products [e.g., tetracylines, epinephrine and epinephrine-like drugs, large doses of vitamin B complex, MAO inhibitors, nalidixic acid (NegGram), aspirin, methyldopa (Aldomet), levodopa (L-Dopa)]; and in uremia when the test method is based on fluorescence.

VMA DECREASED IN:

1. *Some cases of familial dysautomomia*—Riley-Day syndrome.
2. *False reaction* in some patients taking clofibrate (Atromid-S).

Patient Preparation. No dietary restrictions are necessary if the test is based on the oxidation of VMA to vanillin. Certain chemicals contained in some foods distort tests based on other methods; therefore, dietary restriction of chocolate, coffee, tea, bananas, citrus fruits, nuts, and any foods containing vanilla is maintained for 3 days prior *to the urine collection.*

Specimen Collection

1. *24-hr urine specimens* are collected, usually from 8 a.m. to 8 a.m. The patient should void at 8 a.m. at the beginning of the test, and this urine is discarded. All other urine is collected until 8 a.m. the following day, to include a final 8 a.m. voiding.
2. *The specimen container* should be refrigerated and kept at a pH of 3. In one method 30 ml of 6*N* HC1 is added to the collection bottle before use for this purpose.

Related Tests of Importance or Interest. Plasma catecholamines, urine and serum glucose, and GTT may show a diabetic curve, and plasma renin may be increased.

Homovanillic acid, urine

Synonym: HVA	
Normal Range:	0–15 mg/24 hr

Explanation of the Test. (See also the explanation of test 1 above.) The measurement of HVA is a measurement of the products of dopamine degradation. Dopamine is present in sympathetic nervous tissue as a precursor of norepinephrine. Neuroblastomas and ganglioneuromas usually arise from the adrenal medulla and cause a significant increase in all the urinary catecholamines, including HVA. The increase in HVA helps to distinguish the neural crest tumors from pheochromocytoma.

HVA INCREASED IN:

Neural crest tumors (neuroblastoma, ganglioneuroma). Such tumors should not be ruled out without at least one estimation of HVA. In certain cases of neurological tumors the urinary abnormality consists almost entirely of excessive dopamine secretion and its metabolite, HVA.

HVA DECREASED IN:

None.

Patient Preparation

1. *Drugs known to interfere* with the test (diuretics, nerve blockers, tranquilizers, aspirin, levodopa, reserpine, quinine, valium, and Antabuse) are held for at least 3 days before the test—optimum time is 7 days.
2. *Although there is no actual dietary restriction,* restraint is urged in the use of vitamin B-rich foods, coffee, alcohol, or foods high in salt or vanilla.

Related Tests of Importance or Interest. VMA; urinary and plasma total catecholamines and metanephrines.

Catecholamines, total, urine

Synonyms: adrenalin, noradrenaline, total, urine

Normal Ranges

24-hr urine	0–103 μg/24 hr
Random urine	0– 18 μg/24 hr

Explanation of the Test. This test measures the 1 to 5% of epinephrine and norepinephrine that is excreted unchanged in the urine. Increases in the degraded metabolites (VMA, HVA) correlate well with measurement of the catecholamines themselves. This urine test can be used to confirm the results of the VMA or the HVA, but is not usually available in all laboratories.

Random urine total catecholamine measurements provide little useful information because of the diurnal variation in excretion.

CATECHOLAMINE INCREASED IN:

1. *See also* "VMA Increased in," test 1 above.
2. *Periods of sleep,* to a marked degree.
3. *Periods following vigorous exercise,* as much as sevenfold.

CATECHOLAMINE DECREASED IN:

1. *See also* "VMA Decreased in," test 1 above, item 1.
2. *Malnutrition,* due to decreased catecholamine production.

3. *Transection of the cervical spinal cord,* probably due to the loss of excitatory and inhibitory inputs, which are believed to mediate the stress response and hormone production at the hypothalmic level (Henry, 1979).

Patient Preparation

1. *No dietary restriction.*
2. *Vigorous exercise* prior to, or during urine collection for the 24-hr specimen, is to be discouraged.

Related Tests. See VMA, test 1 above.

Catecholamine fractionation, plasma

Synonyms: epinephrine, norepinephrine fractionation, plasma; adrenalin, noradrenaline fractionation, plasma

*Normal Ranges**

	Norepinephrine (ng/L)	Epinephrine (ng/L)
Supine normotensive	103–193	0–150
Standing normotensive	293–489	0–150
Supine hypertensive	145–339	0–150
Standing hypertensive	396–606	0–150

*Total catecholamine levels greater than 1000 ng/mL are suggestive of pheochromocytoma. Values above 2000 ng/mL are presumptive of it. Values in the range 700 to 1000 ng/mL are to be evaluated further. Patients with the tumor, but normotensive at the time of sample taking, can fall in this range.

Explanation of the Test. This test measures the plasma catecholamine levels individually. It is a difficult test and is not done in most laboratories. The only information available from it that cannot be gained using the VMA or total urine catecholamines is that of the individual catecholamine levels. This information can be helpful in determining whether a pheochromocytoma is renal or extrarenal in origin. Adrenal tumors secrete both norepinephrine and epinephrine, so both values would be increased. Extrarenal tumors are often secretors of norepinephrine alone.

PLASMA CATECHOLAMINE INCREASED IN:

See VMA, test 1 above.

PLASMA CATECHOLAMINE DECREASED IN:

See tests 1 and 3 above.

Patient Preparation

1. *All antihypertensive agents,* diuretics, and sympathomimetic drugs must be discontinued 5 days before the test.
2. *Diet for 3 days* before the test must contain a normal daily intake of sodium. Low- or high-sodium diets affect catecholamine secretion.
3. *Physiologic variables* such as activity, stress, and posture affect catecholamine secretion. The patient must therefore be recumbent in a quiet environment with as many stressors removed as can be identified. He or she should be in this stressless state for 30 min prior to the test.
4. *The test should not be done* for at least 30 days after the use of radiopaque iodine, as that substance interferes with enzyme activity necessary to produce catecholamines.
5. *Smoking* should be discontinued for a minimum of 15 min prior to the test, as nicotine promotes catecholamine release.

Related Tests. See VMA, test 1 above.

8.1.2 Adrenocortical Hormones

A. Laboratory and clinical indications of adrenocortical hormone dysfunction

Since the adrenal cortex secretes more than 50 hormones or their precursors, some identical to substances secreted elsewhere in the body (e.g., gonads also secrete androgens), this section must be limited. The hormones of most importance in maintaining life and health are cortisol and aldosterone. They will be covered in this discussion, with some discussion of androgens. Other sex steroid hormones are discussed in Section 8.6.

1. *Serum glucose:* fasting increased; GTT diabetic in pattern.
2. *Electrolytes:*
   a. Plasma sodium increased; serum calcium increased.
   b. Plasma potassium decreased (a few persons may actually demonstrate hypokalemic alkalosis, in which case blood gases would also be altered; from screening tests only CO_2 –

venous—is available, which would be increased as it represents body base); urine potassium and calcium, increased; urine sodium decreased.

3. *WBC.* Leukocytosis with a relative lymphopenia and decreased eosinophils.

B. Tests of adrenocortical function

17-Hydroxycorticosteroids, urine

Synonyms: Porter-Silber test; 17-OHCS; 17-hydroxysteroids

Normal Ranges

Female	2– 8 mg/24 hr
Male	3–12 mg/24 hr

Explanation of the Test. 17-OHCS are the metabolites, or breakdown products, of hydrocortisone, cortisone, and some small amounts of aldosterone. Thus the urinary levels of these products can be used to estimate the level of cortisone and hydrocortisone production in the body. 17-OHCS can be measured in plasma as well, a more difficult procedure. The urine test is a 24-hr test because of the diurnal secretion of glucocorticoids.

Terms Used Synonymously in Glucocorticoid Terminology

1. Glucocorticoids = C_{21} steroids; corticosteroids.
2. Cortisol = compound F; hydrocortisone (the most potent glucocorticoid).
3. Cortisone = compound E (an active glucocorticoid, formed from adrenal cortisol in the liver).
4. Corticosterone = compound B.
5. 11-Deoxycortisone = compound S.

17-OHCS INCREASED IN:

Any condition that increases cortisone and hydrocortisone production, such as:

1. *Basophilic pituitary adenoma,* due to increased ACTH secretion.
2. *Cushing's syndrome,* due to adrenocortical hyperplasia.

3. *Polycystic ovaries* (Stein-Leventhal syndrome), due to adrenal hyperplasia or ovarian secretion.
4. *Late in pregnancy,* due to placental secretion of glucocorticoids.
5. *Adrenal cancer.*
6. *Individuals receiving therapeutic estrogen.*
7. *Extreme stress.* Moderate elevations can occur even with less than extreme stress.
8. *Certain nonrenal tumors* (e.g., lung "oat-cell" carcinoma), due to secretion of ACTH-like substance, known as "ectopic ACTH syndrome."

17-OHCS DECREASED IN:

Any conditions that decrease cortisone and hydrocortisone production, such as:

1. *Addison's disease,* due to adrenal atrophy.
2. *Hypopituitarism,* due to lack of ACTH to stimulate production.
3. *Rarely in eclampsia and pancreatitis.*

Patient Preparation

1. *As a general rule, all medications* are discontinued if possible several days before the test, as there are many that interfere with the accuracy of the test. In particular these include iodides, paraldehyde, chlorohydrate, Furadantin, coffee, colchicine, sulfa drugs, chlorophenothiazines, spirolactones, quinine, and Darvon.
2. *Patient instruction* in 24-hr urine collection and refrigeration of the urine during collection are necessary.

17-Ketogenic steroids, urine

Synonyms: 17 KGS; total 17-OH corticosteroids

Normal Ranges

	Female	Male
Under 1 year	0– 1 mg/24 hr	0– 1 mg/24 hr
Up to 10 years	0– 5 mg/24 hr	0– 5 mg/24 hr
Adults	3–15 mg/24 hr	5–23 mg/24 hr
Senior adult	3–12 mg/24 hr	3–12 mg/24 hr

Explanation of the Test. This test is very similar to the 17-OHCS and is the newer of the two. It measures the 17-OHCS, which can be chemically changed or converted to 17-ketosteroids (KS). It is used as an assessment of adrenocortical secretion even though the products measured are not metabolites of cortisone and hydrocortisone. This test is sensitive to the 17-hydroxycorticoids such as prenantriol, not picked up by the 17-OHCS test and frequently seen in andrenogenital syndromes. In such cases steroid synthesis is shifted toward androgen, rather than cortisone, production.

17-KGS INCREASED IN:

1. *Any conditions that increase* cortisone and hydrocortisone levels (see 17-OHCS test 1 above.)
2. *Andrenogenital syndrome.*

17 KGS DECREASED IN:

No known conditions in which decrease has clinical significance.

Patient Preparation. Although there are several compounds, including medications, that interfere with the test, no special preparation is taken prior to testing other than the necessary instruction in 24-hr urine collection.

17-Ketosteroids, urine

Synonym: 17-KS

*Normal Ranges**

Adult	
Males	9–22 mg/day
Females	6–15 mg/day
Senior adult	
Values progressively decline after 60	
Pediatric	
Under 1 year	0– 1 mg/day
1–4 years	0– 2 mg/day
5–8 years	0– 3 mg/day
9–12 years	3–10 mg/day
13-16 years	5–12 mg/day

*There are marked daily variations in 17-KS secretion.

Explanation of the Test. This is a 24-hr urine test. It measures metabolites of testosterone (approximately 25% of the total 17-KS) and metabolites of androgens other than testosterone. This second group includes nearly 50 different compounds, the measurement of which is quite useful in androgenic and adrenal function evaluation. The adrenal cortex in the male produces some 70% of the 17-KS; the rest are produced in the testes. In the female the adrenal cortex produces almost all of the 17-KS. Testosterone itself is not a 17-KS. The major compound of the 17-KS group is a substance called dehydroepiandrosterone, or DHA, formed in the adrenal gland and having a slight androgenic effect, which accounts for virilization syndromes in females with some adrenal tumors.

17-KS INCREASED IN:

1. *Adrenogenital syndromes,* due to adrenocortical hyperplasia. In babies the condition is usually congenital. In older children and adults the syndrome is usually due to an adrenal tumor.
2. *Interstitial cell testicular tumors.*
3. *Cushing's disease* at times with slight to moderate increase in androgen secretion, due to adrenal hyperplasia.
4. *Adrenal carcinoma,* due to increased androgen metabolites, DHA.
5. *Severe stress.*
6. *Basophilic adenoma of the pituitary,* due to increased ACTH stimulation of the adrenals.
7. *Some patients with Stein-Leventhal syndrome* (polycystic ovaries), due to adrenal androgenic hypersecretion.

17-KS DECREASED IN:

1. *Conditions causing adrenal insufficiency* due to decreased secretion of androgens and glucocorticoids, such as:
   a. Addison's disease.
   b. Panhypopituitarism.
2. *Pituitary hypogonadism in males,* due to reduced testosterone secretion.
3. *Castrated males,* due to reduced testosterone secretion.
4. *Nephrosis* secondary to depressed urinary steroid excretion. This is not an actual decrease in hormone production, but a diminished excretion by the kidney.

5. *Klinefelter's syndrome* at times, when testosterone production decreases.

Patient Preparation. As for 17-KGS test.

Cortisol, plasma

Synonyms: serum cortisol; compound F; hydrocortisone; plasma cortisol by RIA (radioimmunoassay)

Normal Ranges

8:00 A.M.	8–24 μg/dL
4:00 P.M.	4–12 μg/dL
8:00 P.M.	2–12 μg/dL

Explanation of the Test. The test determines the concentration of cortisol in the blood. Cortisol is the major steroid hormone produced by the adrenal cortex. It exists in two forms in circulation, bound and unbound: the bound being inactive, the unbound "free," analogous to thyroxine. Cortisol production is affected by a diurnal rhythm so that the peak and the nadir of secretion may both need to be determined. It is also of importance to know if the person being tested has a long-term life pattern that differs from the norm (e.g., sleeping other than during the night hours). The diurnal pattern will alter in time, and testing needs to be done at different hours to reflect that person's individual rhythm.

PLASMA CORTISOL INCREASED IN:

Conditions that increase hydrocortisone, or compound F secretion, such as:

1. *Hyperadrenalsim*—Cushing's disease and Cushing's syndrome.
2. *Physiologic increases* occurring, due to stress and/or obesity.
3. *False increases occurring in kidney disease,* due to the lack of excretion of the hormone.
4. *False increases due to increased estrogen* levels in pregnancy or individuals on estrogen therapy, or on birth control pills, due to increased cortisol-binding protein [i.e., globulin (CBG)] levels.
5. *False increases due to hepatic disease,* due to decreased hepatic metabolism.

PLASMA CORTISOL DECREASED IN:

1. *Individuals taking Dilantin,* or on androgen therapy, due to the increase in cortisol-binding protein.
2. *Addison's disease,* due to adrenal atrophy and inadequate response to ACTH stimulation.
3. *Hypopituitarism,* due to decreased adrenal secretion secondary to decreased release of ACTH.

Patient Preparation

1. *Specimens should be drawn* at times in the diurnal rhythm for which normals have been established. Laboratories vary as to what hours are used.
2. *No special patient preparation* is necessary.

Cortisol, urinary, free

Synonym: free Cortisol, urine
Normal Range: 0–10 μg/24 hr

Explanation of the Test. A 24-hr urine specimen is collected for this test. The test measures "free" cortisol (not bound to CBG) in the urine, which is the only form in which cortisol can be filtered through the kidney glomerulus. The test is therefore a highly sensitive one and free urinary cortisol corresponds proportionately with changes in plasma cortisol. The test is primarily a screening one for increased corticosteroids, and low values are not necessarily indicators of adrenal hypofunction.

FREE CORTISOL INCREASED IN:

1. *States with increased CBG,* as seen in pregnancy and estrogen administration.
2. *Cushing's syndrome,* due to adrenal hyperplasia. It is considered by some as the most important test for hypercortisolism.
3. *Emotional stress* with rises of 50 to 250%, due to increased glucocorticoid production.

FREE CORTISOL DECREASED IN:

Not clinically significant.

Patient Preparation. No special preparation is required.

8.1.3 Mineralcorticoid Hormones

A. Laboratory and clinical indications of mineralcorticoid dysfunction

Aldosterone is the major electrolyte-regulating steroid of the adrenal cortex. Indications of aldosterone dysfunctions then are primarily indications of fluid and electrolyte imbalances. Dysfunctions of other adrenalcorticosteroids are frequently coexistent with aldosterone dysfunction.

DECREASED ALDOSTERONE (ADDISON'S DISEASE) MIGHT BE SUSPECTED WITH:

1. *Laboratory findings:*
   a. Serum electrolytes: Decreased Na^+, increased K^+ (aldosterone function causes Na^+ conservation, K^+ excretion); decreased pH, decreased HCO_3 (or venous CO_2)–metabolic alkalosis. Electrocardiographic (ECG) changes in the adult secondary to K^+ imbalance.
   b. 24-hr urine: Increased Na^+ excretion despite decreased serum Na^+ and which persists when salt is restricted.
   c. Serum chemistry: Slight to moderate increase in BUN secondary to chronic hypovolemia.
   d. Evidence of other endocrine deficiency (see other tests).
2. *Clinical findings:*
   a. Hypotension, especially postural hypotension.
   b. Anorexia, nausea, changes in bowel habits, acute or chronic abdominal or back pain, due to loss of aldosterone regulation of intestinal electrolyte balance, hypogradism, hypothyroidism.

INCREASED ALDOSTERONE MIGHT BE SUSPECTED WITH:

1. *Laboratory findings:*
   a. Serum electrolytes: Na^+ normal or slightly increased, K^+ decreased, Cl^- decreased (in response to initiation of diuretics).

K^+ decrease does not respond toward normal with regular diet and K^+ supplements.

b. Serum chemistry: Glucose tolerance test (GTT) abnormal and serum glucose increased secondary to decreased K^+. May have indications of metabolic alkalosis [e.g., increased pH, increased HCO_3 (or venous CO_2)].

c. Urine: Increased 24-hr K^+ excretion which responds to sodium restriction by decreasing amounts excreted. Sodium loading causes increased K^+ loss in urine, decreased plasma K^+. Decreased urine specific gravity.

2. *Clinical findings.* Hypertension, weakness, polyuria.

B. Plasma aldosterone

Synonym: mineralcorticoid

Normal Ranges

	Low Sodium	Normal Sodium Intake
7:00 A.M. recumbent	12– 36 ng/dL	3– 9 ng/dL
9:00 A.M. upright	17–137 ng/dL	4–30 ng/dL

Explanation of the Test. Aldosterone is one of the steroid hormones secreted by the adrenal cortex. Its level in plasma is controlled by three things: ACTH, potassium, and sodium levels, and the enzyme renin. It is also influenced by a circadian rhythm, much like that of cortisol, with low levels (50% decreased) in the afternoon. It functions primarily on the distal convoluted tubule to promote sodium reabsorption and compensatory excretion of potassium and hydrogen. This test measures aldosterone concentration in plasma in order to validate the presence of hyperaldosteronism or hypoaldosteronism. Because the plasma concentration is normally low, it is more difficult to measure than is urinary aldosterone.

Plasma assays can be interpreted more readily when accompanied by a random urine sodium test. For example, a finding of less than 30 mEq/L of urinary sodium in a random sodium test (normal = 30 to 90 mEq/L) with an increased plasma aldosterone measurement indicates a false aldosterone elevation because decreased urine sodium suggests decreased secretion, and therefore implies a sodium deficit in the body.

A plasma renin sample is also frequently taken at the same time to help differentiate primary from secondary hyperaldosteronism (see Section 8.1.3D).

PLASMA ALDOSTERONE INCREASED IN:

1. *Primary aldosteronism* (Conn's syndrome), due to adrenal cortical tumor (adenoma) or hyperplasia, which may be congenital, causing overproduction of aldosterone. The release is not affected by normal feedback systems. Plasma renin will be decreased, an important diagnostic point.
2. *Secondary aldosteronism* due to excessive production of aldosterone by the adrenal glomerulosa itself, but activated by stimuli outside the adrenal, almost always due to increased plasma renin activity. Plasma renin will be increased, an important diagnostic point. Secondary aldosteronism is found secondary to many pathologies, such as cardiac failure, nephrotic syndrome, cirrhosis, renal ischemia of any etiology, essential hypertension, or Bartter's syndrome (renal juxtaglomerular hyperplasia).
3. *Physiologic compensatory responses* as seen in normal persons with increased K^+ intake, sodium restriction (low-salt diet of less than 2 g/day), prolonged standing, diuretic therapy [furosemide (Lasix)], or stress.
4. *States of increased estrogen,* such as persons on estrogen therapy or during pregnancy.
5. *Individuals taking drugs* that increase plasma renin, and thus aldosterone [e.g., hydralzine (Apresoline), diazoxide (Hyperstat), nitroprusside].

PLASMA ALDOSTERONE DECREASED IN:

1. *Addison's disease* (primary adrenal-cortical insufficiency), due to idiopathic atrophy of the adrenal, probably an autoimmune adrenalitis.
2. *Sheehan's syndrome* (postpartum necrosis of the anterior pituitary), due to loss of ACTH stimulus.
3. *Adrenal destruction,* due to granulomatous processes such as tuberculosis, histoplasmosis, and rarely, sarcoidosis.
4. *Salt-losing congenital adrenocorticol hyperplasia,* due to inherited enzyme deficiencies.
5. *Physiologic conditions in healthy subjects,* such as the recumbent position; high-sodium diets; decreased potassium intake; some

instances of aging; and glucose ingestion, which causes a temporary decrease.

Patient Preparation

1. *Steroids and diuretics* discontinued (d.c.'d) 2 weeks prior to testing to establish baseline values.
2. *Stable sodium diet* at known intake for 2 weeks prior to testing (low intake 10 mEq/day; normal intake 135 mEq/day).
3. *Owing to treatment, hypertensive patients* may be sodium-depleted despite normal plasma sodium levels. They may receive a high-sodium diet or salt supplements for several days before specimen collection (*N.B.:* Such salt loading would invalidate a renin assay; therefore, both tests could not be done at the same time.)
4. *NPO except water* for 8 hr prior to testing.
5. *Recumbent position* for 30 min prior to testing.
6. *For an upright,* usually nonfasting, specimen, the person should be *ambulatory* for 30 min prior to sample collection.

C. Urine aldosterone

Synonyms: mineralcorticoids; urine aldosterone by RIA

Normal Range: 2–26 μg/24 hr

Explanation of the Test. Measurement of a 24-hr urine specimen for the aldosterone derivative concentration has the same advantages as does urine testing of other steroid hormone metabolites when done on a 24-hr sample; elimination of the short-term fluctuations occurring in response to circadian rhythms and other controlling factors, such as ACTH, and changes in sodium or potassium levels. There is also less overlap between normal and abnormal ranges.

Comparisons of urinary aldosterone and plasma or urinary electrolytes are usually done with this test to validate the findings. (Aldosterone deficiency = hyponatremia, increased potassium, and low concentrations of urine and plasma aldosterone which do not rise in response to salt deprivation. Primary hyperaldosteronism = normal or slightly increased sodium, decreased potassium, and urine and plasma aldosterone would be increased.)

URINE ALDESTRONE INCREASED IN:

See "Plasma aldosterone increased in" in Section 8.1.3 B.

URINE ALDOSTERONE DECREASED IN:

See "Plasma aldosterone decreased in" in Section 8.1.3 B.

Patient Preparation. No special preparation is necessary since a full 24 hr of aldosterone excretion into urine is being assayed. The patient should be instructed in the specimen collection procedure.

D. Plasma renin

Synonyms: plasma renin activity; PRA; peripheral renin

Normal Range: 75–275 ng (of angiotensin liberated/mL/hr).

Synonyms: plasma renin concentration; PRC

Normal Range: 0.6×10^{-4} GU/dL* (Berman and Vertes, 1973)

*When expressed in Goldblatt units/dL (GU/dL) can be compared among laboratories.

Description of the Tests. Renin is an enzyme and cannot be measured directly. Measurement of renin is even more complex than other enzymes in that the substrate that is affected by its presence also cannot be measured directly. Renin is also extremely labile and requires careful laboratory handling. Renin is closely associated with aldosterone through the renin-angiotensin system. Both renin and aldosterone production are stimulated by decreased intravascular volumes secondary to sodium depletion. Also, the angiotensin II produced by the release of renin is itself a strong stimulus for aldosterone release from the adrenal cortex. Increased renin plasma levels are thought to be the major cause of secondary aldosteronism. Renin also increases secondary to sympathetic nerve stimuli and possibly the osmolality of urine.

Frequently, plasma renin is reported with a simultaneous 24-hr urine sodium measurement (*renin, urine sodium correlation test*). When kidney function is normal, urinary sodium excretion is related to the ECF volume and inversely related to the plasma concentration of renin. This information helps identify low-renin hypertensive persons (see Section 8.1.3 E).

Normal Ranges 24-Hr Urine Sodium and Potassium

Urine sodium	43–217 mEq/24 hr
Urine potassium	26–123 mEq/24 hr

INAPPROPRIATE RENIN INCREASES OCCUR IN:

1. *Malignant hypertension* (50% increase or more), due to probable kidney damage and consequent inability of kidney to induce sodium retention.
2. *Secondary aldosteronism.* Renin is almost always the cause of increased aldosterone in this condition.
3. *Individuals on oral contraceptives* with increased blood pressure (with PRA method only), due to an increase in plasma renin substrate. Returns to normal levels about 4 months after the medication is discontinued.
4. *Administration of various drugs* (e.g., vasodilating antihypertensives and several diuretics).

APPROPRIATE PHYSIOLOGICAL INCREASES OCCUR IN:

1. *Prolonged upright posture or low-sodium diets.*

INAPPROPRIATE RENIN DECREASES OCCUR IN:

1. *Primary aldosteronism* (Conn's syndrome), due to autonomous aldosterone production.
2. *"Low-renin" essential hypertension,* cause unknown.
3. *Cushing's syndrome.*
4. *Administration of various drugs* [e.g., methylodopa (Aldomet), guanethidine, levodopa, propranolol].
5. *Tourniquet stasis* with sample collection.

APPROPRIATE RENIN DECREASES OCCUR IN:

Physiologic conditions such as high-salt diet, excess licorice ingestion, and decreased potassium.

Patient Preparation (for PRA Method)

1. *Prior to test.* 6 weeks to 2 months, estrogen or birth control medication to be discontinued; 1 week, diuretics and antihypertensive drugs discontinued and low-salt diet changed to regular diet; 4 to 8 hr prior to test, NPO except for water; 2 to 3 hr prior to test, ambulatory.
2. *If a 24-hr urine sodium is being done,* the usual instructions as to urine collection procedure are needed. Also, the patient should drink three large glasses of water immediately after emptying his or her bladder at the start of the test. Timing of start and completion of test is extremely important.

E. Adrenal stimulation and suppression tests

Because measurement of aldosterone and renin have been technically difficult, many tests have been developed to either hasten the procedure, screen for primary hyperaldosteronism, or to replace renin determinations. With the advent of simpler and more reliable aldosterone and renin measurement, the stimulation and suppression tests are less often used. The test still in fairly frequent use is the furosemide test in the diagnosis of primary aldosteronism, in which the demonstration of increased aldosterone with a low or hyporesponsive PRA are criteria.

Stimulation Tests

1. *Furosemide (Lasix) test* for aldosterone and renin (see "Patient Preparation" in Section 8.1.3 B). Renin and aldosterone secretion are stimulated by an oral dose of 80 mg of furosemide to produce acute volume depletion. Patient is kept in erect position for 3 to 4 hr. A blood specimen is then taken and measured for plasma aldosterone and plasma renin activity (PRA). In primary hyperaldosteronism plasma aldosterone will be inappropriately high in relation to the increase in PRA—hyporesponsiveness.
2. *Simplified furosemide renin stimulation test.* Patient fasting, given 40 mg of furosemide IV. 30 min in upright position. Plasma renin then determined. Low-renin, hypertensive patients unable to increase secretion to level of reference norm (less than 1.0 ng/mL/hr, white race; 0.5 ng/mL/hr, black race).
3. *ACTH stimulation test.* See Section 8.1.4 D.

Suppression Tests. These are more numerous, more time consuming, and in most cases even less frequently used. They will be listed here by name and purpose only. For further information the reader is referred to Henry (1979) or Ravel (1978).

1. *Deoxycorticosterone* (DOCA). To demonstrate relative autonomy of aldosterone secretion in Conn's aldosteronism–nonsuppressed.
2. *Fludrocortisone* (Florinef). Aldosterone loading; similar to DOCA.
3. *Saline infusion.* Also similar to DOCA in purpose.
4. *Spironalactone* (aldosterone antagonist). Measures urinary K^+ for changes in clearance related with aldosterone suppression.
5. *Saralasin test.* Renin suppression measured by decrease in blood pressure in renin-produced hypertension. Normals or nonresin hypertension do not decrease blood pressure.

8.1.4 Tests of Pituitary Feedback Mechanism

A. Laboratory and clinical indications of pituitary feedback dysfunction

Any disturbance of a hormone stimulated by pituitary stimulating hormones can be investigated by testing the negative feedback axis between the pituitary and the target organ. The investigation can look at pituitary production of the organ-specific stimulating hormone, or at the response of the target organ to the stimulation. Tests given under each endocrine gland test the response of the organ. This section looks at the response of the pituitary to stimulation or suppression, as well as measurement of plasma stimulating hormone concentrations. Signs and symptoms of target organ dysfunction are the indicators for pituitary investigation.

B. Dexamethasone suppression tests

Synonyms: None

Normal Ranges

Overnight screening test (single dose):	8:00 A.M. plasma cortisol suppressed to less than 5 μg/dL (Cushing's syndrome greater than 10 μg/dL)
Low-dose test	Urinary free cortisol suppressed to less than 20 μg/24 hr Urine 17-OHCS suppressed to less than 2.5 mg/g of creatinine second day of test
High-dose test	Urinary free cortisol suppressed to less than 20 μg/24 hr Urine 17-OHCS suppressed to less than 2.5 mg/g of creatinine second day of test

Explanation of the Test. Dexamethasone (Decadron) is a highly potent synthetic steroid, similar to cortisone in action, and some 30 times more active. The small dosage used (2 mg/day, low dose; 8 mg/day, high dose) suppresses ACTH production from the pituitary but has little if any effect on increasing the glucocorticoid measurements. There are three approaches to the test.

Overnight (single dose). An accurate and simple screening procedure to differentiate Cushing's disease and Cushing's syndrome, and can be done on an outpatient basis. (See Appendix E for definitions of the difference between the two dysfunctions.) A single low dose of dexamethasone is given by mouth at 11 P.M. and the plasma cortisol is measured between 8 and 9 A.M. If Cushing's syndrome is present, the plasma cortisol will not suppress and will exceed 10 μg/dL. If suppression is normal, Cushing's syndrome is ruled out.

Low-dose test. This test is widely used as a confirmatory test when the overnight test produces no suppression and Cushing's syndrome is suspected. It is usually done in the hospital to control the accuracy of medicine administration and the 24-hr urine collection. A dose of 0.5 mg of dexamethasone is given orally (or the dose is calculated by body weight: 5 μg/kg/6 hr) every 6 hr for 2 days. The 24-hr urine is checked each day for urinary free cortisol, 17-OHCS, and creatinine. The excretion of corticosteroids is expressed in mg/g of creatinine to better discriminate between Cushing's and normals, as the creatinine indicates whether renal function is normal or not. If urine free cortisol or urine 17-OHCS does not suppress, the diagnosis of Cushing's syndrome secondary to any etiology is definitely established. The suppression has been found to be abnormal in 99% of patients with Cushing's syndrome.

High-dose test. This test has been found valuable in identifying the lesion responsible for Cushing's syndrome. A dose of 2 mg of dexamethasone is given every 6 hr for 2 days and the same testing as for the low-dose test is done. If the urinary cortisol or 17-OHCS does not suppress adequately, the probability is that an autonomous adrenal adenoma or carcinoma exists, or the ectopic ACTH syndrome is functioning. (Ectopic ACTH syndrome involves the presence of an ACTH-like hormone being produced by a tumor in tissue not considered endocrine by nature—frequently an oatcell tumor of the lung.) Cushing's disease is identified by this test (i.e., it does not suppress with low-dosc tcst and suppresses to less than 50% of the baseline values of urinary free cortisol and 17-OHCS in the high-dose test).

FAILURE TO SUPPRESS CAN OCCUR IN:

Conditions other than Cushing's, such as:

1. *Hyperthyroidism,* due to the high metabolic clearance of dexamethasone.
2. *Individuals on estrogen therapy,* due to increased levels of transcortin (serum transport protein for cortisol).
3. *Obese individuals.* They fail to suppress in the overnight test but will suppress urinary free cortisol and serum cortisol with the low-dose test. 17-OHCS remain increased.
4. *Seriously stressed,* or seriously ill individuals, due to the glucocorticoid response (see Appendix B).
5. *Severe mental depression* and other like psychiatric disorders, due to unexplained biochemical abnormalities. Level of suppression is greater, however, than that found with ectopic ACTH syndrome. 17-OHCS are elevated, and plasma ACTH and cortisol lack diurnal variation.
6. *Individuals on Dilantin therapy,* due to increased metabolism of dexamethasone.

Patient Preparation. No special preparation other than an explanation of the test. Stress can negate the suppressive effects with small- or low-dose dexamethasone, and barbiturates may be given prior to the test for that reason.

C. Plasma ACTH

Synonyms: corticotropin; adrenocorticotrophic hormone; ACTH level

Normal Ranges

8 A.M. fasting	20–100 pg/mL
4 P.M. nonfasting	10– 50 pg/mL

Explanation of the Test. Measurement of plasma ACTH, a polypeptide secreted by the anterior pituitary gland, can be done to further differentiate the lesion responsible for Cushing's syndrome by identifying ectopic ACTH syndrome as opposed to adrenal adenomas or carcinomas. It is also used to establish a baseline prior to suppressive tests. The test is done using a radioimmunoassay technique which is usually available only through a reference laboratory. An understanding of the pituitary-adrenal axis negative feedback system is necessary to interpret the results.

ACTH INCREASED IN:

1. *Primary adrenal insufficiency* (Addison's disease), due to a decreased plasma cortisol concentration stimulating ACTH secretion.
2. *Ectopic ACTH syndrome* to very high levels, due to the production of ACTH-like substance by nonendocrine malignancies which are independent of negative feedback control and thus do not respond to increased cortisol concentrations. Ectopic focus frequently is an oatcell carcinoma of the lung. (Plasma ACTH may be done to confirm that diagnosis when tissue confirmation is not available.) Plasma levels are greater than 200 pg/mL and serum cortisol will also be above normal.
3. *Stress* due to increased release of glucocorticoids.

NORMAL TO LOW NORMAL ACTH CONCENTRATIONS IN:

Individuals with Cushing's disease—pituitary-dependent adrenal hyperplasia. The plasma levels are inappropropriately high for the levels of plasma cortisol, which are usually high normals. ACTH does not show diurnal variation and remains increased throughout the 24-hr cycle.

DECREASED ACTH LEVELS IN:

1. *Pituitary insufficiency* (hypopituitarism), usually less than 75 pg/mL. Serum cortisol is also depressed. The best discrimination between normal individuals and those with adrenal insufficiency is obtained from the 8 (or 10) A.M. test.
2. *Adrenal adenomas or carcinomas* (Cushing's syndrome), due to increased levels of plasma cortisol, which suppress ACTH production.
3. *Persons receiving glucocorticoids* therapeutically (for the same reason as given in item 2 above).

Patient Preparation. NPO except for water for 8 hr prior to the test except when a 4 P.M. sample is requested.

D. ACTH stimulation test

Synonyms modified thorn test; ACTH infusion test; provocative ACTH test

Normal Ranges

8-hr infusion test (modified Thorn test)	Two- to fourfold increase in plasma cortisol, 17-KS, and/or 17-OHCS levels over baseline determinations
Screening test	30⁻, 60⁻ and/or 120-min plasma cortisol should double over baseline and/or increase 10μg/dL within 60 min (if ACTH given IM, the peak effect will be delayed)
5-day test	Plasma cortisol levels more than double baseline determinations

Description of the Test. The test is not frequently used since reliable direct measurements of plasma ACTH have become available. It is useful as an adequate demonstration of reduced hydrocortisone production, but is not felt to add any significant information in the definition of causes for Cushing's syndrome (Conn and Conn, 1979).

The Thorn test was the original stimulation test and relied on eosinophil depression in response to ACTH-stimulated cortisone production. The more current tests are modifications of that test, using measurement of urinary metabolites of cortisone and cortisol, and/or plasma cortisol, in response to measured amounts of ACTH administered. ACTH can be given in multiple ways: as a single injection, either IV or IM (screening test); 8-hr IV infusion; continuous IV infusion; IM injections of depot ACTH for slow release; or subcutaneously. The test in its various forms can be completed in a matter of hours or continue for up to 5 days.

PLASMA CORTISOL OR URINARY METABOLITES INCREASED ABOVE NORMAL RANGE IN:

1. *Pituitary insufficiency* (secondary adrenal insufficiency).

2. *Individuals with some types of adrenal adenomas* and adrenal cortical hyperplasia, the increase being persistent beyond 24 hr after the day of the test.

PLASMA CORTISOL OR URINARY METABOLITES DECREASED IN:

1. *Some cases of pituitary insufficiency;* in many cases aldosterone is measured as well. Aldosterone should increase in concentration with ACTH stimulation, but it will not rise in primary adrenal failure.
2. *Adrenal insufficiency* (Addison's disease), due to adrenal atrophy.

DELAYED RESPONSE FOUND IN:

Long-term adrenal suppression secondary to the administration of substantial doses of steroid. Given a normal adrenal gland, it will eventually respond to the stimulus.

Patient Preparation. There is no special preparation or time of day necessary for doing this test.

E. Metyrapone test

Synonyms: Metopirone response [when plasma cortisol and urinary metabolites are both used to evaluate results, the test may also be called cortisol/compound-S Metopirone (metyrapone) combination; compound-S Metopirone/cortisol combination; cortisol/11-deoxycortisol]

Normal Ranges

Compound-S baseline	Less than 1 μg/dL
Post Metopirone	Greater than 7 μg/dL (or two- to fourfold increase in urinary 17-OHCS)
Cortisol	
A.M.	7–18 μg/dL
P.M.	2– 9 μg/dL

Description of the Test. Metyrapone (Metopirone) blocks the synthesis of cortisol within the adrenal gland at the stage where compound-S, a precursor of cortisol, has been produced. Usually, compound-S (11-deoxycortisone) is found in very low levels in the blood.

After metyrapone is given, ordinarily at bedtime and blood tested the next morning, compound-S concentration greatly increases and plasma cortisol concentration decreases. The cortisol decrease breaks the negative feedback to the pituitary, and ACTH secretion increases.

The purpose of this test is to identify pituitary-dependent bilateral adrenal hyperplasia (Cushing's disease) and to differentiate it from Cushing's syndrome due to ectopic ACTH syndrome, since both have increased ACTH levels. This is accomplished by measuring plasma cortisol by RIA, which does not include compound-S, included in many other cortisol measurements.

The test can also be used to indicate pituitary reserve. A 2-day test is done. The normal response indicating adequate pituitary reserve is production of plasma cortisol within normal range on the second day—when the adrenal overcomes the metyrapone block—responding to increased secretion of ACTH. The 2-day test has several disadvantages. It can provoke acute adrenal insufficiency in persons with decreased pituitary reserve, and it is time consuming. The single-dose-overnight procedure is the one most often used.

RESPONSES RELATED TO PATHOLOGIC CONDITIONS:

1. *Increased compound-S,* decreased cortisol = normal response.
2. *Exaggerated increase in compound-S, decreased cortisol* = Cushing's disease—pituitary-dependent adrenal hyperplasia.
3. *No increase in compound-S, normal cortisol* = Cushing's syndrome due to adrenal carcinoma, autonomous adrenal function, or androgenital syndrome.
4. *No increase in compound-S with a low baseline plasma cortisol* = pituitary or hypothalamic failure.

Patient Preparation. No special preparation for the overnight procedure. For the 2-day procedure, glucocorticoids may be provided during the testing if decreased pituitary reserve is suspected, to prevent acute adrenal insufficiency.

8.2 THE PITUITARY GLAND

8.2.1 Antidiuretic hormone (ADH)

A. Laboratory and Clinical Indications of ADH Dysfunction

A deficiency in ADH has some relatively obvious signs and symptoms to alert one to deficiencies. The syndrome of inappropriate ADH secretion (SIADH) is less distinguishable. Both, however, require knowledge of both clinical and laboratory findings and the ability to see relationships between them.

ADH DEFICIENCY MIGHT BE SUSPECTED WITH:

1. *Laboratory findings.* Low morning urine specific gravity, less than 1.007 usually; high plasma sodium concentration; absence of indication of renal disease (e.g., normal BUN, plasma creatinine, potassium, serum calcium, and proteins). (Hypernatremic dehydration can occur in infants, causing an increased BUN.)
2. *Clinical findings.* Persistent and massive diuresis (up to 12 to 15/L/day, normal being 6/L/day); polyuria; polydipsia; nocturia; and thirst that wakens the person at night.

SIADH MIGHT BE SUSPECTED WITH:

1. *Laboratory findings.* Decreased plasma sodium and chloride; increased urinary sodium due to water retention; dilutional changes in other values (e.g., decreased hematocrit, increased MCV, decreased MCHC).
2. *Clinical findings.* Urinary output less than intake; weight gain—often 1 lb or more a day; history of trauma, surgery, cerebral lesion, lung carcinoma, or other known precipitants of SIADH.

B. Serum and urine osmolality

Synonyms: plasma and urine osmolality

Normal Ranges

Serum	275–295 mOsm/kg of water
Urine	300–1000 mOsm/kg of water (also expressed as mOsm/L)

Explanation of the Tests. Osmolality is the measurement of the number of dissolved solute particles in a solution. It is the preferred unit of measurement for body fluids, over specific gravity or osmolarity, since it is a constant weight-to-weight relationship. Osmolarity varies with fluid volume, the expanding effect on the solution of dissolved solute, and the temperature of the solution. Specific gravity requires correction for the presence of glucose or protein as well as temperature. Osmolality can be measured over a wider range than specific gravity, and with greater accuracy.

Urine osmolality gives information about a number of things: the ability of the kidney tubules to concentrate or dilute urine; the presence or absence of ADH (presumptive) for renal tubular reabsorption of water; an indication of plasma osmolality; and assistance in the diagnosis of certain fluid and electrolyte problems, as well as control of therapy. More information is available when urine osmolality is compared to plasma osmolality (U/P); electrolytes can also be compared in both solutions (U/P normal range: 0.2 to 4.7). Comparison of plasma sodium concentration to plasma osmolality is another fruitful way to utilize knowledge of osmolality. (Plasma sodium/plasma osmolality normal range = 0.43 to 0.40 and remains unchanged in many dilutional and dehydration states.)

Changes in Osmolality

Condition	Urine	Plasma
Hypernatremia (increased plasma sodium without water increase)	Increased	Increased
Hyperosmolar nonketotic hyperglycemia	Isoosmolar or decreased	Increased
Hyperglycemia	Isoosmolar or decreased	Increased
Uremia	Isoosmolar	Increased
Diabetes insipidus	Decreased	Increased
Hypercalcemia	Decreased	Increased
Excess fluid intake (compulsive drinking)	Decreased	Decreased
SIADH	Increased	Decreased
Renal tubular necrosis	Decreased	Increased
Severe pyelonephritis	Decreased	Increased
Acidosis	Increased	Increased
Shock	Increased	Increased

Patient Preparation. No special preparation is necessary. The first voided specimen in the morning is most likely to demonstrate maximum concentrating ability of the kidney.

C. Water deprivation tests

Synonyms: Mosenthal test (24 hr); Fishberg test (12 hr); renal concentration test; 14-hr deprivation test; 8-hr deprivation test

Normal Ranges

Urine osmolality greater than 800 mOsm/kg of water

Urine osmolality greater than serum osmolality

Serum osmolality unchanged

Explanation of the Tests. Water deprivation of normal persons stimulates ADH secretion through osmolar and volume stimuli. Such deprivation can be used when it is necessary to differentiate among possible causes of polyuria, particularly between nephrogenic diabetes insipidus (DI)—the inability of the tubules to respond to ADH—and neurohypophyseal DI—inadequate or absent ADH secretion. It also establishes the patient's ability to produce ADH.

As indicated by the number of synonyms given above, there are many slightly different approaches to this test, all of which share common principles. The test is based on deprivation of *any* fluid intake; over a specified length of time; or until a given outcome occurs as evidenced by change in urine osmolality to a normal concentration; or to the point of a specific weight loss (e.g., greater than 3% of body weight); or to the point where 2- or 3-hr urine osmolality tests indicate about equal osmolality—a plateau. If the response is abnormal with inadequate concentration, the test can be followed by an injection of vasopressin (exogenous ADH). This will indicate whether the cause is ADH deficiency or nonresponsive kidney tubule.

The shorter tests are more frequently used because individuals with DI and polyuria exceeding 5 L/day usually reach their optimum concentrating ability, the plateau, in 4 to 8 hr, whereas normal individuals may require up to 14 hr. Plasma osmolality, plasma sodium, urine volume, and urine osmolality are checked at the beginning and end of the test. Urine osmolality may be checked every hour, or any variation of timing, and weight is usually taken at the beginning and end, as well as when indicated during the test.

Responses to Water Deprivation Tests

Condition	Osmolality response to H_2O deprivation	Osmolality response to vasopressin
Compulsive water drinking (primary polydipsia)	Normal urine and plasma osmolality	Normal; urine osmolality increases no more than 5%
Neurohypophyseal DI	Urine osmolality less than plasma; plasma osmolality greater than 300 mOsm	Increased to greater than 50% of baseline and greater than plasma osmolality
Nephrogenic DI	Urine osmolality less than plasma; plasma osmolality often greater than 300 mOsm	No response

Source: Data from Henry, 1979 and Conn and Conn, 1979.

Patient Preparation

1. *Conditions such as diabetes mellitus, hypercalcemia, and hyperkalemia* must be ruled out by appropriate tests prior to starting water deprivaton.
2. *The possibility of vascular collapse* with water deprivation is high and close observation is imperative.
3. *Careful instruction and monitoring* is necessary to prevent any fluid intake that would invalidate the test.

D. Water loading tests

Synonyms: water challenge; saline challenge; water load; Hickey-Hare osmolality test

Normal Ranges

Decrease in urine volume (flow rate in ml/min)

Urine osmolality = equal to or greater than 600 mOsm/kg (level obtained when exogenous vasopressin given)

Explanation of the Test. The purpose of this test is to establish the patient's ability to produce ADH. Some authorities believe that the information is more simply acquired by the water deprivation test (Harvey et al., 1976). Water loading is sometimes useful in the diagnosis of inappropriate ADH (IADH), but it is a dangerous test in patients with hyponatremia (less than 125 mEq/L).

The test is based on the principle that a rise in serum osmolality will stimulate ADH release, the effects of which can be measured in the increased urine concentration. Unlike water deprivation, this test also increases blood volume expansion, which alters ADH release and is a conflicting stimulus to that of increased serum osmolality.

Generally, the test is carried out as follows. Diuresis is established by either having the patient drink a 20-ml/kg load of water in 15 min, or by IV infusion of 5% glucose at 8 to 10 ml/min, leading to an increased glomerular filtration rate (GFR) with hypotonic fluid. When urine flow is 5 ml/min, or when over 50% of the initial water load is excreted, or when 1 hr has passed, an IV of 2.5% saline solution (isotonic saline is 0.9%) is started and run at 0.25 ml/kg/min for 45 min. Serum osmolality is measured before and after the hypertonic IV is given, and urine is collected every hour for 4 hr with the volume and osmolality measured.

Vasopressin may be given as a follow-up to differentiate between the two types of DI (see the explanation in Section 8.2.1C).

Responses to Water Loading Tests

Condition	Response
Compulsive water drinking (primary polydipsia)	Normal (see "Normal Ranges")
DI, neurohypophyseal	No antidiuresis–urine osmolality unchanged
DI, nephrogenic	No antidiuresis–urine osmolality unchanged

Patient Preparation

1. *The test is risky* for patients with cardiac disease.
2. *Plasma sodium* should be determined prior to the test. In some instances sodium replacement is done prior to the test to bring plasma levels up to the minimum safe level (125 mEq/L).

E. Direct measurement of serum and urine ADH

Radioimmunoassays are available to measure ADH in serum and urine, and are now sensitive enough to detect basal ADH levels. The tests are not as yet available routinely, even in reference laboratories, but are in use primarily in experimental work (Conn and Conn, 1979).

8.2.2 Growth Hormone (GH)

A. Laboratory and clinical indications of GH dysfunction

Indications of secreting pituitary tumors are the decrease in all but one hormone function, most often GH or ACTH, and that function shows a marked increase. Congenital, or genetic "idiopathic" pituitary deficiencies, which are presumably hypothalamic in origin, often involve GH or the gonadotropins alone.

GH DEFICIENCIES MIGHT BE SUSPECTED WITH:

1. *Clinical findings. Children:* failure to grow, with impaired linear growth within the first few months of life, delayed bone

maturation; no obvious physical abnormalities other than small size. *Adults:* there are no known physical abnormalities associated with deficiency after attainment of full height.

2. *Laboratory findings.* Usual screening tests are normal.

GH EXCESS MIGHT BE SUSPECTED WITH:

1. *Clinical findings. Children:* gigantism = overgrowth of skeleton and soft tissues with proportional overgrowth of long bones; weight and height are in proportion; may have headaches if pituitary tumor is cause. *Adults:* early signs of acromegaly include increased size of hands, head, feet (may be noticed by gloves, hat, or shoes being too small), and facial changes [e.g., increased nose size, enlargement of forehead, jaw (dentures do not fit)]; voice changes—increased resonance, lower pitch; constant perspiration; coarsening of skin; enlargement of tongue with slurring of speech; arthritic complaints.
2. *Laboratory findings. Children:* increased serum glucose; diabetic glucose tolerance test (GTT) curve; untreated = decreased TSH. *Adults:* increased serum inorganic phosphorous (prior to GH by RIA, this was felt to be the most helpful test for acromegaly; relationship to increased GH not established, but inorganic phosphorus is also increased in growing children); increased calcium, serum, and urine; serum glucose and GTT as for child. *Related tests:* basal metabolic rate increased; increased serum prolactin, at times urine 17-KS, 17-OHCS, or 17-KGS are increased despite normal plasma cortisol; TSH may increase.

B. Serum growth hormone, RIA

Synonyms: GH; human growth hormone: HGH; somatotropin hormone; SH; STH

Normal Ranges

Adult	0– 8 ng/mL
Children	0–10 ng/mL

Explanation of the Test. At the present time, assay of GH is the single most important test in evaluation of GH. GH can now be directly measured in the blood by radioimmunoassay, and can be measured equally well in either serum or plasma. Although many hormones are necessary for growth, GH is the most important. In its absence children's growth rate is decreased by from one-half to one-third. As yet the normal function of GH in the adult has not been identified. Measurement of GH gives information not only about its deficit or excess, but also is frequently used as a guide to pituitary dysfunction, since decreases in GH values often indicate pituitary tumors (Henry, 1979).

Normal values of GH have wide variation due to the rather sporadic bursts of secretion. Levels in normal persons are often very low, less than 3 ng/mL, and may actually be undetectable. Short bursts occur, not consistent with any pattern, but their presence is fairly consistent day to day in a given individual. A rise in concentration occurs early in sleep (with the exception of some adults over 50 years of age). Because of the consistent secretion with sleep, basal levels would be drawn in the morning when they are most likely to be detectable—after awakening, but before arising, and while fasting.

Because of the overlap between the basal normal range of GH and values consistent with hypopituitarism, a definite normal is required to rule out hyposecretion of GH. This usually requires a stimulation test (see Section 8.2.2C).

INCREASED SECRETION OF GH ASSOCIATED WITH:

1. *Acromegaly in the adult,* usually due to a pituitary tumor.
2. *Gigantism in children* under age of puberty, a rare occurrence that may be acquired due to a pituitary tumor, or congenital "idiopathic" causes.
3. *Bronchogenic or gastric cancer* in very rare instances due to ectopic GH secretion by tumors.
4. *Infants with psychosocial deprivation syndrome* (e.g., nutritional and emotional deprivation leading to peculiar eating and drinking habits) (Conn and Conn, 1979).
5. *Hypoglycemia.*
6. *Physiological responses* such as:
   a. Sleep. Substantial increases early in sleep with a peak occurring between the first and second hours. May peak two to three times during one night.

b. Exercise of any type, especially when fasting. 15 min of exercise in a fasting patient makes a good, easily performed, and inexpensive stimulation screening test in children of short stature (Conn and Conn, 1979).
c. Increased levels of human placental lactogen in pregnant women.
d. After protein ingestion (e.g., a pure beefsteak meal) or the infusion of certain amino acids such as arginine.
e. Stress such as major surgery. GH levels can increase then, even in the face of hyperglycemia.

7. *Iatrogenic causes* as with:
   a. Therapeutic administration of estrogen elevating basal secretion concentration.
   b. Drugs such as *L*-dopa. However, *L*-dopa can also cause a paradoxical fall of GH levels in acromegalic patients.

DECREASED SECRETION OF GH ASSOCIATED WITH:

1. *Ateliotic (pituitary) dwarfism in children* due to multiple, not well understood causes, such as decreased secretion of GH releasing factor; lesion of the pituitary; decreased ability of the body to respond to GH—end-organ unresponsiveness—which may in turn be due to defects in generation of somatomedin (the GH-dependent substance in plasma that stimulates growth in responsive tissue) (Henry, 1979).
2. *Older children with psychosocial deprivation syndrome* (see "Increased Secretion" above, item 4, for definition) in response to stimulation testing. Basal levels may be normal.
3. *Ingestion of a glucose load hyperglycemia.*
4. *Pharmacologic doses of glucocorticoid.*

Patient Preparation

1. *NPO for 8 hr* prior to the test.
2. *In some methods* the patient is kept recumbent for 30 min prior to blood taking to eliminate GH bursts due to exercise.

C. Growth hormone stimulation tests

Synonyms: insulin tolerance test; ITT; GH provocation test (see names of other types of stimulation tests in body of explanation)

Normal Response Ranges

Consistent rise in GH levels to over 20 ng/mL (blood glucose must decrease to less than 40 mg/dL, or less than 50% basal fasting level for test to accurately assess GH reserve)

Pediatric: children may have no response even though GH is adequate; the combination of ITT and arginine infusion stimulation test is felt to be the most definitive test for GH deficiency in children

Normal response to arginine test: GH level rises to 7 ng/mL

Explanation of the Test. The ITT is only one of a rather large group of stimulation tests (e.g., vasopressin, glucagon, *L*-dopa, tolbutamide, and exercise (see "Increased Secretion in GH," in Section 8.2.2B, item 6b), all of which are undertaken with the same idea in mind, to maximally stimulate GH secretion. When one stimulation test does not provide a rise in GH, another one is frequently tried. Other substances are combined at times to improve GH response (e.g., propranolol is felt to enhance action of glucagon; estrogen is often given with arginine). Insulin-induced hypoglycemia and the arginine infusion test are the two most frequently used tests, although *L*-dopa has strong proponents.

Stimulation tests are frequently necessary in the evaluation of GH secretion, as the normal basal level can be so low as to be undetectable. It is then necessary to stimulate secretion in order to detect a clearly normal result, to rule out hyposecretion. Only GH values well within normal limits can separate pituitary dwarfism from small stature due to other causes.

Stimulation tests also provide information about the reserve capacity of GH because they stress the production ability. Even though serum levels of GH may be within normal limits, the ability to react adequately with increased need, as with the stress of surgery, may be absent.

The ITT is contraindicated in persons with a history of ischemic heart disease, evidence of a myocardial infarction, cerebrovascular disease, epilepsy, or low basal plasma cortisol levels.

Test Procedure. Basal blood sample taken on fasting patient for serum glucose, cortisol, and GH. Insulin given IV, dosage based on 0.1 to 0.15 IU/kg of body weight, except in children, who have a tendency to severe hypoglycemia if deficient in GH. Dosage is calculated on approximately half of the adult dose in such cases. Blood tests as above are taken every 15 min for the first hour, minimum every 30 min, and every 30 min thereafter for 2 hr. The test is terminated immediately if any serious signs related to hypoglycemia occur (fainting, chest pain). Other tests may be run on the blood sample as well to help confirm or rule out a diagnosis.

1. *Prolactin* (LTH)—most secreting tumors and half the nonsecreting tumors induce increased prolactin levels.
2. *Follicle stimulating hormone* (FSH)—measured when a stimulator such as clomiphene has been used, becuase it induces an increase in FSH normally, which does not occur in pituitary failure.
3. *Thyroid stimulating hormone* (TSH)—hypothyroidism is often associated with short stature. GH cannot be assessed properly unless the patient has been euthyroid for a considerable time.

"Failure of GH concentration to rise above the set limit after at least two stimulating tests is indicative of GH deficiency" (Henry, 1979).

Conditions Causing Possible Alterations of Results. (Henry, 1979)

Increased GH response	Decreased GH response
Starvation—in arginine test	Diabetes mellitus
Hyperthyroidism	Cirrhosis
	Hypothyroidism
	Obesity

Patient Preparation

1. *NPO 8 hr* prior to the test.
2. *Screen* for conditions contraindicating the test (see test explanation above).

D. Growth hormone suppression test

Synonyms: glucose loading test; glucose tolerance test

Normal Response

Basal level GH	Less than 10 ng/mL
Suppressed	Less than 5 ng/mL sometime during test

Abnormal Response: found in active acromegaly or gigantism

Basal level GH	Less than 5 ng/mL
With suppression	Does not suppress below 5 ng/mL

Explanation of the Test. This test is a controlled effort to cause GH levels to decrease in response to administration of glucose, a normal physiologic response. The test procedure is not unlike that of the standard glucose tolerance test (see Section 8.4.3) except that GH levels are the substance change evaluated. Suppression tests can be helpful in revealing abnormalities in physiologic function and control. The lack of suppression of GH in conditions of hypersecretion with gigantism and acromegaly is a good example of this. Suppression testing is used less frequently than stimulation testing in the evaluation of GH.

NONSUPPRESSION OCCURRING IN CONDITIONS OTHER THAN INCREASED GH INCLUDES:

1. *Known decreases in somatomedin* (the GH-dependent substance in plasma that stimulates growth in responsive tissue), occurring in renal insufficiency and kwashiorkor.
2. *Renal failure.*
3. *Cirrhosis.*
4. *Starvation.*

8.3 THE THYROID GLAND

8.3.1 Laboratory and Clinical Indications of Thyroid Dysfunction

A. Hyperthyroidism

Clinical Findings (Adults). Usually highly nonspecific, but if "classic" findings are present (exophthalmos, pretibial myxedema, thyroid enlargement), the diagnosis is obvious. Early symptoms include nervousness, fatigue, weight loss, and palpitations. Later–cardiovascular: angina, dyspnea, peripheral edema; emotional: instability, irritability, insomnia; GI: usually increased appetite and food intake in face of weight loss, increased number of defecations, which can progress to true diarrhea; heat intolerance, increased perspiration; changes in menstrual cycle, metorrhagia, amenorrhea; muscle weakness noted particularly in stair climbing, getting out of tub, or combing hair; tremors of hands; hair fine and limp; eye changes in Graves' disease, periorbital edema, prominent stare due to lid retraction or exophthalmos, lid lag, difficulty with vision–double vision, photophobia. After age 50 findings are less obvious, appetite may decrease, cardiovascular symptoms predominate (apathetic hyperthyroidism). See Section 1.13.

Laboratory Findings. Also nonspecific and variable. WBC may have slight increase, lymphocytes increase, mild anemia, mild hypercalcemia (to 11.5 mg/dL) in younger people, as well as an increase in alkaline phosphatase. Tests other than screening tests: creatine clearance may increase; tendency to glucose intolerance (abnormal GTT).

B. Hypothyroidism

Clinical Findings. Infants: often associated with hyaline membrane disease in full-term infant; protuberant abdomen, umbilical herniation, large tongue, hoarse cry, growth failure, and mental retardation if not treated. Not usually obese. *Adults:* nonpitting periorbital edema, and edema of the face and extremities. Hair coarse, dry, loss of outer one-third of eyebrow; mild enlargement of tongue; cold dry skin and cold intolerance (mottled skin); lethargy and lethargic appearance, personality change–dulled, slowed mentation; menstrual changes with menorrhagia; cardiac enlargement, bradycardia; generalized weakness; entrapment neuropathy (carpal tunnel syndrome); anorexia which may be concomitant with weight gain, constipation.

Laboratory Findings. Infants: prolonged physiologic indirect hyperbilirubinemia, plus most of findings in adults. *Adults:* increased serum cholesterol and triglycerides; anemia in 50% of patients, which can be macrocytic at times as well as normochromic or hypochromic. *Tests other than screening tests:* ECG changes with low voltage and flattened or inverted T waves.

8.3.2 Measurements of Thyroxine, Total (T_4)

T_4 RIA Serum thyroxine by radioimmunoassay; the test of choice with satisfactory specificity and very sensitive

Normal Range: 4.5 to 12.5 μg/dL

T_4(D) (Also given as T_4D; T_4 Murphy-Patee) Serum thyroxine by displacement; independent of iodine content–therefore, a better choice for testing than the following tests, which are dependent on iodine content or interfered with because of iodine contamination

Normal Ranges

Neonate	10.1–20.0 μg/dL
1– 6 years	5.6–12.6 μg/dL
6–10 years	4.9–11.7 μg/dL
Adult	4.7–11.1 μg/dL

PBI Protein-bound iodine, a measurement of all PBI, not just that bound to thyroxine; rarely used

Normal Range: 4–8 μg/dL

BEI Butanol extractable iodine; thyroxine measured as PBI after removal of extraneous organically bound iodine; still altered by iodine contamination, and by alterations in carrier protein levels; rarely used.

T_4(C) [Also given as T_4I(C) and T_4 by column] Thyroxine measured as PBI after removal of extraneous organically bound iodine; limitations as for BEI

Explanation of the Test. Determination of total thyroxine is the initial screening test for most suspected thyroid disorders, particularly hyperthyroidism (see Fig. 8.1). These tests all measure total thyroxine, that is, both bound and "free" thyroxine, and are therefore altered by conditions altering thyroid binding globulin (TBG). T_4 accounts for 95% of total thyroid hormone output. Approximately 20% of T_4 produced is ultimately converted to T_3 in peripheral tissues. For some time it has been questioned whether T_4 is biologically active. Evidence indicates that it indeed is, but to a lesser degree than is T_3. Evidently, T_4 accounts for only about one-third of the total biologic effect of thyroid (Farese, 1980).

T_4 exists primarily bound to TBG or in a lesser amount to thyroxine binding prealbumin (TBPA). It is more firmly bound than

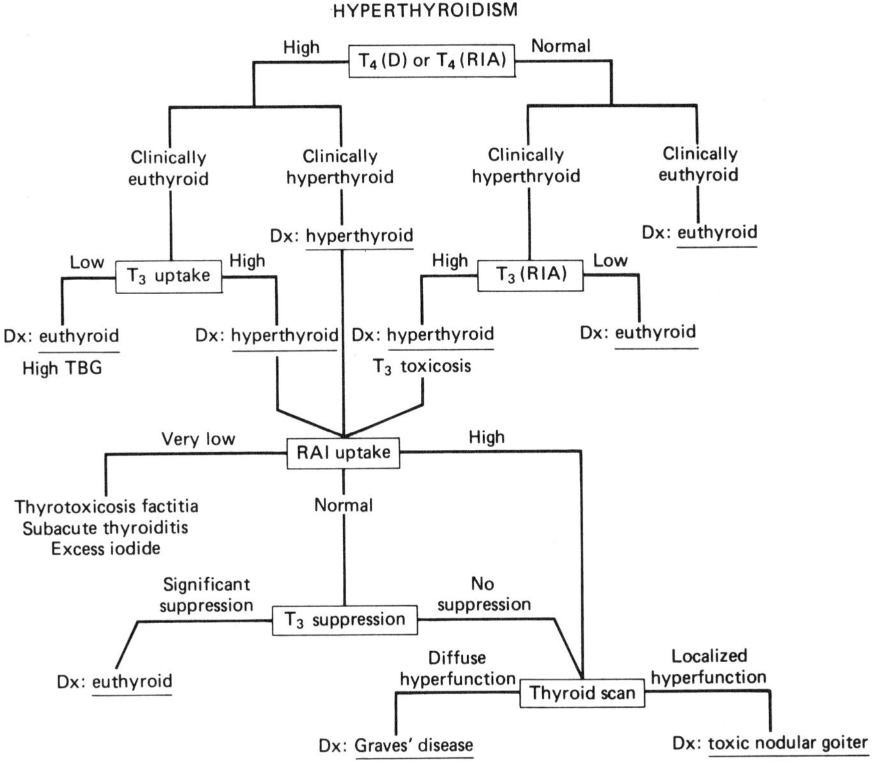

FIGURE 8.1 Laboratory evaluation of hyperthyroidism. T_4 is the initial screening test. If it is high in a clinically euthyroid patient, a T_3U should be done. Either the T_3U will show that an elevated TBG level is the cause of the high T_4, or it will support hyperthyroidism. If the T_4 is normal in a clinically hyperthyroid patient, a T_3 (RIA) will indicate whether T_3 toxicosis is present. Once the serum hormone confirmation of hyperthyroidism is completed, the RAIU will separate the various causes. If the RAIU is normal in a case of suspected Graves' disease, a T_3 suppression test should be performed. Finally, the pattern of uptake on the thyroid scan will indicate whether toxic nodular goiter or Graves' disease is the cause of the elevated or nonsuppressible RAIU. [From Paul L. Marguilies and David V. Becker, "Hyperthyroidism," in Howard F. Conn and Rex B. Conn, *Current Diagnosis 5* (Philadelphia: W. B. Saunders Company, 1977) p. 774.]

T_3, which accounts, in part, for the fact that T_4 is found in higher concentrations in the plasma than is T_3.

PBI, BEI, and T_4(C) tests measure thyroxine by measuring the amount of iodine present. They are then indirect estimations of thyroxine, thus tend to have frequent alterations due to ingested iodine or contamination by extraneous iodine during test procedure. They are altered as well by changes in TBG. For these reasons their use has been generally supplanted by the RIA test.

T_4 INCREASED IN:

1. *Dysfunctions of thyroid production,* as in hyperthyroidism and acute and subacute thyroiditis.
2. *Conditions that increase concentration* or binding capacity of thyroxine binding globulin (TBG), a transport protein for thyroid hormone, such as:
   a. Increased estrogen levels found in pregnancy, use of birth control pills.
   b. Liver disease (e.g., acute viral hepatitis).
   c. Congenital increases found in familial idiopathic dysproteinemia.
   d. Newborn infants.
   e. Acute intermittent porphyria.
   f. Some instances of hypothyroidism.

T_4 DECREASED IN:

1. *Dysfunctions of thyroid production,* as in cretinism of infants and children myxedema, chronic thyroiditis, and occasionally in subacute thyroiditis.
2. *Conditions that decrease concentration* or binding capacity of TBG, such as:
   a. Increased steroid serum levels (Cushing's disease/syndrome, therapeutic administration of glucocorticoids).
   b. Administration of androgens therapeutically.
   c. Chronic debilitating illness (multiple myeloma, leukemia, Hodgkin's disease, active acromegaly, nephrotic syndrome, nephrosis).
   d. Acute illness, or with surgical stress due to increased glucocorticoid production.
3. *Conditions that require the administration of certain drugs* which either decrease T_4 synthesis (salicylates, sulfonamides), increase T_4 destruction (Reserpine), or displace T_4 from binding sites (aspirin, heparin).
4. *Patients treated with T_3 alone and euthyroid* (no clinical signs or symptoms of abnormal thyroid function, and free thyroid index within normal limits).
5. *Hashimoto's thyroiditis, radiation damage, thyroid dysgenesis.* The patients may be euthyroid, however, due to increased T_3 secretion.

Patient Preparation. No special preparation is needed.

8.3.3 Measurements of Triiodothyronine, Total (T_3)

Synonyms: T_3 RIA; T_3 by radioimmunoassay; T_3 (RIA)

Normal Ranges

Adult	80–200 ng/dL (declining by 10% every 10 years)
Pediatric	
Neonate	140 ± 6 ng/dL
1–2 years	124 ± 8 ng/dL
3–10 years	136 ± 5 ng/dL
Adolescent	129 ± 5 ng/dL

Explanation of the Test. This is a measurement of the most metabolically active segment of thyroid hormone. Like the thyroxine test given previously, this measures both protein bound and free portions of T_3 and is therefore affected by alterations in TBG and TBPA. The measurement of T_3 is felt by some authorities to be the most sensitive test for thyrotoxicosis (Ravel, 1978). It is seldom used for the detection of hypothyroidism because of the overlap between the low-normal range and hypothyroid conditions. It is therefore not reliable for distinguishing between normal and hypothyroid states.

T_3 INCREASED IN:

1. *See* Section 8.3.2. Over 90% of all hyperthyroid patients have increases in both T_3 and T_4 and the increase in T_3 is often greater than that of T_4. T_3 may be the better diagnostic test in hyperthyroid states.
2. *Thyrotoxicosis,* even before T_4 levels have reached upper limits of normal.
3. *T_3 toxicosis.* A significant minority of hyperthyroid patients with a normal T_4, but increased T_3 occur, especially early in the course of toxic nodular goiter, in relapses following treatment of Graves' disease, and in regions of iodine deficiency.
4. *Overdosage with T_3 replacement.* Known time of dosage administration is important for accurate interpretation of T_3 levels, as

the exogenous hormone has serum level peaks about 4 hr after administration.

5. *Hashimoto's thyroiditis,* radiation damage of thyroid and thyroid dysgenesis. T_3 may be secreted in preference to T_4. The patient may be euthyroid.

T_3 DECREASED IN:

1. *See* Section 8.3.2.
2. *The "euthyroid sick,"* in which T_4 is converted to a metabolically inert substance called "reverse T_3" instead of active T_3 in the periphery. Reverse T_3 does not measure as T_3, thus decreasing the level (Farese, 1980). Seen in debilitating disease such as chronic renal failure or cirrhosis; persons being treated with glucocorticoids; gravely ill patients from any cause; in starvation or during fasting; in the newborn period and in the elderly.
3. *Persons being treated with T_4.*
4. *Persons with acute illness,* and after surgery, due to stress effect.

Patient Preparation. No special preparation is necessary.

8.3.4 Measurement of Thyroid Binding Globulin (TBG) Binding Sites: Resin Uptake

Synonyms: Resin T_3 uptake; T_3U; RT_3 U

Normal Range: Each method and each laboratory has its own normal range, which are not comparable; the results should be expressed as a ratio

Explanation of the Test. This is *not* a test of T_3 concentration. The term T_3 as used in this title refers to the radioactive labeled T_3 used in the test, *not* T_3 measurement. RT_3U is a measurement, or estimate, of TBG binding capacity, or free binding sites. It provides a means for correcting T_4 values to compensate to TBG alterations. It is not useful as a screening test, but is used when a serum T_4 level does not correspond with the patient's clinical status. RT_3U is inversely related to the TBG, so that all the factors listed under thyroxine tests that decrease TBG will cause an increase in the RT_3U value, and vice versa (see Fig. 8.1).

RT_3U values are determined and reported in many different ways. When calculated with the total thyroxine, it provides a free triiodothyronine (T_3) index, or a free thyroxine index when calculated with total triiodothyronine (see measurements of "free" thyroid hormone). Each laboratory has its own methods and reporting systems which the reader should use for normal ranges.

TBG can be measured by assay as well.

TBG INCREASED IN:

1. *All items listed* under decreased thyroxine (T_4) test related to TBG.
2. *Hyperthyroidism* due to decreased available binding sites.

TBG DECREASED IN:

1. *All items listed* under increased T_4 test related to TBG.
2. *Hypothyroidism* due to increased available binding sites.

Patient Preparation. No special preparation is required.

8.3.5. Measurement of "Free" Thyroid Hormone

1. *By dialysis:* free thyroxine (FT_4) and free triiodothyronine (FT_3).
2. *Free thyroxin index* [FTI; FT_4 index; T_4 RIA, or T_4(D), and T_3U ratio], and *free triiodothyronine index* (FT_3I; FT_3 index; T_3 RIA and T_3U ratio). (Both tests, when combined and reported together, are called T_7 by some laboratories. T_7 is the product of the T_4 or T_3 and the T_3U resin uptake.)

Explanation of the Tests

Dialysis. It is possible, but costly and time consuming, to obtain accurate measurements of free T_4 and T_3. One method is equilibrium dialysis, in which radioactively labeled T_4 is added to serum as a tracer. The free T_4 (or T_3) is then separated from the bound T_4 and the radioactivity of the dialysate is measured. Comparable information is available from the less expensive and more available tests, and computations of the free thyroid hormone index tests.

Free thyroxin/triiodothyronine index. T_4 and T_3 are present in the circulation primarily in the bound state (99.77% and 97.0%, respectively). The biological activity of both factions corresponds better with the free serum levels of the hormones because the free fractions are not tied to protein and can be used immediately. They can maintain an individual in a euthyroid state despite variations in available binding sites.

Free thyroid hormone fractions are directly proportional to the RT_3U and inversely proportional to TBG, as seen in the discussion of total thyroid hormone measurement. Usually, T_4 and T_3 fluctuate together and it is not necessary to determine both levels. In some instances (e.g., hypothyroidism), T_3 may be disproportionately high. The calculation called the free thyroxin (or triiodothyronine) index is done according to this formula: total T_4 RIA (or T_4(D) × RT_3U = free T_4 index or total T_3 RIA × RT_3U = free T_3. Calculation of this index gives a true picture of the patient status by compensating for TBG alterations and describing the metabolically active part of the hormone.

A method of calculating mean absolute free level of the hormone fractions makes use of the known approximate percentages of free versus bound hormone [e.g., (T_4 mean total level μg/dL = 7.0) × (percent free = 0.03%) = mean absolute free level in ng/dL = 2.1].

INCREASES AND DECREASES OF TEST VALUES:

These parallel those for T_4 and T_3 RIA but eliminate changes due to alterations in TBG.

Preparation for test. No special preparations necessary.

8.3.6 Thyroid Stimulating Hormone (RIA)—Serum

Synonyms: TSH: human thyroid stimulating hormone; HTSH

Normal Range: 2–10 μIU/mL

Explanation of the test. This is not a basic thyroid diagnostic test, but one that is helpful in special circumstances. Circulating serum concentrations of free thyroid hormones T_4 and T_3 regulate TSH secretion and release from the anterior pituitary by way of a negative feedback cycle (e.g., increased T_3 and T_4 cause decreased TSH, and vice versa). A second regulatory control on TSH production is from thyrotropin releasing factor (TRF) or hormone (TRH) produced in the hypothalamus. Knowledge of the circulating levels of TSH can help especially to differentiate between primary and secondary hypothyroidism, particularly in the milder cases. Primary hypothyroidism refers to thyroid gland defect–hypofunction or nonfunction–and is indicated by increased TSH levels (increased stimulation of the thyroid) due to the decreased circulating levels of thyroid hormone. Secondary hypothyroidism refers to a pituitary (or hypothalamic) hypofunction or nonfunction, and is indicated by a decreased TSH level due to the inability of the pituitary to produce adequate hormone. T_3 and T_4 levels have no effect in this instance. The TSH is considered the single best test to confirm the diagnosis of hypothyroidism and to localize the level of dysfunction–pituitary, hypothalamic, or thyroid failure (Conn and Conn, 1979).

TSH can be stimulated to test its function by giving TRF, thyroid releasing factor, now available commercially as Thypinone, and its pituitary reserve measured by the increase, or lack thereof, of TSH.

Very few changes occur in TSH due to outside influences, making it a quite specific test.

TSH INCREASED IN:

1. *Primary hypothyroidism,* generally over twice normal.
2. *Exaggerated increases* may occur when TRF is used to stimulate. The response may also be delayed.
3. *Clinically euthyroid persons* with Hashimoto's thyroiditis.
4. *Physiologic states* such as the neonatal period. Usually, a euthyroid state, but which may ultimately raise both T_3 and T_4 levels for several weeks.
5. *Moderate or high levels* in compensated dysfunction of the thyroid (5 to 10 μIU/mL). Levels may become excessively high prior to failure in risk patients (goiter, chronic lymphocytic thyroiditis, after thyroidectomy or ablation of the thyroid by x-ray or radioactive iodine).

TSH LOW NORMAL OR DECREASED IN:

1. *Secondary hypothyroidism.* An important condition to distinguish since secondary hypothyroidism almost always requires adrenal replacement as well. ACTH should also be evaluated. If only the thyroid dysfunction is treated, the patient may well go into adrenal crisis.

2. *Multinodular goiter.* On rare occasions elevations do occur.
3. *Overdosage* with thyroid replacement hormone.

Patient Preparation. No special preparation is necessary.

8.3.7 Thyroid Suppression Test

Synonym: T_3 suppression

Normal Response

TSH levels suppress below basal value

T_4 will suppress to less than 50% basal value

Explanation of the Test. The test is based on the principle that in hyperthyroidism thyroid production and release is autonomous and will continue to manufacture hormone despite the administration of oral T_3 (the most active metabolic form of the hormone) in a standard dose daily over 1 week's time. It is a useful test in confirming the diagnosis of borderline hyperthyroidism. It is less used now than in the past because of the availability of T_3 RIA and TRF tests, which help define borderline cases and cause no danger to the patient. Administration of T_3 is not advised in the elderly, particularly those with cardiac disease, or any person with cardiac disease, or high plasma thyroid. If done, extreme caution must be used.

FAILURE TO SUPPRESS OCCURS IN:

Primary hyperthyroidism (e.g., multinodular goiter, Graves' disease).

Patient Preparation. No special preparation is necessary.

8.3.8 Thyrotropin Releasing Factor Test

Synonyms: TRH; TRF; thyrotropic releasing hormone; TSH stimulation test

Normal Ranges:

Prompt rise in TSH, peaking in 15–30 min

Women	Peak value: 16–26 μIU/mL from base of 6 μIU/mL
Men	Slightly lower

(Serum T_3 increases 70% above baseline 1 to 4 hr after test, but is not usually measured)

Explanation of the Test. The principle on which this test is based is that TRF controls pituitary production of TSH. It is therefore primarily a pituitary stimulation test. The test is done to differentiate between hypothalamic and pituitary insufficiency in the patient with hypothyroidism and low TSH. An intact pituitary will respond by increasing TSH when TRF is given.

The test supplants the T_3 suppression test in many laboratories, as the outcomes compare well with that test and avoids the administration of T_3, which can be dangerous in the elderly, those with cardiac disease, or in those with already high levels of circulating thyroid hormone.

NO RESPONSE IN:

1. *Hypothyroidism due to pituitary failure.*
2. *Hyperthyroidism due to functional autonomy of the thyroid,* as in toxic goiter.

RESPONSE LESS THAN NORMAL IN:

1. *Patients who have been withdrawn* from long-term thyroid therapy for a considerable time.
2. *Patients who have been on prolonged administration* of corticosteroids, *L*-dopa, or aspirin.
3. *Persons with multinodular goiter.*
4. *Euthyroid persons post-treatment* of Graves' disease.

NORMAL RESPONSE IN:

1. *Primary hyperthyroidism.*
2. *Hypothyroidism due to deficiency,* but not absence of pituitary or hypothalamic function. The peak will most likely be delayed by 45 to 90 min.

Patient Preparation. No special preparation is necessary.

8.3.9 Thyroid Circulating Antibody Tests

A. Antimicrosomal antibody

Synonyms: microsomal antibody; antithyroid microsomal antibody
Normal Range: 0–100

B. Antithyroglobin antibody titer

> *Synonyms:* Thyroid auto-antibody; TAA
>
> *Normal Range:* 0–20

Explanation of the Tests. There is strong evidence that the immunologic system plays a role in Hashimoto's disease (thyroiditis) and in Graves' disease. Such immunologic traits are definitely genetic in Hashimoto's disease and the probability is for genetic etiology in Graves' disease. The immunoglobulins produced are thought to be antibody to the TSH receptor. Some of the antibodies have been identified and are fairly widely known, such as the long-acting thyroid stimulator (LATS), LATS-protector (LATS-P), and human thyroid stimulator. [LATS at one time was thought to be implicated in the exophthalamos of Graves' disease; that belief is now uncertain at best (Soll and Cohen, 1978).] Four separate organ-specific antigen-antibody systems have been identified in human thyroiditis.

The two tests listed above help diagnose the autoimmune thyroid conditions, which also include lymphadenoid goiter, and can be useful in following treatment responses. Several different types or organ-specific autoantibodies exist in almost all patients with thyroid disease, and some nonsymptomatic, but genetically related, individuals. Extremely high titers are inconsistent with most thyroid diagnoses other than Hashimoto's thyroiditis, Graves' disease, and lymphadenoid goiter. Lymph node enlargement and lymphocytosis are frequent concomitant signs occurring with Graves' disease which reinforce its autoimmune origin.

HIGH TITERS OCCUR IN:

Hashimoto's and Graves' diseases, primarily.

LOW TITERS OCCUR IN:

1. *Almost all thyroid disorders* and in some nonaffected but related persons. The elevations are due principally to an increase in antithyroglobulin antibody.
2. *Some patients with pernicious anemia* and myasthenia gravis, with some regularity, and without evidence of thyroid dysfunction. Over 50% of all patients with pernicious anemia tested demonstrated detectable thyroid antibodies (Seigler, 1978).
3. *Approximately 10% of all persons with juvenile-onset diabetes.*

4. *Patients with primary myxedema* (hypothyroidism), primarily of the antithyroid antibody.

Patient Preparation. No special preparation is necessary.

8.4 THE PANCREAS

The pancreas functions in a dual role, one of which is endocrine and produces the hormones glucagon and insulin, and which is the focus of this section. The second role is as an exocrine organ, producing digestive enzymes (amylase, lipase, and trypsin), which is discussed in Chapter 10.

8.4.1 Laboratory and Clinical Indications of Pancreatic Endocrine Dysfunction

A. Hyposecretion of insulin

(Hyperglycemia may be due to other than the direct effect of decreased insulin, but insulin change is the major offender.)

Laboratory Findings. Fasting serum glucose more than 110 mg/dL, or 2 hr postprandial (p.p.) between 120 and 140 mg/dL; glycosuria occurring in the presence of "normal" fasting blood sugar (FBS); glycosuria or hyperglycemia with stress (surgery, trauma, stroke, MI, adrenal steroid administration; hyperlipoproteinemia (lactescent serum); ketonuria; increased serum cholesterol; increased serum uric acid; presence of gallstones (cholelithiasis); presence of Charcot joint (a neuropathic arthropathy with degeneration of bone and cartilage of a joint with hypertrophic changes at the joint edge, causing deformity and instability of the joint; found most commonly in diabetic polyneuritis, syringomyelia, and tabes dorsalis).

Clinical Findings. Other than the most obvious signs and symptoms of polyuria, polydipsia, and polyphagia, there are: family history of diabetes mellitus; personal history of hypoglycemia, vascular disease, pruritis, and/or impotence; in females having been pregnant or borne children or a history of spontaneous abortion, toxemia, hydramnios, or congenital defects in an infant; in adults: obesity, orthostatic hypotension; eye changes—cataracts, retinopathy; frequent infections; vascular disease (peripheral, coronary, or cerebral); sensory changes primarily in the feet or hands (glove and stocking); plantar abcesses; peridontal disease.

B. Hypersecretion of insulin

(Hypoglycemia may be due to other than the direct effect of increased insulin, but insulin change is the major offender.)

Laboratory Findings. Serum glucose less than 60 mg/dL (by more recent and liberal standards less than 46 mg/dL is the criterion), either fasting or p.p. Can occur in infants or adults; usually transient when postprandial.

Clinical Findings. *Infants:* risk groups include low birthweight; diabetic mother; many hereditary conditions, such as galactosemia. *Adults:* signs and symptoms related to increased epinephrine release, frequently postprandial (e.g., hunger, nervousness, feelings of anxiety, tachycardia); signs and symptoms related to CNS response (e.g., decreased attention span, headache, bizarre behavior, convulsions). Although an individual patient may have any or all of the possible signs and symptoms, the same set of symptoms tend to recur in the same individual.

8.4.2 Glycosylated Hemoglobin

Synonyms: total fast Hb, HbA_{1c}

Normal Range: 4.82–5.09% of total hemoglobin

Explanation of the Test. HbA_{1c} is a minor component of hemoglobin (Hb) found in normal individuals, but elevated two- to threefold in patients with diabetes mellitus. The component increases at a slow and constant rate in response to physiologic occurrences of hyperglycemia during the 120-day life span of the red cell. Measurement of the component provides a picture of the state of hyperglycemia over time in the individual (the life span of the red blood cell), and correlates with glucose intolerance in diabetics. With good diabetic control the concentration of HbA_{1c} returns to the normal range, as the RBCs with increased concentrations die off.

The test is based on the principle that the individual red cell accumulates more and more HbA_{1c} throughout its life span, and that increased glycosylation reaction occurs in the diabetic person. This accelerated reaction in diabetics may not only help evaluate the effectiveness of their therapeutic control, it may in time supplant blood, urine glucose determinations, and glucose tolerance tests. It may also prove to be a tool to help understand the basic pathogenesis of diabetes. Relationships have already been shown in the literature between the increase of HbA_{1c} and basement membrane thickening, functional abnormalities of leukocytes and platelets, and the increased incidence of infection, lipoproteinemia, and thrombotic complications in diabetics (Peterson et al., 1977; Koenig et al., 1976, 1977; Coller et al., 1978).

The total fast hemoglobin (Hb) test measures all three components: HbA_{1a}, HbA_{1b}, HbA_{1c}. Some laboratories use this more complex test. However, most use the HbA_{1c}. HbA_{1c} assays the substance of the single hemoglobin component peak, that of HbA_{1c}, instead of all three components.

HbA_{1c} INCREASED IN:

Hyperglycemia. There appear to be no other conditions that are reflected by an increase in HbA_{1c}.

HbA_{1c} DECREASED IN:

Hemolytic states due to loss of hemoglobin rather than actual decreased production (see "Hemoglobin Decreased in" in Section 2.1.2).

Patient Preparation. No special preparation is required.

8.4.3 Glucose Tolerance Tests

Synonyms: oral glucose tolerance test: GTT; intravenous glucose tolerance test: GTT, IV; IVGTT

Normal Ranges: the glucose curves of both tests are very similar; IVGTT tends to have a higher 30 min concentration than does the oral

	Serum	Blood, Whole[a]
Adult		
Fasting	60–110 mg/dL	60–100 mg/dL
30 min	110–160 mg/dL[b]	Less than 160
(IVGTT)	110–200 mg/dL	Less than 170 mg/dL
1 hr	90–150 mg/dL	Less than 145
2–6 hr	60–110 mg/dL	Less than 120
Senior adult	Add 1 mg/dL/yr over age 50 to each nonfasting value	
Urine	Glycosuria may occur at 30 min; negative at other sampling times	

[a]Whole blood determinations are approximately 15% less in glucose concentration than serum or plasma (Conn and Conn, 1979).

[b]30-min concentrations can rise as high as 300 to 400 mg/dL. The height of the curve has little or no significance (Ravel, 1979).

TABLE 8.1 *Criteria for diagnosis of chemical diabetes by oral glucose tolerance*

	Plasma glucose (mg/dL)	Diagnostic criteria
Fajans and Conn[a]—1.75 g/kg	1-hr > 185 1½-hr > 160 2-hr > 140	All three values abnormal
United States Public Health Service (USPHS), Wilkerson[b]—100 g	Fasting > 130 = 1 point 1-hr > 195 = ½ point 2-hr > 140 = ½ point 3-hr > 130 = 1 point	Two points or more
O'Sullivan and Mahon[c] (for use in pregnancy)—100 g	Fasting > 110 1-hr > 195 2-hr > 175 3-hr > 150	Two or more values abnormal
ADA (American Diabetes Association)[d]—40 g/m[b]	Fasting > 115 1-hr > 185 1½-hr > 165 2-hr > 140	Elevated fasting or all three post-test values abnormal
Danowski: Glucose tolerance sum[e]—1.75 g/kg	*Venous whole blood*	Sum = fasting + 1 hr + 2 hr + 3 hr *Adults* / *Children* Normal <450 / <450 Borderline 450–700 / 450–700 Diabetic >700 / >650
Seltzer:[f] for children—1.75 g/kg	*Capillary whole blood* Fasting > 115 1-hr > 175 2-hr > 140 3-hr > 125	Elevated fasting or two of three post-test values abnormal

[a]*Ann. N.Y. Acad. Sci.,* 82 (1959), 208.
[b]*J. Chronic Dis.,* 13 (1961), 6.
[c]*Diabetes,* 13 (1964), 278.
[d]*Diabetes,* 18 (1969), 299.
[e]*Metabolism,* 22 (1973), 295.
[f]*In Diabetes Mellitus: Theory and Practice,* M. Ellenberg and H. Rifkin, eds. (New York: McGraw-Hill, 1970), p. 480.

Source: Joseph C. Shipp, and Fred C. Lovrien, "Diabetes Mellitus," in Howard F. Conn, and Rex B. Conn, eds. *Current Diagnosis 5* (Philadelphia: W. B. Saunders Company, 1977), p. 734.

Interpretation of the Tests. Most of the criteria for glucose tolerance tests are based on data from measurements of whole blood glucose. The test as given here is that done on serum glucose. Serum and plasma glucose are the more often used. There are therefore small changes in comparative glucose values which can confuse understanding of results. There are many different measurement systems, each of which has differing criteria for a diagnosis of diabetes mellitus to be made. Table 8.1 provides some clarification of this subject. The reader should determine the method and criteria used in his or her facility.

Explanation of the Tests. Glucose tolerance tests are provocative, or stimulating tests, in which large doses of glucose are given, orally or by IV, and the rise and fall (the "curve") of the blood glucose, and in many cases urine glucose, are checked at timed intervals. The assumption is that the decrease that occurs after the initial rise of the blood glucose level is due to stimulation and release of insulin by the induced hyperglycemia. The diabetic, having either inadequate or ineffective insulin, will show a "typical diabetic curve"; that is, the blood glucose elevation is prolonged and will not return to fasting levels in the expected 1 to 2 hr. A "flat" curve has also been noted [blood glucose rise of less than 25 mg/dL above fasting blood sugar (FBS) level], but no specific significance is attached to it; it may well be normal (Henry, 1979).

Unfortunately, the GTT, although very sensitive, lacks specificity. A wide number of diseases and other variables such as diet cause abnormal responses–diabetic curves. Therefore, interpretation, to be accurate, must control the variables and retest those with interferring disease when the disease is quiescent or cured, if at all possible. The American Diabetes Association (ADA) has developed standardized conditions under which the procedure must be performed for accuracy (see "Patient Preparation and Test Procedure" below). It must be recognized that any variation from the procedural conditions, or the presence of an interfering disease, will produce widely varied results which cannot be accurately interpreted.

The most widely used of the two tests is the oral method. The IVGTT is felt to be a poor method for estimating glucose disposal, but it does have the advantage of overcoming variability of glucose absorption found in the oral method. The IVGTT may be used when the results of the oral test are uncertain.

Because it is a provocative test, the GTT has been used to identify early diabetes mellitus. However, some authorities feel that the diagnosis is too often incorrect and that the delay in diagnosis does not affect morbidity from the disease. They, in fact, recommend abandoning the test because of its questionable outcomes and potential for misdiagnosis. Some suggest it be used only in the management of obese or pregnant patients; to provide stimulus for weight reduction in the one, and to improve the rate of fetal survival for gestational diabetics in the other (Henry, 1979).

DECREASED GLUCOSE TOLERANCE FOUND IN (DIABETIC-TYPE CURVE):

1. *Diabetes mellitus,* assuming that all variables are controlled.
2. *Physiologic conditions* such as:
   a. Inadequate carbohydrate intake prior to the test; more than 150 g is necessary for accurate testing conditions in persons

of normal bodyweight (not obese) due to peripheral resistance to insulin secondary to increases in growth hormone (GH) and catecholamine output.

b. Increased age. Otherwise, normal individuals' GTT will increase approximately 1 mg/dL/yr or 7 mg/dL/decade from ages 20 to 80. The degree of the abnormality is not severe enough to affect the fasting serum glucose.
c. Inactivity–bedrest.
d. Obesity.
e. Fever.
f. Diurnal variation with decreased carbohydrate tolerance in the afternoon and normal tolerance in the morning.
g. Emotional stress, probably due to catecholamine release and steroid glyconeogenesis.
h. Pregnancy, due to increased estrogen and progesterone levels; the mechanism is unclear. IVGTT is normal.
i. Race. Oriental races have significantly higher glucose levels than either white or black races.

3. *Individuals receiving a number of different drugs* (e.g., xanthines, nicotine); diuretics, especially thiazides, furosemide, and ethacrynic acid; hormones (oral contraceptives–adrenal corticol steroids–excessive thyroid dosage); nicotinic acid; chlorpromazine; diphylhydantoid (Dilantin); sympathomimetic amines (epinephrine, ephredrine, most decongestants); diazoxide (Hyperstat) and salicylates.

4. *Other diseases,* such as:

   a. Adrenal, thyroid, and pituitary dysfunctions due to hormonal influence on tissue response to changes in serum glucose concentrations; for example:
      (1) Cushing's syndrome, due to increased gluconeogenesis.
      (2) Pheochromocytoma, due to epinephrine production increase.
      (3) Primary aldosteronism, due to potassium (K^+) depletion, which affects pancreatic beta-cell response to hyperglycemia, mechanism unknown. This mechanism relates also to thiazide's effect on glucose tolerance (item 3, above).
      (4) Hyperthyroidism with variable effect, and without relation to the severity of the hyperthyroidism, due in part to increased glucose absorption. The IVGTT is normal.
      (5) Hypothyroidism with variable effect, from a diabetic curve to a "flat" oral GTT.

(6) Hyperpituitarism, especially acromegaly, due to increased GH.

b. Pancreatitis; abnormal GTT extremely common due to beta-cell dysfunction.
c. Chronic renal disease with azotemia, reason not known.
d. Cerebral lesions, mechanisms not known, possibly due to the presence of a medullary glucose regulation center that is injured.
e. Severe carbon monoxide poisoning, due to direct cerebral effect.
f. Malignancies, may be due to secondary effects of the malignancy (e.g., fever, starvation, inactivity or liver dysfunction).
g. Liver disease (e.g., cirrhosis). GTT abnormality correlates with the severity of the disease, due to the amount of disruption of glucose homeostasis.
h. Stressful or stress-related conditions such as myocardial infarct (MI), surgery, "strokes."

INCREASED GLUCOSE TOLERANCE IN (FLAT CURVE):

1. *Some cases of hypothyroidism.*
2. *Any condition that decreases glucose absorption* from the GI tract (e.g., severe diarrhea–infectious or stress-related).
3. *The black race,* who tend to have lower glucose values than the white race.
4. *Idiopathic.*

Patient Preparation and Test Procedure

1. *Diet pretest* should contain adequate carbohydrate (CHO). May be prepared with a 3-day high-CHO diet. If patient is not eating or is vomiting, test should be delayed.
2. *Screen for any illness present,* or present during preceding 2 weeks.
3. *NPO other than water* 8 to 12 hr prior to the test.
4. *Done in morning*–7 to 9 A.M.–normalize diurnal rhythm.
5. *Ambulatory* but without even mild exercise prior to the test–normalize decreased glucose tolerance due to inactivity. At rest 30 min before first sample taken.

6. *No eating, drinking, or smoking* during test, (nicotine decreases GT).
7. *Fasting glucose sample taken,* and urine sample if it is to be tested.
8. *Glucose administered orally or IV.* Glucose load determined by formula, which varies with the facility. (ADA formula: 40 g/m^2 of body surface. This translates roughly to between 0.5 g/kg of body weight to 1.75 g/kg of body weight. Oral glucose load administered over 5 min; IV load over 30 min.)
9. *Blood specimens and urine specimens* (if required) collected at specified times (e.g., in 30 min, 1 hr, and hourly thereafter as long as required; see Table 8.1).
10. *If nausea, fainting, sweating,* or other indications of autonomic nervous system overstimulation occur, glucose specimen is drawn stat and the procedure terminated with carbohydrates and protein supplied stat. (Beware of hyperventilation, which can mimic hypoglycemia and terminate the test before it is valid.)
11. *The test is usually continued* for 4 hr, but can be more or less depending on the physician's requirements. Diabetic curves, as described previously, remain high—above fasting level—longer than normal. Hypoglycemic curves may be high or normal initially but eventually fall to low levels (e.g., less than 46 mg/dL).

8.4.4 Serum Insulin

Synonyms: plasma insulin; immunoreactive insulin; IRI; insulin assay

Normal Range: 4–24 microunits (μIU)/mL

Explanation of the Test. Insulin was the first substance successfully measured in radioisotope immunoassay. It is a small polypeptide hormone, produced by the pancreatic beta cells in response to increased blood glucose levels. During fasting states, serum insulin levels decline.

Serum insulin determinations are used as the diagnostic tool of choice in evaluating fasting hypoglycemia. They are of little value in diagnosis of postprandial (p.p.) or reactive hypoglycemia. Insulin concentrations may be more useful there in looking at groups of people, rather than individuals, because of the variability of normal response. Serum insulin is not used at present in the diagnosis of diabetes mellitus, probably for the same reason.

Insulin assay can be used with the glucose tolerance test (GTT), showing characteristic curves in given conditions (e.g., juvenile-onset diabetes mellitus, (JODM)—flat curve—little or no increase in insulin concentrations; mild diabetes—delayed rise in insulin). The insulin GTT has been found no more efficient than the serum glucose GTT in diagnosis of subclinical diabetes.

Ratio of insulin to glucose (IRI/G). The insulin/glucose ratio is important in defining inappropriate insulin secretions and may be the most valid use of insulin assay. The normal ratio is usually less than 0.30 μIU of insulin to 1 mg of glucose in normal, nonobese, fasting individuals. In obese persons the ratio is abnormal if greater than 0.3 μIU compared to a serum glucose below 60 mg/dL. Inappropriate insulin secretion is most often due to the presence of an insulinoma [a pancreatic beta (islet) cell tumor]. Even with an insulinoma, actual insulin serum concentrations may be within the normal range. They will be excessively high for the degree of hypoglycemia present, however, which demonstrates the usefulness of the IRI/G.

Insulin secretion from normal beta cells is at basal level (4 μIU/mL) in the presence of hypoglycemia in the normal person. When glucose concentrations decline to a value of 30 mg/dL, insulin levels cannot be detected by RIA. Thus in making the equation for the IRI/G, a value of 30 mg/dL is subtracted from the glucose level. The IRI/G is then calculated by this formula (Henry, 1979):

$$\frac{100 \times \text{insulin level } (\mu\text{IU/mL})}{\text{glucose (mg/dL)} - 30 \text{ mg/dL}} = \frac{\text{IRI}}{\text{G}}$$

SERUM INSULIN LEVELS DECREASED IN:

1. *Juvenile-onset diabetes mellitus* (JODM) and may be nondetectable.
2. *Adult-onset diabetes mellitus* (AODM).
3. *Obesity.* The decrease may be relative, however, not necessarily an absolute deficiency: that is, the insulin is low in comparison to the amount of glucose present; the insulin/glucose ratio is out of balance.
4. *Some persons being treated with insulin* for a period greater than 6 weeks. The formation of insulin antibodies interferes by competing with insulin antibodies used in the RIA test. Depending on the method used for testing, the insulin level can be either falsely decreased or falsely increased (see below).

SERUM INSULIN LEVELS INCREASED IN:

1. *Insulinoma,* insulin-producing tumor. Such tumors can produce insulin to a concentration of 20 to 30 μIU/mL when serum glucose is less than 50 mg/dL (inappropriate insulin secretion).
2. *Conditions causing reactive hypoglycemia*—postprandial—such as:
   a. Early diabetes, mild adult-onset diabetes.
   b. Alimentary hypoglycemia, most frequently found after gastric surgery.
   c. Idiopathic (functional) hypoglycemia. Insulin secretory patterns vary widely in these conditions and may be normal despite hypoglycemic symptoms. May be due to early, subclinical diabetes, an alimentary disorder, or psychologic problems, in which case the symptoms are usually due to stress response rather than true hypoglycemia. A combination of causes can also occur (Permutt, 1980).

      Idiopathic hypoglycemia of childhood is often considered a separate nonreactive hypoglycemia.
   d. Abrupt termination of prolonged glucose infusion.
   e. Following ingestion of alcohol. Alcohol can potentiate hypoglycemia, even in normal subjects.
3. *Persons being treated with insulin* for a period greater than 6 weeks. Insulin antibodies developed in the body may not be distinguished from those used in the insulin RIA test (see "Serum Insulin Levels Decreased in" above, item 4).

Patient Preparation. NPO except for water for 8 hr prior to blood sampling.

8.4.5 Tolbutamide Tolerance Test

Synonyms: insulin tolerance; orinase diagnostic; TTT; insulin stimulation

Normal Ranges

Maximum fall of serum glucose at 30 to 45 min, usually to slightly higher than 50% of FBS level.

Serum glucose returns to fasting, basal values in 1½ to 3 hr.

Serum insulin decreases to basal level (4 μIU/mL) or lower depending on the degree of hypoglycemia.

Explanation of the Test. Tolbutamide (Orinase) is a sulfonylurea drug that apparently stimulates insulin production from the pancreatic beta cells. The drug is used therapeutically in the treatment of many cases of adult-onset diabetes mellitus (AODM), in which pancreatic function exists but is reduced. In this test it is used to stimulate insulin secretion, the levels and effects of which can be measured. The test is thought by some to be one of the more specific tests for diabetes mellitus. Others feel there exist too many false-positive responses. The TTT has been found to be somewhat less sensitive than the oral GTT. The TTT has been used most frequently in determining the presence of insulinoma. Manifestations of inappropriate insulin release are exaggerated in response to tolbutamide. Diagnostic criteria for the presence of an insulinoma are: serum glucose decreased more than 65%, or to less than 30 mg/dL; glucose depression persisting up to 2 hr or longer; serum insulin levels increased beyond upper limits of normal (over 24 μIU/mL) (Henry, 1979). The persistence of the hypoglycemia is thought more diagnostic than its level of decrease, and the decrease frequently persists over 3 hr.

The test process begins with a FBS sample taken and 1 g of a special water-soluble tolbutamide given rapidly by IV. The response to the tolbutamide stimulus is followed by taking blood samples for glucose and/or insulin determinations every 15 min for the first hour and every 30 min thereafter. The test is discontinued when severe hypoglycemic symptoms occur and IV glucose is administered to reverse the process. (*Caution:* Differentiate between hypoglycemia symptoms and symptoms due to hyperventilation.)

Diabetic response is identified by a diminished response to the tolbutamide. Maximum serum glucose decreases are also delayed, occurring after 45 min. There is, however, considerable overlap between mild diabetic and normal response.

FALSE-POSITIVE RESPONSES OCCUR IN:

1. *Functional hypoglycemia,* although the blood glucose returns to 80% of normal in 3 hr.
2. *Adrenal insufficiency* with an initial decrease as low as that in insulinoma, but the serum glucose returns to 80% of normal in 3 hr.
3. *Some types of liver disease,* although the occurrence is rare. The pattern is very similar to that of an insulinoma.
4. *Obese individuals.*
5. *Conditions of starvation and alcoholism.*

FALSE-NEGATIVE RESPONSES OCCUR IN:

Approximately 50% of patients with insulinomas.

Patient Preparation

1. *A high-carbohydrate diet* (150 to 300 g/day) for 3 days prior to the test.
2. *NPO except for water* for 8 hr prior to the test.
3. *No smoking, drinking, or eating* for the duration of the test.
4. *Physician should administer the tolbutamide* and supervise during the test, assuming responsibility for the effects of the tolbutamide.
5. *The test is not used,* or used with extreme caution in the last trimester of pregnancy, with individuals having a history of heart disease, in the elderly, and in many severe acute illnesses, or chronic disease. Hypoglycemia resulting from IV tolbutamide can be fatal.

8.5 THE PARATHYROID GLANDS

8.5.1 Laboratory and Clinical Indications of Parathyroid Dysfunction

A. Hyperfunction

Laboratory Findings. Serum calcium increased (serum calcium and phosphorus are often found in screening tests; see SMA-12 Survey Model in Table 1.3). Decreased serum inorganic phosphate, uric acid may increase, increased alkaline phosphatase; BUN, hematology normal (anemia may occur and BUN increase with long-standing hyperfunction). Urine calcium increased in 24-hr sample—hypercalciuria.

Clinical Findings. Many nonspecific and variable findings. (Clinical pearl: bones, groans, stones, psychiatric overtones.) Hypertension; recent weight loss; dry skin; mental changes (depression, anxiety, emotional lability); neurological changes (increased fatigability, proximal muscle weakness, hypotonia, slight to moderate muscle wasting, hyperreflexia, loss of vibratory sense in the feet); if on digitalis, incidence of intoxication increased; renal symptoms (polyuria, nocturia, renal colic with renal stones); polydipsia; skeletal symptoms (bone pain, joint pain, tooth loss, bone cysts, arthritis, arthralgia); may have symptoms of peptic ulcer.

B. Hypofunction

Laboratory Findings. Serum calcium decreased; increased serum inorganic phosphorus; BUN and total protein or serum albumin normal (important to differential diagnosis). Other pertinent tests: Normal serum magnesium (Mg). Urine calcium decreased (hypocalciuria).

Clinical Findings. Increased muscle tone and irritability—may be slight or overt. Latent symptoms: elicited spasm (Chvostek's sign: twitching of facial muscle when facial nerve is tapped; Trousseau's sign: carpopedal spasm with inflation of blood pressure cuff above systolic pressure for 3 min); early symptoms = neuromuscular irritability, feelings of "needles and pins" in extremities or circumoral, twitching, muscle spasms causing laryngeal stridor, dysphagia, wheezing (bronchospasm), carpopedal spasm, photophobia, blepharospasm. General symptoms: lenticular cataracts common, skin coarse, scaley, may have patches of brown pigmentation, exfoliative dermatitis. Fingernails brittle, horizontally ridged. Moniliasis common. ECG if done may show prolonged ST segment. In infants and young children, teeth may be hypoplastic with enamel deficits. Presenting symptom may be bowed legs only.

8.5.2 Serum Calcium

Synonyms: Ca, serum; calcium, total serum

Normal Ranges

Adult (less than 50 years)	9.0–10.5 mg/dL
Senior adult (over 50 years)	8.5–10.5 mg/dL
Pediatric	9.5–11.5 mg/dL
Newborn	7.5–13.9 mg/dL
Infant	9.0–11.0 mg/dL

Explanation of the Test. This measurement of serum calcium includes both the active fraction (ionized calcium), approximately 50% of total calcium, and the inactive fraction bound to protein, also about 50% of total. The serum levels then are dependent in part on the serum levels of protein, particularly albumin. When calcium concentration decreases secondary to a decrease in serum protein, tetany rarely occurs, since such a decrease involves only the metabolically inactive fraction, or bound calcium. Ionized serum calcium (Ca^{2+}) levels are not affected. An increase in total protein (as in some cases of multiple myeloma or sarcoidosis) will increase the total serum calcium but will not significantly alter the amount of ionized calcium present. Therefore, it is important to know the total protein values of serum in order to interpret results of total serum calcium tests.

Calcium levels are regulated and influenced by several things, the major regulator being parathyroid hormone (PTH). Increased amounts of PTH will increase serum calcium levels. If renal function is normal, an increase in serum calcium levels will be accompanied by a decrease in serum inorganic phosphate, and vice versa.

SERUM CALCIUM INCREASED IN:

1. *Primary hyperparathyroidism,* due to (in order of frequency of occurrence) single parathyroid adenoma, multiple adenomas, and hyperplasia.
2. *Conditions causing increased concentrations of total protein/albumin* (a fairly rare occurrence), such as multiple myeloma, sarcoidosis.
3. *Conditions causing increased bony resorption* (osteoclasis), such as (a) invasive bone disease; (b) disuse atrophy of bone; (c) osteoporosis or osteomalacia. Over time the presence of increased serum calcium can also *cause* so-called "renal rickets," leading to osteoporosis and osteomalacia.
4. *Excess intake of vitamin A,* which increases bone resorption.
5. *Excess intake or absorption of vitamin D,* which increases calcium absorption from the gut.
6. *Carcinoma with metastases to the bone,* particularly in the elderly, due to increased bony breakdown.
7. *Carcinoma with PTH-like production from the tumor* (ectopic PTH syndrome), found most frequently in cancers of the lung.
8. *Milk-alkali syndrome* (Burnett's syndrome), due to intensive antacid therapy and milk ingestion. Infrequent cause now.
9. *Physiologic causes* such as dehydration (relative increase) or prolonged use of a tourniquet when drawing blood (hemoconcentration).

SERUM CALCIUM DECREASED IN:

1. *Hypoparathyroidism.* Primary—due to postthyroidectomy, temporary probably due to gland injury, or permanent due to total removal, and due to idiopathic cause—hereditary, rare. Secondary—severe hypomagnesemia, which decreases body tissues' ability to respond to PTH and ultimately parathyroid loss of

capacity to produce/release PTH; other causes of secondary hypoparathyroidism include postirradiation; hypoalbuminemia (nephrotic syndrome, starvation, cachexia, celiac disease, cystic fibrosis of the pancreas); chronic renal disease with uremia and/or azotemia with phosphate retention and decreased production of the active metabolite of vitamin D by the kidney; vitamin D-deficiency rickets (rickets of childhood); De Fanconi syndrome, due to renal tubular defect; and hyperinsulinism.

2. *Conditions causing increased osteoblastic* (bone building) *activity,* such as with healing of fractures.
3. *Physiologic conditions,* such as recumbent posture; insufficient ingestion of calcium or vitamin D (late pregnancy).
4. *Neonates whose mothers have hyperparathyroidism,* due to suppression of fetal parathyroid activity.
5. *Individuals on long-term therapy with phenytoin* (Dilantin) by increasing metabolic inactivaton of vitamin D.

Patient Preparation. Depending on the laboratory being used, there may be no special preparaton, or the patient may be required to fast for 12 hr prior to the test. In either case it is important that the blood sample be removed with minimal venous stasis and/or hemolysis.

8.5.3 Serum Calcium, Ionized

Synonyms: Ca, I; Ca^{2+}; Ca^{++}

Normal Ranges

Adult	1.90–2.25 mEq/L at pH 7.5 and 37°C
Child	2.10–2.60 mEq/L

Explanation of the Test. Measurement of this relatively stable, metabolically active fraction of serum calcium is believed to be a better indicator of calcium metabolism than total serum calcium and is not influenced by changes in total protein or serum albumin levels. Ionized calcium fraction is pH-dependent, however, whereas protein-bound calcium is not. (Increase in pH = decrease in ionized calcium, and vice versa.) Very slight variations in serum pH will produce changes in ionized calcium concentrations (e.g., hyperventilation sufficient to increase serum pH 0.1 to 0.2 pH units of blood pH will cause up to a 10% decrease in ionized calcium concentration) (Henry, 1979).

This test is more specific for metabolically active calcium than the total serum calcium test.

SERUM CALCIUM INCREASED IN:

1. *All conditions listed under total serum calcium except* those related to increased serum total protein or albumin concentrations.
2. *Acidotic conditions* (e.g., diabetic ketoacidosis, hyperosmolar nonketotic acidosis, respiratory acidosis, renal acidosis).

SERUM CALCIUM DECREASED IN:

1. *All conditions listed under total serum calcium except* those related to decreased serum total protein or albumin concentrations.
2. *Alkalotic conditions,* metabolic or respiratory, which cause ionized serum calcium to become bound to protein in greater concentrations.
3. *Serum samples exposed to air* or allowed to stand.

Patient Preparation. As for total serum calcium.

8.5.4 Serum Phosphorus

Synonyms: inorganic phosphorus; phosphate

Normal Ranges

Adult	2.3–4.3 mg/dL
Pediatric	4.0–7.0 mg/dL
Newborn	3.5–8.6 mg/dL
Infants	4.5–6.7 mg/dL
Child	4.5–5.5 mg/dL
Thereafter	2.5–4.8 mg/dL

Explanation of the Test. Under optimum conditions ionized calcium and serum phosphorus exist in a reciprocal balance. Increases in calcium due to increased release of PTH result in decreases of serum inorganic phosphorus, and vice versa. The balance is evidently maintained by selective reabsorption or filtration and excretion of phosphorus by the renal tubules under the influence of PTH. Excretion is also increased or decreased by the level of calcium mobilization from other causes. The excretion of phosphorus is referred to as a phosphate diuresis (Kagan, 1979).

SERUM PHOSPHORUS INCREASED IN:

1. *Any chronic renal failure,* most commonly chronic glomerulonephritis.
2. *Hypoparathyroidism,* primary or secondary (see serum total calcium decreased in), due to increased renal reabsorption of phosphate.
3. *Prolonged or massive administration* of antacids, vitamin D, heparin, tetracycline, pituitrin, and Methicillin.
4. In growth hormone excess (e.g., gigantism).

SERUM PHOSPHORUS DECREASED IN:

1. *See* "Serum Calcium increased in" in Section 8.5.2.
2. *Women during menstrual periods.*
3. *Periods immediately following meals.*
4. *Persons receiving aluminum hydroxide, epinephrine, insulin,* or after having had a general anesthesia.

Patient Preparation. NPO except for water for 8 hr prior to taking blood sample.

8.5.5 Parathyroid Hormone

Synonyms: PTH; parathormone

Two tests are now in more general use than any others and use the two most available antisera (see Table 8.2). The parathyroids secrete intact hormone, which is metabolized into smaller fragments. The following tests react with two of these smaller fragments: N-terminal amine PTH, which is thought to be metabolically active but is rapidly cleared from the system; C-terminal PTH, an inactive fragment. An ionized Ca^{2+} test is often done at the same time as the PTH.

Explanation of the Test. Both of these tests are done by RIA. The direct measurement of PTH is relatively new, at least in terms of being clinically available. Theoretically, the test should differentiate

TABLE 8.2 *Tests for parathyroid hormone*

Test name	Reacts with:	Recommended usage	Normal range
C-terminal PTH	C-terminal carboxyl PTH (anti-C)	Conditions causing gradual changes in PTH, or chronic overproduction; measures long-duration hormone	From less than 150 to 375 pg Eq/mL; values under 150 are not detectable by this method
Intact PTH	Terminal amine PTH (anti-N)	Conditions causing acute changes in PTH secretion, or when samples are taken from selective venous catheterization (neck veins); measures long-duration PTH	163–347 pg Eq/mL; this normal depends on the serum total calcium level: it is inversely correlated with serum total calcium

Source: Data from SHMC, 1978, and Ravel, 1979.

parathyroid tumor from other causes of hypercalcemia by virtue of demonstrating increased PTH with increased serum calcium. Unfortunately, PTH assays are not yet specific enough or sensitive enough to be relied on totally. "Ectopic PTH" secreted by tumors not in the parathyroid gland cannot be distinguished from true PTH by this test. Other factors that confuse interpretation of results include "inappropriate" levels of PTH to serum calcium, neither being out of normal range, but one being inappropriately high or low compared to the other. Authorities are divided as to whether to consider such results as pathologic (Conn and Conn, 1979). Some laboratories prepare graphs or nomograms of the various antisera in relation to serum calcium levels to assist in that differentiation.

Another approach to determining whether PTH arises from an ectopic focus or from the parathyroid glands, which can also indicate the gland that is secreting excess hormone, involves catheterization of the small veins draining the parathyroids bilaterally. Blood samples are taken from each, proximally and distally, and a concentration gradient of PTH determined for each side. Normally, the gradient is higher at the proximal sites, lower at distal sites, and relatively equal on both sides. With a parathyroid adenoma the gradient is sharply increased on the side with the tumor (at least a fivefold difference) and diminished, or even absent, on the unaffected side (twofold or less difference) due to suppression of that gland by the increased circulating calcium. Interpretation of results from this approach is not yet totally standardized, however (Ravel, 1979).

Usefulness of PTH measurement is debatable at this point. If used, periodic reassay of equivocal results is suggested (Henry, 1979).

PTH INCREASED IN:

1. *Hyperparathyroidism,* due to parathyroid tumor or hyperplasia.
2. *Cross-reaction responses,* due to certain tumors which secrete a PTH-like substance, especially tumors of the lung (bronchus). Other sites include kidney, ovary, and colon.

PTH DECREASED IN:

1. *Post-thyroidectomy,* probably due to transient trauma to the parathyroid.
2. *Postparathyroidectomy:* intentional—for removal of a tumor or to control calcium levels in some forms of renal disease; accidental—with thyroidectomy.
3. *The morning hours,* due to the normal diurnal rhythm.

Patient Preparation:

1. *NPO except for water* for 8 hr prior to testing.
2. *Sample should be drawn* in the morning, as normals are usually calculated for that time.

8.5.6 Tubular Phosphate Reabsorption

Synonyms: TPR; parathyroid function test; tubular reabsorption of phosphate; TRP

Normal Ranges

TRP*	78 – 90%
Serum creatinine	0.7– 1.5 mg/dL
Serum phosphorus	2.3– 4.3 mg/dL
Creatinine clearance	70 – 130 mL clearance/min
Phosphate excretion index (PEI)	0±0.12%

*TRP is calculated using serum creatinine, serum phosphorus, and the creatinine clearance rate. A rough formula can approximate the process (Ravel, 1979):

$$\%TRP = \frac{\text{urine } PO_4 \text{ concentration} \times \text{serum creatinine concentration}}{\text{urine creatinine concentration} \times \text{serum } PO_4 \text{ concentration}} \times 100$$

Explanation of the Test. This is an indirect measurement of PTH by measuring its effect on phosphate reabsorption; it is done to help distinguish hypercalcemia due to hyperparathyroidism from that due to other etiologies by demonstrating the presence or absence of a phosphate diuresis. Normally, about two-thirds of dietary phosphate appears in the urine (5 to 15 mg/min) except when intake is low. Phosphate clearance and reabsorption is not solely under the control of PTH; serum calcium levels, potassium depletion, calcitonin secretion, changes in certain hormone levels (estrogen, adrenal steroids, GH), and renal defects also play roles.

Despite the many variables and related problems (inability to void, inability to completely empty the bladder, timing inaccuracies of sample collection) the TRP seems to be one of the better simple diagnostic tests for primary hyperparathyroidism.

The test can be done in two ways—using a 24-hr urine specimen or by taking an hourly sample. The 24-hr test is preferred by many facilities because it eliminates many of the inaccuracies inherent in the need for precise timing of the hourly test. However, the hourly test can be done more easily on an outpatient basis.

LOW TRP INDEX VALUES (LESS THAN 80%) OCCUR IN
(INCREASED SERUM PTH; INCREASED Ca^{2+}; DECREASED PO_4):

1. *Primary hyperparathyroidism.*
2. *Hypercalcemia,* due to PTH-secreting malignancy.
3. *Some patients with sarcoidosis or myeloma.*
4. *Five percent of patients with renal stones* but without parathyroid tumor.
5. *Serum elevations of estrogen or adrenal steroids,* due to disease or administration of the substances therapeutically. Administered calcium has the same effect.
6. *Renal defects* causing increased creatinine clearance. (The test is not reliable in the face of renal insufficiency.)

FALSE NORMAL TRP (OVER 80%) OCCUR IN
(DECREASED PTH; DECREASED Ca^{2+}; INCREASED PO_4–SERUM):

1. *Increased circulating levels of growth hormone or thyroid.*
2. *Prolonged heparin administration.*

Patient Preparation and Test Procedure

1. *Diet.* On normal phosphate (more than 500 mg/day and less than 3000 mg/day). Excessive amounts of coffee, tea, and meat to be avoided for 24 hr before the test.
2. *NPO other than water* for 8 hr prior to blood drawing with 24-hr urine specimen test. The patient is not required to be NPO the full 24 hr. NPO 8 to 12 hr prior to test, beginning with hourly test.
3. *24-hr test.* Follow usual procedure for 24-hr urine collection; urine specimen test. The patient is not required to be NPO the full taken. Sample can be drawn at any time during the 24 hr, but usually done as soon as possible for comfort of the patient.
4. *Hourly test.* Complete emptying of the bladder is essential with each urine collection. Timing of each step of the test must be accurate for the test to be reliable.
   a. Patient drinks two 8-oz glasses of water.
   b. One hour later bladder is emptied and another full glass of water is taken. Time of voiding must be noted exactly and lab notified. Urine discarded.
   c. One hour after first voiding, patient voids completely again and exact time is noted. Urine saved (in some facilities the urine is sent to the lab with each voiding; others are sent only at the end of the test). If urine volume less than 120 mL, test should be restarted. Full glass of water taken.
   d. One hour later (2 hr after first voiding), patient completely empties bladder, urine saved (exact time noted), drinks full glass of water, and a blood sample is taken.
   e. Again in 1 hr, patient voids completely, drinks a full glass of water, blood sample is taken, and the test is complete. All urine is examined for urine creatinine and phosphorus; blood sample examined for serum creatinine and phosphorus. Urine volume is also measured.

8.5.7 Urine Calcium

A. Calcium, qualitative, urine

> *Synonym:* Sulkowitch qualitative test, urine
>
> *Normal Range:* 1+ – 2+
>
> (also reported as negative, moderately positive, and strong positive)

Explanation of the Test. A substance called Sulkowitch reagent is used to test the urine for calcium, hence the test name. It is a quick, simple precipitation test that is relatively inexpensive and is often used instead of the more complex and costly urine calcium test, especially in medical offices and clinics.

Under normal conditions calcium is excreted in the urine at about 2.5 to 15 mEq/day. That output depends upon the intake of calcium, skeletal weight, and many endocrine factors. Given a normal physiologic state, with adequate calcium intake and adequate renal function, urine calcium concentrations reflect serum calcium levels. If serum calcium falls to 7.5 mg/dL or below, almost none is excreted in the urine.

URINE CALCIUM INCREASED IN:

1. *Physiologic conditions* such as concentrated urine.
2. *Hyperparathyroidism.*
3. *Conditions causing bony reabsorption* without repair, such as osteolytic bone disease and osteoporosis.
4. *Renal tubular acidosis.*
5. *Hyperthyroidism.*
6. *Vitamin D intoxication.*

URINE CALCIUM DECREASED IN:

1. *Physiologic conditions* such as dilute urine.
2. *Hypoparathyroidism.*
3. *Malabsorption disorders* such as steatorrhea, due to inadequate calcium or vitamin D absorption, even with normal intake.
4. *Vitamin D deficiency,* due to the need for the vitamin in the absorption of calcium in the gut.

Patient Preparation. No special preparation is necessary.

B. Urine calcium

Synonym: Ca, urine

Normal Range: 0.1–0.3 g/24 hr

Explanation of the Test. This is a quantitative test used when knowledge of the precise amount of calcium being excreted is important. It requires collection of a 24-hr urine specimen.

INCREASED IN/DECREASED IN:

Changes in values are the same as those given in the Sulkowitch test except that large amounts of phosphate in the urine can lower the values.

Patient Preparation

1. *Because a more precise measurement of calcium* is needed, the patient is usually placed on a controlled diet of 100 mg calcium for 3 days prior to testing.
2. *The 24-hr urine specimen container* should be kept at room temperature rather than refrigerated, to prevent insoluble calcium sediment from precipitating. The urine is preserved with 6 *N* HC1, a strong acid; caution in handling is advised.

8.5.8 Serum Magnesium/Urine Magnesium

Synonym: Mg

Normal Ranges

Serum	1.5–1.95 mEq/L
Urine	1.0–24.0 mEq/L

Explanation of the Test. This test fits equally well with a number of systems (neural, gastrointestinal), but is placed with the endocrine parathyroid section because deficiencies of the substance produce a tetany that cannot be differentiated from hypocalcemic tetany except by laboratory examination. Although the test itself is relatively expensive and not applicable to many other laboratory tests, the occurrence of magnesium deficiency in the hospitalized surgical patient is frequent enough to warrant attention being directed to it. Also of importance because of the increasing use of total parenteral nutrition (TPN)—hyperalimentation. Deficiencies occur more frequently than excesses.

Magnesium (Mg) is the second most plentiful intracellular cation after potassium. It works primarily as an activator of various enzymes and is essential to the preservation of DNA/RNA structure. It is absorbed in the intestine and excreted in the urine, so that defects in those systems can cause changes in the body's concentration of magnesium. Preservation of serum levels is accomplished by renal tubular reabsorption.

Mg INCREASED IN (RARELY ENCOUNTERED):

1. *Serum:*

   a. Renal retention due to any number of renal defects and is the more frequent cause for serum increases.
   b. Physiologic conditions such as dehydration.
   c. Overadministration therapeutically.
   d. Untreated diabetic coma.

2. *Urine.* Rarely demonstrates increased levels.

Mg DECREASED IN:

Relatively uncommon but clinically more significant than increases. Signs and symptoms do not usually occur until the serum level is less than 1 mEq/L.

1. *Serum:*

   a. Patients on TPN. Mg concentrations must be followed intermittently.
   b. Malabsorption problems such as steatorrhea.
   c. Rapid transit of chyme through intestine (e.g., diarrhea).
   d. Patients having nasogastric suction and fluid replacement without magnesium replacement, usually postoperatively.
   e. Conditions interfering with metabolism of magnesium, such as hepatic cirrhosis and pancreatitis.
   f. Excessive excretion, as in early chronic renal disease (diuretic stage) and diuretic therapy.
   g. Response to effects of hormonal influence [e.g., hypoparathyroidism, hyperaldosteronism, syndrome of inappropriate antidiuretic hormone (SIADH) with porphyria].

2. *Urine:*

   a. Serum magnesium deficiency = urine magnesium deficiency.
   b. Conditions that destroy renal glomerular function.

Patient Preparation. No special preparation is necessary.

8.6 REPRODUCTIVE HORMONES: GONADAL FUNCTION

The term *gonad* refers to a sex gland, the ovary in the female, the testis in the male. The ovary produces ova, and the testis produces spermatozoa. Gonadal function is not limited to reproduction. Both sex glands produce hormones that control sexual maturation, pubertal reproductive organ development, and physical traits that define femininity and masculinity (e.g., voice pitch, body form, muscular development, hair growth patterns). The principal hormones produced are estrogen and progesterone by the ovary and testosterone by the testis.

Gonadal function is under the control of the pituitary [luteinizing hormone (LH) and follicle stimulating hormone, (FSH)] and there is evidence to suggest that the hypothalamus secretes a single peptide releasing hormone that controls secretion of both gonadotropins. This factor is known by several names [e.g., luteinizing releasing hormone (LRH); LH/FSH releasing hormone (RH); or gonadotropin releasing hormone (GnRH)]. LH is sometimes called interstitial cell stimulating hormone (ICSH) in males (see Fig. 8.2).

Another hormone of importance in reproduction is the human chorionic gonadotropin hormone (hCG), a so-called "hormone of pregnancy," produced by the placenta. The placenta also produces estrogen and progesterone, increasing those serum levels during pregnancy.

8.6.1 Laboratory and Clinical Indications of Gonadal Dysfunction

Laboratory Findings. Screening tests do not provide indicators of congenital gonadal dysfunction other than a marked increase in urinary 17-KS, a test that is rarely done in screening. In acquired dysfunction the screening tests reflect the primary disorder without specific clues to gonadal dysfunction.

Clinical Findings. Adolescent failure to develop appropriate, or any, secondary sex characteristics; the presence in the infant or young child of intersex genitalia, hypospadias, clitoral enlargement, webbing of the neck, lymphedema; in adult women, menstrual disorders, such as abnormal uterine bleeding, absence of menarche, amenorrhea, painful menses, signs of pregnancy; hirsutism; virilization; in men or women evidence of infertility; adult males, hypogonadism, change in body hair patterns, impotency.

8.6.2 Tests of Gonadal Function

Table 8.3 lists the normal ranges, uses, and characteristics of major gonadal function tests.

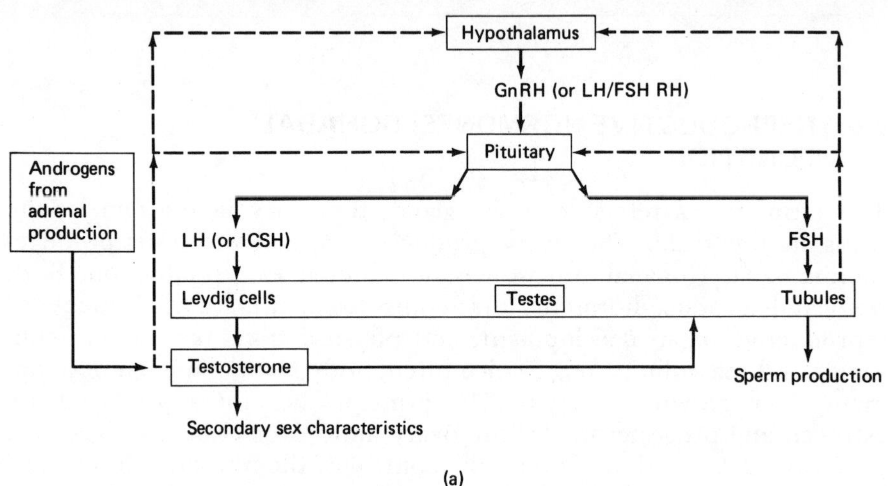

(a)

Hypothalamus

GnRH

Pituitary

Peripheral conversion of adrenal andro-stenediene to estrone. Estrone + testosterone + androstene-diene = estra-diol.

LH

FSH

Corpus luteum

Ovary

Follicle

Progesterone

Estrogen

(Estradiol, E_2)

Serum

Ovulation

Secondary sex characteristics

Pregnancy

Menses

Placenta

Estrogen

hCG

Progesterone

(b)

— — = negative feedback

—— = positive feedback

FIGURE 8.2 Gonadal function: (a) male; (b) female.

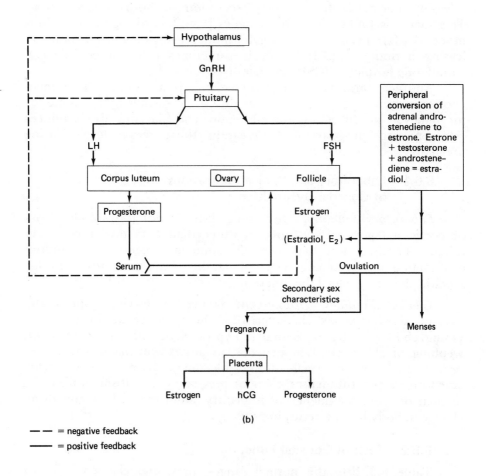

TABLE 8.3 *Tests of gonadal function*

Name of test	Normal range	Comments	Purpose/increases/decreases
1. Estrogen tests			
a. Estradiol (E_2) serum	Adult female Follicular phase: 3–10 ng/dL Luteal phase: 7–10 ng/dL Adult male: 0.8–3.0 ng/dL Pediatrics: 2–10 years: 0–1.0 ng/dL	Estradiol is the most potent estrogen in human serum; an RIA test with no special patient preparation	Used to detect secondary ovarian failure due to decreased pituitary gonadotropins; primary ovarian failure due to premature menopause (failure due to ovarian dysgenesis); disorders of follicular maturation; a more accurate monitor of ovarian function than urine total estrogen
b. Estriol (E_3) serum (free estriol)	6–34 ng/mL (first detectable at 9 weeks' gestation; usually reported by reference graph comparing previous values/week of gestation and a "normal" curve) *Reference values* Week of Gestation — Estriol Range (ng/mL) 30 — 3.3– 8.7 31 — 3.3–10.8 32 — 3.3–14.5 33 — 3.8–14.0 34 — 5.0–15.0 35 — 5.0–18.3 36 — 5.3–19.8 37 — 5.7–24.1 38 — 5.0–28.0 39 — 5.4–29.0 40 — 6.4–31.8	An RIA test; no special patient preparation necessary; continued production of estriol depends on having a living fetus and functioning placenta; should be sampled serially to establish baseline and trend	E^3 arises from the placenta and is used to monitor fetal and placental function Decreased in: Fetal death—sharp drop within 1–2 hr Low levels with fetal adrenal hyperplasia Hydatidiform mole Placental dysfunction secondary to maternal diabetes, hypertension Last 6 weeks of pregnancy to less than 4 ng/mL usually indicates fetal distress

(An assay for progesterone receptors is also available and used for much the same purpose, but a normal range has not been established)

TABLE 8.3 *Tests of gonadal function (cont.)*

Name of test	Normal range	Comments	Purpose/increases/decreases
c. Estriol, urine (pregnancy urine for estriol; E_3 urine)	Normal value depends on week of gestation	A 24-hr urine specimen; no special patient preparation; if the patient is diabetic, presence of urinary sugar will interfere with test result	Used as an indicator of placental function and fetal status (estriol is the major urinary estrogen and secreted during pregnancy by the placenta) Decreased in: Fetal distress; placental insufficiency; a marked decline from previous values, especially if sustained, indicates high probability of fetal distress Fetal adrenal atrophy with anacephaly Increased in: Erythroblastosis fetalis but does not correlate with this disease, nor with maternal ecclampsia
d. Estrogen, urine fractionation (estrogen by Brown fractionation)	Total estrogen Female: 4–60 μg/24 hr Male: 4–24 μg/24 hr E_1 (female only); estrone: 2–25 μg/24 hr E_2 (estradiol): 0–10 μg/24 hr E_3 (estriol): 2–30 μg/24 hr	Includes all three estrogen components, E_1, E_2, E_3, requires a 24-hr urine specimen but no special patient preparation; increases in urine urobilinogen can falsely increase values	Decreased in absence or deficiency of ovarian hormones Increased in pregnancy or with ovarian or adrenal-corticol tumors Used in diagnosis or management of female infertility or diagnosis of tumors listed above
2. Serum progesterone	Male: less than 20 ng/dL Female Follicular phase: less than 100 ng/dL Luteal phase: more than 400 ng/dL Pregnancy: more than 800 ng/dL	An RIA test; no special patient preparation	Used in diagnosis of some congenital gonadal disorders, trophoblastic tumors, and evaluation of placental function Increased in: Pregnancy after week 10, levels to 10,000–30,000 ng/dL Along with 17-hydroxyprogesterone and compound-S in adrenogenital syndrome Nonaborted hydatidiform moles up to week 20

Name of test	Normal range	Comments	Purpose/increases/decreases
			Choriocarcinoma, along with increased estradiol-17-beta and decreased urine prenanediol Decreased in: impending abortion to levels below 1000 ng/dL at 10–12 weeks
3. Serum testosterone	Female: 25–100 ng/dL Male: 300–800 ng/dL	An RIA test; no special patient preparation; testosterone is produced by both the ovary and the adrenal glands in females	Used in diagnosis of congenital and acquired gonadal disorders; used to evaluate premature or delayed puberty, hypogonadism in males, and to differentiate certain testicular tumors Increased in: Polycystic ovary—virilizing syndrome in females Adrenogenital syndrome Precocious maturity in males Decreased in: Delayed puberty in males Male hypogonadism (Klinefelter's syndrome, idiopathic gonadal failure) —LH and FSH usually increased Some patients with cirrhosis Secondary hypogonadism (pituitary or hypothalamic failure); LH decreased
4. FSH, serum (follicle stimulating hormone)	Male: 3–17 mIU/ml (mIU = milli International unit) Female Follicular phase: 3–20 mIU/ml Ovulatory peak: 4–35 mIU/mL Luteal: 2–11 mIU/mL Postmenopausal: 40–200 mIU/mL Pediatric: children: up to 12 mIU/ml	An RIA test; no special patient preparation for baseline evaluation; if used with a stimulation test (Clomiphene), lab should be informed of expected high values; also, if a gonadotropin producing neoplasm is suspected (clomiphene will increase FSH normally but not in pituitary failure; normal response = 85% over baseline)	Used for diagnosis of ectopic tumor as well as disorders of the hypothalmic–pituitary–gonadal axis (e.g., delayed puberty, testicular failure—primary, precocious puberty) Increased in primary gonadal failure Decreased in hypothalamic or pituitary failure

TABLE 8.3 *Tests of gonadal function (cont.)*

Name of test	Normal range	Comments	Purpose/increases/decreases
5. FSH, urine (prolan A: pituitary gonadotropins: follicle stimulating hormone)	Adults: approx. 6–50 mUU (mouse uterine units)/24 hr Pediatrics: prepubertal: 2 years to puberty = less than 6 mUU/24 hr Postmenopausal females: greater than 50 mUU/24 hr (fluctuations occur in women during menstrual cycle, peak at midcycle)	A bioassay; no special patient preparation 24-hr urine collection; not used greatly now; serum assay thought to be more reliable	Useful in evaluation of gonadal dysfunction Increased in primary gonadal failure (e.g., ovarian agenesis, seminiferous tubular failure, anorchia, Klinefelter's syndrome) Decreased after administration of estrogen; with androgen secreting tumors; after primary pituitary failure
6. LH, serum (luteinizing hormone)	Adult Male: 6–30 mIU/mL Female: Follicular = 2–30 mIU/mL Ovulatory = 40–200 mIU/mL Luteal = 0–20 mIU/mL Postmenopausal = 35–300 mIU/mL Pediatric: 2 years to puberty: 4–20 mIU/mL [Episodic in adult male; peaks at midcycle (ovulation) in females]	RIA test with no special patient preparation for baseline test (see serum FSH regarding expected high values, stimulation tests)	Used generally the same as the FSH test (see test 5 above); this test tends to cross-react with hCG and thus can be useful in detecting increased hCG levels produced with certain trophoblastic tumors (Henry, 1979); sometimes used to establish exact time of ovulation with menstrual cycle Increased in: Primary gonadal failure With estrogen administration (see Fig. 8.2) Turner's syndrome, although can be normal (primary hypogonadism) Decreased in: hypothalamic/pituitary failure
7. Prolactin, serum (PRL; lactogenic hormone; luteotropin; mamotropin)	8 A.M. fasting Adult Female: 6–30 ng/mL Male: 5–18 ng/mL Pediatric: neonate levels are elevated with progressive decrease to normal by 6 weeks	RIA test; hormone has a diurnal variation similar to GH with levels increased during sleep; sample should be taken at time determined by lab's reference normal, usually 8 A.M.; no food or drink other than water for 8 hr prior to test	Differs from other anterior pituitary hormones since control is maintained by an inhibitory factor from hypothalamus Rarely decreased—pituitary necrosis or infarction Increased in most cases of amenorrhea and galactorrhea; hypothalamic and some pituitary tumors; primary

Name of test	Normal range	Comments	Purpose/increases/decreases
			hypothroidism; with administration of many drugs, notably estrogen, phenothiazines, reserpine, oral contraceptives causing galactorrhea; and in physiologic states of stress, pregnancy, lactation, exercise, sleep
8. Human chorionic gonadotropin assay (hCG assay; "pregnancy tests")	*General comments:* The placenta secretes hCG. There are four general methods to measure hCG activity: bioassay, immunoassay (hemagglutination inhibition–HAI, latex particles agglutination inhibition–LAI, direct agglutination of latex particles), RIA, and radio receptor assay–RRA. The immunoassay methods include many rapid, relatively simple tests, frequently used for pregnancy evaluation, which are given briefly below. Two other tests, more complex and done primarily by laboratories, are also given, as they are either semiquantitative or quantitative and can be used in diagnosis and follow-up of trophoblastic or hCG-producing ectopic tumors.		
a. Qualitative urine pregnancy tests	Reported as negative or positive		False negatives occur in HAI, LAI, and direct agglutination tests in early pregnancy due to low hCG levels; may also occur with ectopic pregnancy or threatened abortion
HAI tube tests: Pregnosticon[a] (Organon)	Slide tests: Pregnosticon (Organon)[b]		
UCG (Walpole)[a]	UCG (Walpole)[b]	These tests are primarily screening tests	False positives occur due to: Increased LH levels at midcycle peak, in menopausal patient, with administration of hCG, ectopic LH production with certain tumors [nontrophoblastic tumors such as carcinoma of the lung, testicular tumors, ovarian cysts; and trophoblastic neoplasma (e.g., hydatidiform mole, choriocarcinomal)]
Gravindex (Ortho)[a]	Gravindex (Ortho)[b]		
LAI: Placentex (Roche)[a]	Pregnosis (Roche)[b]		
Direct latex agglutination	DAP test (Walpole)[b]	The DAP test is the only one of the tests given here that can be used for both serum and urine	

(cont.)

TABLE 8.3 *Tests of gonadal function (cont.)*

Name of test	Normal range	Comments	Purpose/increases/decreases
			Increased LH excretion with administration of phenothiazine drugs Tubo-ovarian abcess Proteinuria greater than 1.0 g/24 hr
b. hCG, serum semiquantitative screen (human chorionic gonadotropin)	Detectable levels with 24 hr after implantation; 5 mIU/mL; peak levels vary; can reach 500 mIU/mL There is a wide variation in levels in second and third trimesters	No special patient preparation in pregnancy, sequential assays follow a normal curve; rapid rise to peak first 70 days after last menses (LMP); direct latex agglutination test Peak is followed by a rapid fall, plateauing at 5–10 mIU/mL at about 120 days after LMP	Used for diagnosis of pregnancy, differential diagnosis of trophoblastic disease, and follow-up after treatment of such disease Low levels occur with a dying trophoblast and could indicate a threatened abortion Cross-reacts with LH as given under pregnancy tests above
c. hCG beta subunit by RIA, serum (human chorionic gonadotropin)	0–3 mIU/mL	No special patient preparation. The beta subunit of hCG is functional unit of human hCG. The test is then highly specific and is also more sensitive than are standard pregnancy tests	Because the test is function-specific, there are no false positives or false negative due to functionally inactive hCG; can be used to diagnose pregnancy as early as 8 days after LMP; it is the more accurate test in diagnosis of ectopic pregnancy and trophoblastic and hCG-producing ectopic tumors; used to follow up on treatment for such conditions as well
d. Chemical hCG tests: Twentisec, urine; LPT, urine	*General comments:* these are qualitative tests, more recently developed, based on color change with positive reactions. As yet, there are few data regarding possible false positives and negatives, or how the tests are affected by such cross-reacting material as protein.		

[a], [b]Incubation time for these pregnancy tests varies from 1 to 2 hr[a] to 1 to 2 min[b].

Source: Data from SHMC, 1978; Henry, 1979; and Ravel, 1979.

8.6.3 Associated Tests

A. Buccal smear

Synonyms: Barr test; sex chromatin test; S-chromatin study

Reported Results (normal)

Female	Barr body positive, single (20–40% of cells)
Male	Barr body negative

Indications for Use. Ambiguous or abnormal genitalia; male or female infertility without other known cause; symptoms suggestive of Turner's or Klinefelter's syndromes.

Explanation of the Test. This is primarily a screening test for the purpose of visualizing Barr bodies. The nuclei of various body cells contain a stable chromatin mass (Barr body). The Barr body is derived from one entire X chromosome. Males have a single X chromosome per cell (XY) and therefore normally do not have Barr bodies. Females carry XX chromosomes. The Barr body appears normally in females since, in the presence of more than one X chromosome in a cell, all but one will become inactivated (i.e., a Barr body). As only one chromosome is necessary to transfer genetic information, the presence of an inactivated X chromosome in a cell causes no difficulty. The X chromosome inactivated can be of either paternal or maternal origin—the process is entirely random and occurs at the time of embryonic implantation in the uterus. However, all cells descending from a specific cell will each have the same X inactivated (Henry, 1979). The Barr body appears in certain sex chromosomal abnormalities. Presumptive diagnosis of these abnormalities can be made by comparison of the results of the buccal smear test with the individual's genitalia and secondary sex characteristics. The buccal smear test does not indicate true genetic sex; it only shows the number of female (X) chromosomes present. Confirmation of presumptive diagnoses can be done by chromosome karyotyping.

Special staining techniques of buccal smear cells are necessary to use the smear in defining gonosomal intersexuality (mixed gonadal dysgenesis) or Y chromosome abnormalities such as the XYY or "supermale" condition. Karyotyping is preferable and usually necessary in any case.

The Barr test can also be done on epithelial cells of vaginal smears, urinary sediment, or amniotic fluid. Any sex chromosomal abnormality can be diagnosed by amniocentesis at 15 to 16 weeks gestation and karyotyping.

Note: Inaccurate reports of the Barr test can occur. Poor slide preparation or degenerating cells can cause false negative reports. Artifacts such as bacteria can cause false-positive reports. Only 40 to 60% of normal female cells contain identifiable Barr bodies, so a sufficient number, usually at least 100, must be examined.

Patient Preparation

1. *Buccal smears* should not be done during the first week of life or during adrenal corticosteroid or estrogen treatment. False decreases in the incidence of Barr bodies occur.
2. *The outermost layer of epithelium* does not demonstrate Barr bodies and must be removed prior to collecting the specimen. Specimen collection is probably best done by a cytotechnologist.
3. *Several slides* should be prepared and must be immersed immediately after collection in fixative (Pap test fixative), as the Barr bodies fade rapidly when exposed to air.

B. Semen analysis

Synonym: semen examination

Normal Ranges (complete test)

pH	7 –8.5 (less than 7 abnormal)
Volume	1.5–5.0 mL (infertile males tend to have increased volume)
Count	60 – 150 million/mL (less than 20 million is abnormal
Motility	60% motile at 3 hr 50% motile at 6 hr
Morphology	At least 70% of sperm normally formed
Microscopic	No RBC; none to occasional WBC; occasional to few cells; no crystals

Explanation of the Test. Usually this test is part of a thorough work-up of both partners to investigate fertility, or it may be done to check the outcomes of a vasectomy.

Patient Preparation

1. *Varying periods of continence* are suggested prior to sample collection (3 days or a period equal to usual frequency of coitus for the couple).

2. *Collection is most satisfactory* if done as near as possible to the facility where it will be examined.
3. *Specimens must be kept* at a constant body temperature after collection, with no extreme changes, until examined.
4. *Time of collection* must be known and be accurate. After 2 hr the sample should not be used for full examination. Postvasectomy (microscopic only) can be done on 2-hr specimens, but the fresher the sample, the more accurate the test.

C. Serum alkaline phosphatase

(See Section 1.12.1 for more detailed information on this test.) Marked elevations of heat-stable alkaline phosphatase occur in the third trimester of pregnancy. Used as a placental function test in the past, it is no longer an important test in pregnancy. Plasma and urinary estriol have replaced it. It can serve as a useful tumor "marker" for a wide variety of neoplasms, but clinical values have not been well established for this.

D. Pregnancy-associated plasma proteins (PAPP), serum

Alpha and beta globulins appearing with a specificity comparable to hCG are now called pregnancy-associated plasma proteins. Clinical values have not yet been established, but in time it might be expected these proteins will be used to diagnose first-trimester pregnancy and evaluate placental function (Henry, 1979).

The Renal System

chapter **9**

The evaluation of kidney function is still relatively crude, relying as it does on measurement of what passes into and out of the kidney. What goes on inside the kidney can only be speculated upon. Such speculation requires careful correlation with other clinical and laboratory data and a thorough understanding of the actual physiologic basis for each test. (See also Section 4.1 for physiology of urine production.)

Renal function tests look at two specific areas of the kidney nephron:

1. *The glomerulus.* A tuft of capillaries invaginated into the dilated, blind end of the nephron (Bowman's capsule), whose purpose is to filter water and solutes from the blood plasma presented to it. Normal glomerular filtration depends on adequate hydrostatic pressure in the glomerulus (60 to 70 mmHg), colloid osmotic pressure of plasma proteins (30 mmHg), pressure in the glomerular capsule itself, surrounding the capillaries, (5 to 10 mmHg), and an intact glomerular membrane. Glomerular function tests look at the glomerular filtration rate (GFR), which is the amount of a substance filtered through the glomerulus in a given time. The

normal filtration rate of plasma is approximately 125 mL/min, or 25% of cardiac output. The GFR increases with increased glomerular pressure and decreases with increased colloid osmotic pressure and decreased cardiac output.

2. *The tubules.* Proximal, loop of Henle, and distal portions. Both proximal and distal tubules have convoluted sections. The tubules empty into a collecting duct in the kidney cortex. Tubular function includes active and passive reabsorption of glomerular filtrate from the tubules to systemic circulation, and tubular secretion—active transport from the peritubular capillaries to the tubular lumen—to maintain acid-base, water, and electrolyte balance (see Table 4.1 and Fig. 4.1).

9.1 TESTS OF GLOMERULAR FUNCTION

9.1.1 Laboratory and Clinical Indications of Glomerular Dysfunction

Laboratory Findings. *Urine:* Major clue is the presence of proteinuria, which may include hematuria, increased specific gravity, a cloudy or smokey gross appearance of the urine, and increased uric acid (normally the glomerular filter does not allow protein, especially large protein, to pass). Increased numbers of casts of all types, increased WBC, oval fat bodies, and lipiduria may also appear, depending on the cause of glomerular dysfunction. *Blood:* Hypoalbuminemia, due to loss in urine; dilutional anemia due to decreased glomerular filtration of water; electrolytes usually within normal limits (WNL), but total serum calcium may be decreased (lost with protein); ionized calcium will be normal. Increased total cholesterol; hyperlipidemia and cholesterolemia; increased BUN; true anemia with severe renal insufficiency due to decreased erythropoietin (normocytic, normochronic); and the hallmark of severe renal disease, increased serum creatinine.

Clinical Findings. Depends in part on the cause of glomerular function loss, and in part on the total renal status. Most common symptoms of glomerulopathies are slight to moderate hypertension, edema, and oliguria. Headache may occur. Edema often periorbital, especially in the morning, later dependent edema. Urine excessively foamy; growth failure in children; vague signs and symptoms of malaise, fatigue, irritability; may have ascites; signs and symptoms of congestive heart failure.

9.1.2 Creatinine Clearance Test

Synonyms: None

Normal Ranges:* 70–130 mL/min

Serum creatinine	
Adult	0.7–1.5 mg/dL
Senior adult	0.6–1.2 mg/dL
Child	0.3–1.1 mg/dL
Urine creatinine	
Adult	
Female	16 –22 mg/kg/24 hr
Male	21 – 26 mg/kg/24 hr

*Clearance rate decreases after approximately 40 years of age, due to decreased GFR and renal plasma flow. In some facilities 10 mL/min is subtracted from the normal for every 10-year period after 40 (Kagan, 1979).

Explanation of the Test. Since there is little tubular reabsorption of creatinine, using creatinine measurements in the blood and in the urine appears to be a valid measure of the GFT. The creatinine clearance test is used most frequently as an indicator of total renal status rather than just glomerular status. The values of creatinine clearance closely parallel the percent of functioning nephrons. Serum creatinine rises when the GFR declines and creatinine clearance into the urine decreases, whereas creatinine clearance increases with increased GFR. The creatinine clearance test has been found to be the most practical of the clearance tests, since creatinine is endogenous to the body and is formed at a fairly constant rate.

The test can be used to evaluate long-term management of patients with chronic disorders of renal function and to determine appropriate fluid and electrolyte replacement therapy.

Clearance is calculated by multiplying the concentration of measured urine creatinine by the volume of urine in a set time interval (converted to mL/min) and dividing the product by the serum concentration of creatinine. The outcome of the calculation is corrected when necessary for differing kidney masses, using a body surface nomogram (Henry, 1979).

Creatinine clearance tests are best compared sequentially in the seriously ill patient with an increased serum creatinine because impaired renal function may be one of the factors increasing plasma levels and absolute normal values may not be an accurate reference for measurement of increased tubular secretion of creatinine (Widmann, 1979).

Urea clearance: Urea is the other endogenous body substance measured by clearance testing. It is used less often because urea concentration in plasma is much more variable, necessitating shorter collection periods. Tubular reabsorption of urea also occurs at normal plasma levels. Urea clearance is a measure of total (glomerular and tubular) renal function. Normal range is 64 to 99 mL/min—maximal clearance (C_m) at urine flow rate of 2 mL/min or greater. At flow rates less than 2 mL/min, normal is 41 to 69 mL/min—standard clearance (C_s).

CREATININE CLEARANCE RATES DECREASED IN:

1. *False low values* due to nonrefrigerated specimens, or specimens tested over 24 hr after collection.
2. *Glomerulonephritis.*
3. *Nephrosis.*
4. *Any significant renal disease,* regardless of cause, can diminish the glomerular filtration rate (Sodeman and Sodeman, 1979).
5. *Nonrenal conditions* that impair microcirculation to the kidney (e.g., congestive heart failure, cirrhosis with ascites, shock, dehydration). (With a normal BUN, normal blood pressure and absence of anemia, diffuse bilateral renal disease is suspect; with an increased BUN, prognosis is guarded.)

Patient Preparation

1. *The test can be done* as an hourly, 12-hr, or 24-hr test. The 24-hr test is preferred. The hourly test requires extreme accuracy in timing, complete collection of urine specimens, and adequate hydration and renal blood flow.
2. *The process for hourly collection of urine and blood sampling* is the same as that described for the tubular phosphate reabsorption test. For the hourly and 24-hr test, the patient should be fasting (see "Patient Preparation and Test Procedure in Section 8.5.6).
3. *Excessive amounts of tea, coffee, or meat* should be avoided for 24 hr prior to the test.
4. 24-hr test: Time exactly. Have patient void and discard the urine at the start of the test. Save all urine—refrigerate or ice until end of test. A blood specimen can be taken any time during the test.

9.1.3 Inulin Clearance Test

Synonyms: none

Normal Ranges

Adult
- Male: 124 ± 15 mL/min (corrected to 1.73 m^2 of body surface)
- Female: 110 ± 15 mL/min

Lower in children up to 2 years

Explanation of the Test. Inulin is a polysaccharide of fructose which is freely filtered by the glomerulus and neither reabsorbed nor secreted by the tubules. Inulin clearance is therefore equal to the GFR. Since inulin is not normally present in the body, it must be infused to maintain a constant plasma level. It is not used for routine laboratory work because of the need to monitor plasma levels frequently and the need for extremely careful urine collection. The test has, however, provided information in research studies about the relative accuracies or shortcomings of other clearance tests used clinically. It is also used to calculate tubular transport capacity (T_m). See Section 9.2.2A.

INULIN DECREASED IN:

See Section 9.1.2.

Patient Preparation. Not used clinically.

9.2 TESTS OF TUBULAR FUNCTION

9.2.1 Laboratory and Clinical Indications of Tubular Dysfunction

Laboratory Findings. *Urine:* decreased specific gravity and, with severe tubular dysfunction, fixed specific gravity of 1.010; Increased pH–alkaline urine (may be due in part to NH_3 production by urea splitting bacteria–*Proteus*); glycosuria; aminoaciduria (general or specific to a few); WBC casts, pyuria, bacteriuria; increased urinary sodium in salt-losing conditions; increased K^+. *Blood:* increased BUN, increased H^+ (decreased pH), and decreased HCO_3; increased phosphorus and decreased calcium (vice versa in nephrogenic diabetes insipidus); decreased potassium (K^+); decreased sodium in salt-losing conditions, increased in uremia; serum creatinine increased when 50% or more of renal function lost; anemia–normocytic, normochromic.

Clinical Findings. Specific to underlying problems. *Children:* inadequate growth; rickets. *General:* polyuria (nephrogenic diabetes insipidus and acute pyelonephritis); polydypsia; oliguria (with acute tubular necrosis); bruising, purpuric lesions; increased susceptibility to infections; complaints of burning feet, puruitis, nausea; vomiting, diarrhea; changes in level of consciousness; changes in muscle tone and function (twitching, tremors, weakness); functional abnormalities (e.g., urinary incontinence in children); anatomical abnormalities of the genital-urinary tract (e.g., spraying of urinary stream, enuresis).

9.2.2 Excretion Tests

A. Para-aminohippuric acid clearance test, urine

Synonyms: PAH clearance; sodium *p*-aminohippurate clearance

Normal Ranges

Depends on venous plasma PAH concentration–90% clearance

With 0.02 mg/mL venous plasma concentration, 600–700 mL/min; effective renal plasma flow (ERPF): that which is in contact with the tubules; normal RPF would be higher) (Sodeman and Sodeman, 1979).

Explanation of the Test. Para-aminohippuric acid (PAH) is excreted primarily by tubular secretion (that bound by plasma proteins), and to a limited extent by glomerular filtration (unbound PAH). Total urinary excretion is measured and compared to the GFR obtained by inulin clearance. Clearance of PAH from low plasma levels is almost total, but clearance is self-suppressed with high plasma values since the excess saturates the transfer system (plasma proteins).

Because the test is technically and clinically difficult, it is not widely used. When done in a normally functioning kidney with intact tubular function, the test indicates renal plasma flow.

DECREASED IN:

See Section 9.1.2.

Patient Preparation:

1. *A baseline, or control, blood and urine specimen* is collected.
2. *PAH is given* in an IV priming dose and then by slow continuous infusion in low concentration.
3. *Three timed urine specimens* are collected and blood samples are taken at the beginning and end of each urine collection. All three clearance values are averaged.
4. *Adequate hydration* is important.

B. Phenolsulfonphthalein test

Synonyms: PSP test; PSP excretion test

Normal Range

25–35% excretion in 15 min
40–60% total excretion in 1 hr
60–75% total excretion in 2 hr

Explanation of the Test. PSP is an older test of renal function which provides much the same information as the creatinine clearance test and has been mostly replaced by it in practice. Its purpose is to indicate the secretory ability of the renal tubules. 95% of the PSP injected IV is actively secreted by the tubules and cleared (excreted) from the kidney. The excretion is proportional to renal blood flow. It is a simpler measurement of secretory function than the PAH test and has therefore been used more frequently.

Decreased, or depressed, 15-min excretion rates are usually due to impaired renal perfusion rather than decreased tubular function and indicate the need to explore for cardiac failure or renal vascular disease.

PSP INCREASED IN:

1. *False elevations with hypoalbuminemia.* Normally 80% of the PSP is protein-bound and therefore slowed in clearance.
2. *Liver disease with an excess of 90% excretion.* A small percentage is usually excreted by the liver; excess renal excretion may indicate lack of that function by the liver.

PSP DECREASED IN:

1. *Acute tubular necrosis,* idiopathic and acquired.
2. *De Toni-Fanconi's syndrome,* secondary and idiopathic.
3. *Chronic pyelonephritis.*
4. *Galactosemia.*
5. *Idiopathic hypercalcemia.*
6. *Vitamin D-resistant rickets.*
7. *Any severe, diffuse kidney disease.*

Patient Preparation and Test Procedure

1. *Bladder is emptied*—catheterization as necessary if approved by physician in charge.
2. *Hydrate* with 600 to 800 ml of water.
3. *Dye injected* in 20 min, usually by lab personnel.
4. *Postinjection urine samples* collected at 15 and 30 min, and 1 and 2 hr. All urine voided during the time of testing must be saved, collected in separate bottles, and labeled with time of collection.
5. *The test is not used* if the BUN, creatinine, or other indicators of severely diminished renal functions are present because of the danger due to the rapid hydration used with this test.

9.2.3 Concentration Tests

See Section 8.2.1B.

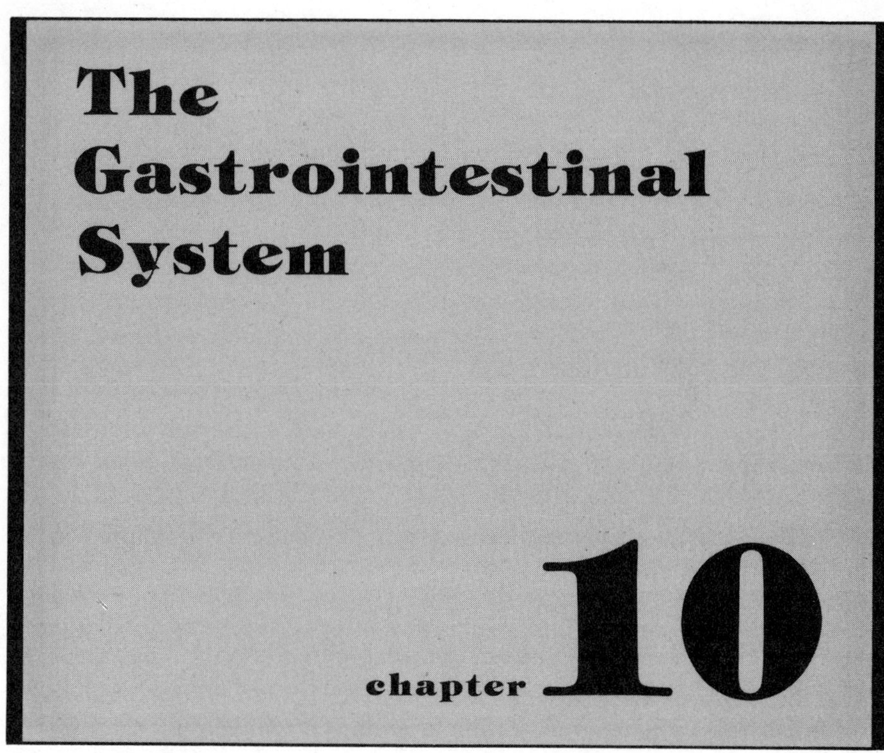

10.1 LABORATORY AND CLINICAL INDICATIONS OF GASTROINTESTINAL DYSFUNCTION

Laboratory Findings. Presence of occult blood in stool; chronic iron-deficiency anemia (hypochromic, microcytic) or macrocytic anemia (normochromic with increased MCV, MCH, and normal MCHC); anisocytosis; poikilocytosis; neutropenia, hypersegmented nuclei (four to six lobes); thrombocytopenia; in many instances increased LDH. Other tests: decreased serum haptoglobin.

Clinical Findings. Complaints of "ulcer-like" pain (pinpoint, periodic—decreased in A.M., increased in P.M., relieved by food, vomiting; return of pain 30 to 90 min after eating); hemoptysis, dark, tarry stools; glossitis (red, smooth, painful tongue); easy bruising; parasthesias; impaired vibratory sense; premature graying; signs and symptoms of anemia (e.g., fatigue, pallor, shortness of breath, lassitude, angina); complaints of indigestion, anorexia; history of recent weight loss (some of these symptoms in persons of Japanese, Finnish, or Icelandic heritage should increase the index of suspicion for gastric cancer). Family history of pernicious anemia, gastric cancer, or gastric/duodenal ulcer; self-history of previous peptic ulcer; consistent use of antacids.

10.2 TESTS OF GASTRIC SECRETION

10.2.1 Gastric Analysis

Synonyms: gastric secretory test; basal gastric secretion; 1-hr morning aspiration

Normal Ranges: 0-5 mEq/hour (females and senior adults tend to be within the lower ranges of normal).

Explanation of the Test. Basal gastric secretion represents the response of the stomach to endogenous stimuli continually present: the test can be used to determine gastric acidity or to obtain material for exfoliative cytology. Differences in basal secretion rates can be helpful in the differential diagnosis of several conditions (gastric versus duodenal ulcer). The test is helpful but not diagnostic, since there is considerable overlap among the responses. No pathognomonic range exists for any of the disease states linked with basal gastric secretion rates, with the exception of the very high acid output of Zollinger-Ellison syndrome. If there is no evidence of basal secretion, or the results of the test are ambiguous, stimulation tests are done.

SIGNIFICANCE OF RESPONSES:

1. *Basal secretion within normal limits* will rule out the presence of pernicious anemia. True achlorhydria exists.
2. *A high basal secretion* (15 to 20 mEq/hr, as high as 60 mEq/hr at times) is strongly suggestive of Zollinger-Ellison syndrome.
3. *Benign gastric ulcers* usually have normal or even low rates. Basal secretion greater than 10 mEq/hr is strong evidence against their existence.
4. *Duodenal ulcers* tend toward basal secretion rates of 5 to 15 mEq/hr. Low acid secretion is evidence against their existence.
5. *Gastric cancer* is often concurrent with somewhat lower than normal basal secretion, or can be suspected with total absence of acid secretion, particularly if pernicious anemia is ruled out.

Patient Preparation and Test Procedure

1. *Any medications or foods* that might influence gastric secretions should be held for 25 hr prior to the test (e.g., anticholinergics, andrenergics, alcohol, corticosteroids, reserpine). No antacids or coffee.
2. *Patient should be fasting* for 12 hr prior to the test.
3. *Water may be taken until* 8 hr prior to intubation.
4. *No smoking* the morning of the test.
5. *Basal physiologic and environmental conditions* maintained; quiet, stress-free environment with no odor or sight of food.
6. *The patient is intubated* and residual stomach volume removed. Gastric juices are continuously collected for 1 hr. Usually, the aspirate is separated into 15-min samples and the volume, pH, titratable acid, and any other requested measurements made on each sample. pH measures can be converted to hydrogen ion concentration in mEq per hour.

10.2.2 Gastric Stimulation Tests

Synonyms: histalog (Betazole); pentagastrin; insulin hypoglycemic test; augmented histamine test

Normal Range

Maximal acid output (MAO)*	1–20 mEq/hr
Peak acid output (PAO)†	1–50 mEq/hr

*MAO is the total acid excreted in 1 hr (four specimens) following stimulation. Some procedures call for 4- to 30-min specimens (Ravel, 1979).

†PAO is the highest acid output for two successive specimens adjusted to the hourly rate—X 2 for 15-min specimens (SHMC, 1978).

Explanation of the Tests. The substances given above are strong stimulants for secretion of gastric acid, pepsin, and intrinsic factor in the stomach. The pentagastrin test has largely replaced the augmented histamine test, as it has far fewer side effects. Generally, the tests are used when there is no basal secretion found with the regular gastric analysis. The histalog or pentagastrin tests are most frequently used for this. The insulin test has been used primarily to assess gastric function following vagotomy, since the major component of gastric secretion stimulus in hypoglycemia is transmitted by the vagus nerve and should be abolished by complete vagotomy. Because the normal range is so broad, only generalizations can be made as to the diagnostic outcomes of the tests.

SIGNIFICANCE OF RESPONSES (MAO):

1. *0 mEq/hr* = true achlorhydria and is compatible with some cases of gastric cancer, gastritis, and pernicious anemia.
2. *1 to 20 mEq/hr* = normal. Can be compatible with gastric ulcer.
3. *20 to 60 mEq/hr* = high normal. Compatible with duodenal ulcer, possibly Zollinger-Ellison syndrome.
4. *Over 60 mEq/hr* = Zollinger-Ellison syndrome. Generally not more than two times basal acid output.

10.2.3 Tubeless Gastric Analysis

Synonym: Diagnex Blue Test

Normal Ranges

A qualitative test (color comparison): presence of the dye in the urine indicates gastric acid secretion

Less than 0.3 mg of azure blue in urine in 2 hr: presumptive anacity (achlorhydria)

Between 0.3 and 0.6: borderline secretion

Greater than 0.6 mg of azure blue in urine: adequate hydrochloric acid secretion

Explanation of the Test. The resin dye and a gastric stimulant, usually caffeine sodium benzoate + histalog, are taken orally. Free hydrochloric acid in the stomach replaces the dye, which is then absorbed and excreted in the urine. This test has been found useful as a screening test in pernicious anemia, since the degree of acid secretion is not of importance in that instance. There exist, however, a high rate of false-negative and false-positive results with the test, and it is not sensitive to diminished secretion. Further, it is thought unreliable in patients with previous gastric surgery (subtotal gastrectomy, gastroenterostomy, pyloroplasty) due to the rapid transit of the dye through the stomach. Although considered a discredited procedure by many gastroenterologists (Henry, 1979), the test is attractive to the general public and some physicians, when compared to the standard gastric analysis, and is still found in use.

Patient Preparation. The patient must be NPO as given under gastric analysis, and fasting throughout the test.

10.2.4 Plasma Gastrin

Synonyms: none

Normal Range: 0–100 pg/mL (a level of 100–150 pg/mL is considered borderline)

Explanation of the Test. This is a fairly new, sensitive, and specific RIA test. Gastrin is a peptide hormone which acts on the parietal cells of the stomach's antral mucosa and that of the duodenum. Measurement of its concentration is of particular use in the diagnosis of Zollinger-Ellison syndrome (Z-E syndrome) and pernicious anemia, both of which are associated with marked increases of gastrin.

PLASMA GASTRIN INCREASED IN:

1. *Peptic ulcer disease* casued by pancreatic islet cell tumors (Z-E syndrome). Serum gastrin may be very high, 800 to 1000 pg/mL. When found in lower ranges, 200 to 400 pg/mL, stimulation by infusion of calcium or secretin will induce high levels.
2. *Pernicious anemia* with very high levels in the presence of achlorhydria.
3. *Gastric ulcer,* gastric carcinoma, and gastrointestinal obstruction with slight to moderate elevations.
4. *Postprandial tests* in some peptic ulcer disease, which show normal fasting gastrin levels.
5. *Aging,* with slight to moderate elevations.

Patient Preparation. No special preparation is required other than NPO for 8 hr prior to the test; may have water.

10.3 TESTS OF DIGESTIVE FUNCTION (PANCREATIC EXOCRINE FUNCTION)

10.3.1 Laboratory and Clinical Indications of Pancreatic Exocrine Dysfunction

Laboratory Findings. Hyperglycemia (moderate to frank diabetes); with acute pancreatitis—moderate leukocytosis with a shift to the left, increased SGOT and alkaline phophatase, transient hyperlipidemia, possible glucose in the urine and aminoaciduria (cystine, lysine); with chronic pancreatitis, postprandial hypoglycemia, decreased serum calcium (may be due to malabsorption of vitamin D and/or increased combining of calcium with fat).

Clinical Findings. *Acute:* severe epigastric pain, sudden onset, radiating; nausea and vomiting; abdominal distention; mild jaundice; decreased urine output, fever, signs of dehydration, hypovolemia, and shock. *Chronic:* steatorrhea, bleeding tendencies, osteomalacia.

10.3.2 Amylase, Serum and Urine

Synonyms: alpha-amylase; diastase; AMY; 1,4-α-D-glucan-glucanohydrolase; ptyalin

Normal Ranges

Serum	20–130 IU/L
Urine	
Adult	3–21 IU/hr
Neonatal	0–1000 IU/hr
Thereafter	700–5200 IU/hr

Explanation of the Test. Amylases are enzymes that catalyze the hydrolysis of polysaccharides. Serum and urine amylase tests are quantitative measurements of the amount of that enzyme found in the blood or urine. This test is most important in evaluating acute pancreatitis. Amylase found in the blood is produced primarily in the salivary glands and the pancreas. Damage to the glandular cells (as in acute pancreatitis) will liberate large amounts of amylase. The enzyme rapidly enters the blood, increasing serum levels. Urine amylase also increases promptly, often within several hours of the serum increase. Urine increase often occurs as the serum levels begin to decrease. The ratio between urine amylase and creatinine clearance (expressed as a percentage or as units per hr) is used diagnostically.

Serial determinations at 4- to 6-hr intervals often provide more helpful information than a single determination.

AMYLASE INCREASED IN:

1. *Acute pancreatitis.* Serum values over five times the upper limit of normal are highly suggestive of this diagnosis. The levels fall abruptly, within 2 to 3 days after onset, even though active in-

flammation persists. Urinary amylase may be diagnostic at such a time. Continued increase in serum levels suggests continuing pancreatic necrosis, or formation of a pseudocyst.

2. *Chronic, relapsing pancreatitis,* but to a much less marked degree. May be associated with trauma, alcohol, viral hepatitis, hyperparathyroidism, or may be idiopathic in origin.
3. *Conditions causing obstruction of the sphincter of Oddi* (e.g., cholecystitis, biliary tract stones, tumor, or spasm secondary to the use of morphine, Demerol, or biliary tract cannulation).
4. *Pancreatic carcinoma,* only late in the progress of the disease, if at all.
5. *Miscellaneous conditions,* such as renal failure due to decreased excretion; pregnancy; burns; drug hypersensitivity (thiazides, ethacrynic acid, oral contraceptives); some 60% of patients with diabetic ketoacidosis (salivary amylase is predominant in this rise—cause not clear).
6. *Some diseases of the parotid glands,* such as mumps. This determination can be useful in diagnosing cases of mumps orchitis or encephalitis, when there is little salivary gland involvement noted.
7. *Conditions causing chemical irritation* of the pancreas, such as peptic ulcer, postoperatively—after gastric resection, intestinal obstruction, mesenteric thrombosis, peritonitis, and ruptured ectopic pregnancy.
8. *Individuals with a protein abnormality* (macroamylasemia). Found in persons with malabsorption and/or alcoholism having normal pancreatic function. Urine levels are normal, however, since the protein is too large to pass the renal glomerulus.

AMYLASE DECREASED IN:

1. *Physiologic situations* such as following a meal or administration of glucose intravenously.
2. *Conditions associated with a decrease of functioning pancreatic cells,* such as some cases of chronic pancreatitis, pancreatic cancer, and massive hemorrhagic pancreatic necrosis.
3. *Infrequently in miscellaneous conditions,* such as congestive heart failure, gastrointestinal cancer, bone fractures, and pleurisy. Due to multiple, and in some cases not clearly understood, mechanisms.

Patient Preparation

1. *No special preparation* is necessary.

2. *Blood should be taken* 1 to 2 hours p.c., and preferably not when IV glucose is being administered.

10.3.3 Serum Lipase

Synonyms: None

Normal Ranges

Adult	1–21 IU/dL
Pediatric	8–35 IU/mL, (olive oil, 37°C)

Explanation of the Test. Lipases are enzymes that hydrolyze (or split) emulsified fats from fatty acids to triglycerides. Bile salts, calcium, and albumin are lipase activators and necessary to that activity. Lipase is found primarily in the pancreas, but is also present in stomach, intestine, WBCs, fat cells, and milk. There are also other related, but different, forms of lipase in the body as well. Measurement of serum lipase is considered more specific, but less sensitive, for pancreatic damage than is amylase. Like amylase, lipase is released into the bloodstream with damage to the pancreatic secretory cell. Its levels rise later than amylase, within 24 to 48 hr, and stay elevated longer, 7 to 10 days, usually peaking on day 4. Urine amylase measurement, although available, is not currently used.

SERUM LIPASE INCREASED IN:

1. *Acute pancreatitis* with levels up to 100 times normal.
2. *Conditions leading to obstruction of the ampulla of Vater* (e.g. some cases of pancreatic carcinoma, carcinoma of the ampulla of Vater, chronic biliary disease).
3. *Some cases of mumps,* when there is significant pancreatic involvement as well.

Patient Preparation. No special preparation is necessary.

10.3.4 Serum Carotene

Synonyms: plasma carotene; serum carotenoids

Normal Range: 50–100 μg/dL

Explanation of the Test. Carotene is a fat-soluble precursor (provitamin) of vitamin A. Its absorption from the intestine depends on the presence of dietary fat and the normal absorption of that fat. It is not stored by the body. Carotene is found in green or yellow vegetables and in some animal protein. Measurement of serum carotene is useful in establishing the presence of intestinal malabsorption conditions, and as a screening test for steatorrhea.

SERUM CAROTENE INCREASED IN:

1. *Excessive intake of carotene* (e.g., carrots).
2. *Increased absorption,* as in pregnancy.
3. *Hyperlipedemia and hypocholesterolemia,* often associated with diabetes mellitus.

SERUM CAROTENE DECREASED IN:

1. *States of lipid malabsorption* (steatorrhea).
2. *Conditions of inadequate intake of either fat* (e.g., individuals on low-fat diets) *or carotene* (green or yellow vegetables).
3. *Severe liver disease.*
4. *States with high fevers.*

10.3.5 Secretin Test

Synonyms: pancreatic stimulation test; stimulated secretin test; augmented secretin test

Normal Ranges (adult)*

	Standard	Augmented
Volume	Increased volume of clear watery secretion; 2 mL/kg of body weight	4.5–8.1 mL/kg
Bicarbonate concentration (HCO_3)	Marked increase; peak of 90–100 mEq/L	93–141 mEq/L
Sodium	Increased	
Chloride	Decreased—reciprocal to HCO_3 increase	
pH	Increased; greater than 8.0	

*Values less than those given are significant of decreased pancreatic activity. Values greater than those given are not useful for determining pancreatic status, as hypersecretion of pancreatic juice is not known.

Explanation of the Test. Secretin is a hormone known to stimulate secretion of pancreatic juice and bile. A standard (1.0 IU/kg) or augmented dose (4.0 to 5.0 IU/kg) of secretin is given IV after the stomach and duodenal contents have been aspirated until clear, via a double lumen tube. Pancreatic secretions are then collected for 60 to 80 min, and the aspirate measured at 20-min intervals for volume, bicarbonate content, and other measurements as dictated by the facility's procedure or doctor's request. There is controversy over the usefulness of the measurement of serum amylase with the stimulation of secretin. Secretin is not known to stimulate release of pancreatic enzymes. Pancreozymin is used for this purpose.

The test is useful in differentiation of causes of malabsorption by designating pancreatic hypofunction. The augmented test is done when the standard test is equivocal.

SECRETION RATE INCREASED IN (HYPERSECRETION RATE NOT KNOWN):

1. *Biliary cirrhosis and nonalcoholic cirrhosis.* Increased volume and high normal bicarbonate secretion occurs.
2. *Zollinger-Ellison syndrome,* hemachromatosis, and alcoholic cirrhosis with a marked volume increase and a lesser increase in bicarbonate secretion.

SECRETION RATE DECREASED IN:

1. *Conditions causing mechanical decrease in excretion of pancreatic juice,* such as cystic fibrosis and edema of the pancreas.
2. *Conditions causing decreased secretion of pancreatic juice* due to cell injury or loss, such as chronic pancreatitis, pancreatic cysts, pancreatic calcification, and cancer of the pancreas.

Patient Preparation

1. *NPO other than water* for 8 hr prior to the test.
2. *All anticholinergic drugs* discontinued 48 hr prior to the test.

10.4 LIVER FUNCTION TESTS

10.4.1 Laboratory and Clinical Indications of Liver Dysfunction

Laboratory Findings: Blood: increased total bilirubin + direct and indirect in most cases; increased serum cholesterol and alkaline phosphatase (especially with biliary obstruction); decreased total protein due to decreased albumin with prolonged disease (total protein could be normal or elevated with increases in gamma globulin fraction); high elevations of SGOT (SAST) and slight increases in LDH; dilutional decrease in serum sodium; serum potassium decreased; with viral hepatitis or cirrhosis, WBCs may be increased with atypical lymphocytes; decreased platelet count; prothrombin time 1 to 2 sec above normal or control; mild to moderate anemia, which may be normocytic to macrocytic, normochromic to hyperchromic. *Urine:* bilirubin increased. *Feces:* may be positive for occult blood; blood streaked due to rupture of hemorroids.

Clinical Findings: Clay-colored stools, jaundice, dark urine, anorexia, fatigue, ascites, edema, spider angiomata, muscle wasting, virilization or feminization with changes in hair pattern, varicose veins of legs and/or periumbilical, increased susceptibility to infections, enlarged, tender liver.

10.4.2 Serum Glutamic Pyruvic-Transaminase

Synonyms: SGPT: alanine aminotransferase; ALT

Normal Range: 1–12 IU/L or 4–24 U/L at 30°C*

Explanation of the Test. Formerly glutamic pyruvic-transaminase or GPT, this enzyme is now referred to as serum alanine transaminase, or ALT, and is found mostly, but not exclusively, in the liver. Because of this, serum increases are seldom seen without involvement of the liver. More severe or more extensive liver damage is necessary to cause abnormal values than is the case with SGOT (now referred to as asparate aminotransferase, or AST). It can be said that the ALT (GPT) test is less sensitive but much more specific than the AST (GOT). Kidney, heart, and skeletal muscle have significant amounts of ALT (GPT), in descending order as listed. ALT (GPT) usually returns to normal* before AST (GOT) in most cases, probably because most tissues containing both enzymes contain proportionately more AST (GOT) than ALT (GPT). It is often helpful to compare the two in differential diagnosis.

---

*Previously the reader has been warned of the danger of comparing reference ranges (normal ranges) when dealing with serum enzymes. Because of the multiple variations in methods of measurement, and the variations intrinsic to even the same methods done in different settings, values are *not* comparable. The reader should use as a guide the normal reference range supplied by the laboratory doing the test. See the discussion in Section 1.12.

SGPT (ALT) INCREASED IN:

1. *Acute heptocellular injury* with a 100-fold increase over normal values. The increase is greater than that of AST (GOT). Seen in viral or toxic hepatitis.
2. *Extrahepatic jaundice* due to biliary obstruction with up to a tenfold increase. AST increased about the same or slightly less.
3. *Primary or secondary carcinoma of the liver* with a fivefold increase. The AST increase is seven- to tenfold.
4. *Primary biliary cirrhosis* with a fivefold increase. The AST increase is about the same.
5. *Alcoholic hepatitis* with a threefold increase. The AST has a five- to sixfold increase.
6. *Alcoholic cirrhosis* with a slight, one- to twofold increase. The AST has a three- to fourfold increase. In fatty liver secondary to alcoholism and without cirrhosis, the rise is very slight, or may be within normal limits. The AST is slightly above normal.
7. *Chronic active hepatitis* with or without cirrhosis with an increase from 1 to 12 times normal. The AST rises to 15 to 75 times normal.
8. *Infectious mononucleosis* with an increase about 15 times normal. The AST rises approximately 10 times normal (Henry, 1979).

Patient Preparation.

1. *If possible* in cases of suspected hepatic disease, hepatotoxic drugs should be withdrawn about 12 hr prior to testing.
2. *See* "Implications for Nursing for SGOT and LDH" in Section 1.12.3.

10.4.3 Gamma-Glutamyl Transferase, Serum*

Synonyms: GGT; gamma-glutamyl transpeptidase; gamma-glutamyl transferase; γ-glutamyl transferase; GGTP

Normal Ranges

Female	8–55 IU/L
Male	10–65 IU/L

*The test can be done on plasma, but serum is preferred.

Explanation of the Test. GGT is a microsomal enzyme. It is found in almost identical intracellular distribution as that of alkaline phosphatase (AP) in the liver, biliary system and pancrcas. The two enzymes rise roughly in parallel in heptobiliary and pancreatic disease. Whereas GGT is found in its greatest concentrations in liver and kidneys, with smaller amounts in heart muscle, that found in circulation derives from cells that line the small branches of the biliary tract. The feature that distinguishes GGT from other enzymes used in assessing liver function is its response to alcohol. Alcohol apparently stimulates rapid GGT elevations (within 18 hr), even with relatively small intake and without other evidence of hepatocellular damage, such as an increase in other liver enzymes. It provides objective evidence of recent drinking. For this reason it has been recommended for use in the evaluation of patients with alcoholism (Henry, 1979). In normal persons the GGT serum level varies little from day to day.

GGT INCREASED IN:

1. *Hepatobiliary obstructive disease* and pancreatic obstructive disease, to their highest recorded levels. Increases in such cases appear to approximate the degree of increase of alkaline phosphatase and serve as an estimate for the level of the hepatic isoenzyme of AP.
2. *Neoplastic or granulomatous hepatic infiltrates,* to levels greater than ten times the upper limit of normal. Some report that it is a more sensitive detector of hepatic metastases than other liver tests (Ravel, 1979).
3. *All diseases with hepatic involvement* (e.g., hepatitis, biliary tract disease, cirrhosis), with early and persistent increases as long as cellular damage exists.
4. *Alcohol ingestion,* elevated before GOT (AST). Usually elevated in 75% of all chronic alcoholics.
5. *Patients receiving certain drugs* [e.g., diphenylhydantoin (Dilantin), phenobarbital], possibly due to the induction of the microsomal enzyme system by such drugs.
6. *Neonates,* to rather high levels. The cause is unknown.
7. *Mild to moderate amounts in renal disease* and congestive heart failure.

GTT NORMAL IN:

Metabolic or bone disease. The test is therefore useful in differentiating bone disease from hepatobiliary disease when AP is increased.

Patient Preparation

1. *The test is not interfered with* by hemolysis as are LDH and AST (GOT).
2. *No special preparation* is necessary.

10.4.4 Serum Ammonia

Synonyms: NH_4; plasma ammonia

Normal Range: 0–150 μg N (nitrogen)/dL (values with plasma are somewhat lower than with serum)

Explanation of the Test. The ammonia found in the blood is derived primarily from bacterial action on nitrogen-containing materials such as food in the intestine. Some ammonia comes from the kidney, from hydrolysis of glutamine—a temporary storage substance for ammonia. Blood ammonia is presumed to be in transit to the liver (Widmann, 1979), where it is synthesized to urea. Elevations do not usually occur without some degree of hepatic failure.

NH_4 INCREASED IN:

1. *Some instances of hepatic cirrhosis,* due to impaired hepatocyte function and shunting of the blood past the liver, secondary to congestion and portal hypertension.
2. *Some instances of hepatitis,* due to incomplete removal of ammonia because of defective urea synthesis.
3. *Gastrointestinal bleeding,* usually from esophagal varices, associated with hepatic cirrhosis, due to an increased load of ammonia being delivered to a compromised liver.
4. *Severe heart failure,* or cor pulmonale, due to hepatic congestion and possible hepatic damage.
5. *Metabolic acidosis with renal failure,* or azotemia, due to decreased excretion of renal hydrogen.
6. *Reye's syndrome,* due to diffuse hepatic dysfunction with peculiar accumulation of microvacuoles of fat (may be viral induced).
7. *Stored blood,* which may reach five to ten times normal ammonia levels. Use of such blood, especially in large volumes, is particularly dangerous in liver disease.

Patient Preparation

1. *NPO other than water* for 8 to 12 hr prior to the test.
2. *Patient activity* should be minimized. Blood should not be drawn following vigorous muscular activity.
3. *Ammonia* is highly unstable. The blood sample must be iced and tested stat.

10.4.5 Hepatitis Tests

Much has been discovered in the fairly recent past about the types of hepatitis in existence, the body's response to the different infections, and the diagnostic approaches to the various types of hepatitis. Much remains to be discovered or clarified. The following definitions may assist the reader in understanding the physiologic basis for the tests to be covered in this section.

Hepatitis A. Previously called "infectious hepatitis," a liver infection of relatively short duration (2 weeks prodromal, 2 weeks after abnormal enzyme peak levels occur), often subclinical (no overt, specific, identifying symptoms), and often transmitted by food or water contamination. There are no known carrier states. Previously diagnosed by ruling out hepatitis B, diagnostic tests have been developed (see below) using the specific hepatitis A antigen and antibody identified.

Anti-HAV (*anti-hepatitis A virus*). A population of antibodies produced in response to an infection with hepatitis A virus and made up of immunoglobulins G and M.

Hepatitis B. Previously called "serum hepatitis." A disease that produces carriers: 90% of persons infected have complete recovery; 10% persist with a chronic active, or chronic persistent hepatitis and are carriers of the infection. Spread by parenteral infection (blood, blood products) primarily, but can also be spread by rather casual contact with the infective agent, (e.g., through mucous membrane, breaks in the skin, and may well be spread by sexual contact). Maternal transmission also occurs to the fetus or newborn. All body secretions have been found to contain the viral surface antigen (see below). The infection may be severe and prolonged.

HB_sAg (*hepatitis B surface antigen*). Antigenic substances that appear after exposure to hepatitis B but before symptoms appear. Found in the cytoplasm of infected cells and detectable in the serum.

HB_cAg (*hepatitis B core antigen*). Antigenic substances that appear in circulation only as part of the Dane particle (see below). Found in the nucleus of the infected cell.

Anti-HB_s (*antibody to hepatitis B surface antigen*). Formed in response to the presence of the surface antigen and provides protection against reinfection.

Anti-HB_c (*anti-hepatitis B core*). An antibody formed in response to HB_c antigen, detectable in the blood.

Dane particle. A term previously used for the complete infectious virions of hepatitis B—the HB virus. Found in the patient's blood and the blood of carriers. A DNA virus with multiple antigenic features (HB_s, HB_c, and HB_e).

HB_e antigen and anti-HB_e. Less often seen than the other HB virus antigens and antibodies. The presence of HB_e antigen may be associated with a higher degree of infectivity in both the acute disease and in chronic carriers (Henry, 1979; Widmann, 1979). The presence of anti-HB_e in carriers implies low infectivity.

A. Anti-HAV

Synonyms: anti-hepatitis A virus: antibody to hepatitis A virus

Reactions Reported

Normal	Negative
Significant	Greater than fourfold rise in titer between acute and convalescent sera (Ackley, 1980)

Explanation of the Test. If the hepatitis A virus (antigen) is present in the patient's serum, antibodies will be produced against the virus. The presence of the antibody IgM and the absence of anti-IgG in the early, acute stage of suspected hepatitis A indicates a presumptive diagnosis of its presence. The presence of anti-HAV in the serum at the start of the illness but without increase in titer throughout the following weeks indicates past infection rather than present infection with HAV (Ackley, 1980).

The test used in most laboratories at this time provides information only about the presence of antibodies to HAV in the serum. The more sophisticated laboratories can also measure anti-HAV titers (Troutman, 1980).

ANTI-HAV PRESENT IN:

1. *Acute hepatitis A* (HAV).
2. *Some patients with past history of hepatitis A* (clinical or subclinical).

Anti-HAV does not appear in hepatitis B or non-A, non-B hepatitis.

Patient Preparation. No special preparation is required.

B. Hepatitis B surface antigen

Synonyms: HB_sAg; HBA_C; hepatitis B associated antigen; serum hepatitis antigen; Australia antigen; HAA

Normal Reaction: Negative

Explanation of the Test. Now usually done by RIA, the tests to detect HB_sAg are the primary laboratory tests for diagnosis of hepatitis B, and differential diagnosis of hepatitis by virtue of their present state of relative availability and accuracy. They are used to detect active infection. HB_sAg appears in the blood approximately 1 to 7 weeks after exposure and before clinical illness is apparent. It usually persists for 1 to 12 weeks. The tests are also used to screen blood donors. HB_sAg is not eliminated in some 10% of infected individuals, and after 6 months such persons are considered carriers. The persons with persistent HB_sAg usually have a chronic form of hepatitis (Ravel, 1979). Screening blood donors is particularly important since hepatitis B is most readily contracted through parenteral administration of blood or blood products, although most post-transmission hepatitis is non-A, non-B (hepatitis C).

Subtyping of HB_sAg is available, but is used primarily for epidemiologic investigations.

HB_sAg PRESENT IN:

1. *Acute hepatitis B.*
2. *Most chronic carriers of hepatitis B.*

HB_sAg does not appear in hepatitis A or hepatitis C (also known as non-A, non-B hepatitis).

Patient Preparation. No special preparation is necessary. Handling of specimens must be done with special care because of the high potential for infection.

C. Hepatitis B surface antigen antibody

Synonyms: anti-HB_s; antibody to hepatitis B surface antigen; HB_sAb

Normal Reaction: none detected

Explanation of the Test. Anti-HB_s is not usually helpful in diagnosis; the antibody appears late (2 to 13 weeks after HB_sAg is first detected), sometimes as late as 6 to 12 months after the acute episode. The test is used primarily to determine past infection and possible immunity in persons exposed to hepatitis B, or those working in high-exposure risk areas (e.g., hemodialysis units). The anti-HB_s remains detectable for differing lengths of time, usually a period of years, but may decrease earlier. Not all persons having had hepatitis B infections have detectable anti-HB_s. The presence of anti-HB_s does not protect against hepatitis A or C (non-A, non-B).

Patient Preparation. No special preparation is necessary.

10.5 TESTS OF GALLBLADDER FUNCTION

10.5.1 Laboratory and Clinical Indications of Gallbladder Dysfunction

Laboratory Findings. In many cases the findings are very similar to dysfunction of the liver; many liver function tests may be abnormal. Increased total bilirubin–increased direct conjugated fraction most frequently; increased WBCs to 12,000 to 15,000 per mm^3 in acute cholecystitis; increased alkaline phosphatase; SGOT (SAST) may be increased; bilirubinuria.

Clinical Findings. Jaundice; right upper quadrant pain/tenderness which may be first noted by noticing decreased respiratory excursion; with acute cholecystitis vomiting may occur, slight temperature elevation which can progress to marked elevation with chills and fever spikes; chronic cholecystitis, dyspepsia, intolerance to fatty foods, heartburn; increased index of suspicion if these symptoms occur in a fair, fat, fortyish female.

10.5.2 Other Tests of Gallbladder Function—Visualization

At present specific diagnostic tests for gallbladder dysfunction tend to fall more in the field of x-ray or other visualizing diagnostic methods. The reader is urged to check any complete medical-surgical text, or other laboratory texts for information on endoscopy, laproscopy, cholangiography, oral and IV cholecystography, ultrasonography, and computerized axial tomography (CAT).

10.5.3 Bromsulphthalein Test

Synonyms: BSP; sodium sulfobromophthalein; BSP retention test; BSP clearance test

Normal Range (usually reported as % retention)

Less than 5% retention in serum at 45 min (or less than 0.5 mg/dL)
Less than 2% retention in serum at 60 min

Explanation of the Test. BSP is a dye that the liver cell transports and excretes exactly as it does bilirubin. Clearance is normal only when there is adequate blood flow to the liver, liver cell function is intact, and the biliary tree (or bile duct excretory channel) is patent. What is actually tested, then, is the status of bilirubin transport, so the BSP test is not limited to evaluation of gallbladder function.

The test is not done when jaundice exists, since bilirubin and BSP use the same transport and the presence of jaundice is an obvious indication that transport is blocked. Results will be increased in any case and provide few hard data for use.

BSP RETENTION INCREASED IN:

1. *Cholelithiasis, cholecystitis, and partial biliary tract obstruction* from whatever cause. Increases occur even before noticeable bilirubin retention occurs.
2. *Beginning viral or toxic hepatitis.*
3. *Portal or nutritional cirrhosis.* Increases may parallel the activity of the disease. Fatty or cirrhotic livers may have increased BSP retention even when other liver function tests are normal.
4. *Conditions causing decreased blood flow to the liver,* such as congestive heart failure, shock, or hepatic vein occlusion.

5. *Invasive disease of the liver,* such as metastatic cancer, sarcoidosis, lymphoma, amyloidosis, or tuberculosis.

BSP FALSE INCREASES OCCUR WITH:

1. *Increased body fat.* BSP dye dosage is weight-adjusted, but fatty tissue has little plasma volume. Therefore, an excessive dose may be given.
2. *Conditions causing increased body metabolic rate,* such as high temperatures (103°F or above).
3. *Upper gastrointestinal bleeding.*

BSP FALSE DECREASES OCCUR WITH:

1. *Individuals who have had cholecystograms* with dye injection. Dye saturates the transport substance (albumin) and the BSP dye may bypass the liver and be excreted in the urine.
2. *Conditions causing low serum albumin* (less than 2.5 g/dL).

Patient Preparation.

1. *The test should not be scheduled* for at least 3 days after gall-bladder x-rays, and preferably before they are done.
2. *The patient should be weighed* and that information provided to the laboratory, as the BSP dose is calculated on weight.
3. *The dye is very irritating* to tissues. Care must be taken to prevent extravasation during intravenous injection.

10.5.4 Urobilinogen, Urine and Fecal

Synonyms: mesobilirubinogen; stercobilinogen

Normal Ranges:

Urine		
	2 hr	0–1.0 EU (Ehrlich units)/2 hr
	24 hr	0–4.0 EU/24 hr (values of 5–10 are borderline)
Fecal		10–250 EU/100 g (values of 250–400 are borderline)

Explanation of the Test. The urobilinogens (mesobilirubin, stercobilinogen, and urobilinogen) are formed from direct, conjugated bilirubin, released as bile into the intestinal tract. Part of the urobilinogen formed is excreted in the feces, and a smaller portion is reabsorbed into portal circulation (see Fig. 1.1). A small portion of that reabsorbed into portal circulation is excreted into the urine. The major portion is extracted by the liver cells and is again excreted as bile. Increases in direct, conjugated bilirubin will increase the amounts excreted into feces and urine. Increases of indirect, unconjugated bilirubin, when due to breakdown of red blood cells only, increase fecal urobilinogen levels only. Other increases of indirect, unconjugated bilirubin cause increased production of conjugated bilirubin, ultimately increasing urobilinogen in both urine and feces.

CHANGES IN UROBILINOGEN LEVELS

	Urine urobilinogen	Fecal urobilinogen
Hemolytic anemia	Normal	Increased
Biliary obstruction	Decreased	Decreased
Liver parenchymal disease	Increased	Normal

Patient Preparation. No special preparation is necessary.

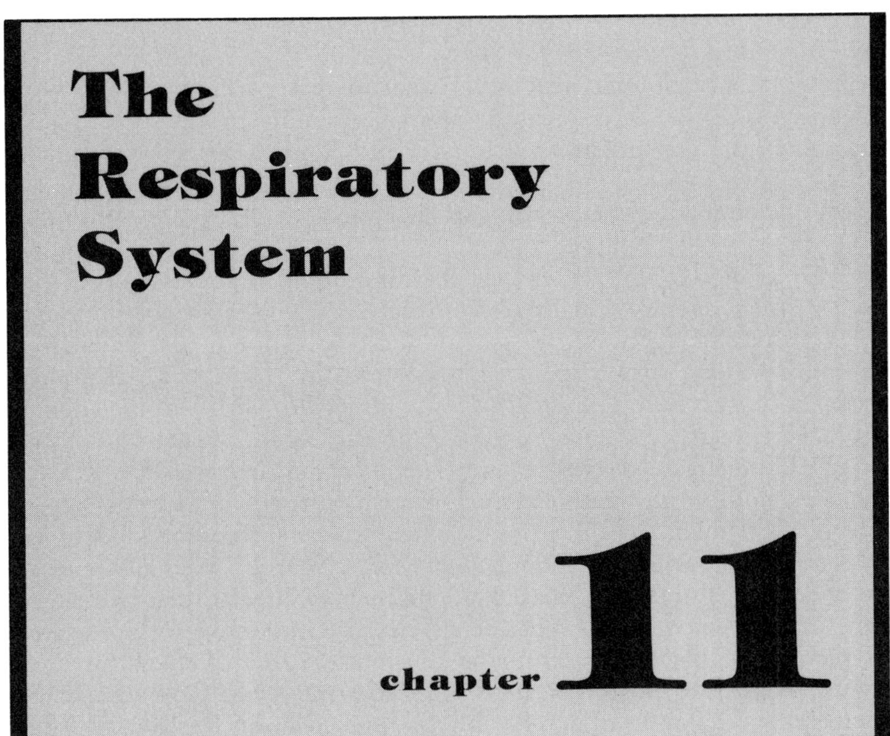

11.1 LABORATORY AND CLINICAL INDICATIONS OF THE RESPIRATORY SYSTEM DYSFUNCTION

Laboratory Findings. Since the respiratory and cardiovascular systems are so closely connected in function, what affects one, in time usually affects the other. There is, therefore, considerable overlap in the clues indicating a need to investigate the function of these systems. *Blood:* increased WBC and slight shift to the left (infectious processes), increased erythrocyte sedimentation rate, eosinophilia with allergic processes (with sputum culture, Gram + organisms such as *Streptococcus pneumoniae* or *Hemophilus influenzae,* and increased WBC on gross examination). Chronic infections may be accompanied by a normochromic, normocytic anemia. Electrolyte imbalances with COPD (e.g., decreased potassium, decreased chloride; venous CO_2 may increase, indicating compensation for respiratory acidosis). Polycythemia secondary to decreased arterial O_2. Increased WBC without a shift to the left found with pulmonary emboli + increased LDH and GOT (AST). Change in total proteins—may decrease in chronic disease with long-term decrease in albumin production; may increase with hypersensitivity pneumonitis, due to increased gamma globulin production. *Urine:* changes in pH dependent on acid-base and compensatory status of the body; changes in volume and specific gravity are dependent on the effect of pulmonary changes on cardiac action.

Clinical Findings. *Changes in respirations:* increased rate, shallow, gasping; asymmetrical chest movement, use of accessory muscles, chest retraction between ribs and at sternal notch—particularly in children—S.O.B., pursed lip breathing, complaint of dyspnea, orthopnea, dyspnea on exertion. *Changes in skin color:* pallor with chronic anemia, lividity with polycythemia, cyanosis with cardiac involvement (may not occur if anemia is severe). *Changes in level of consciousness (LOC):* hyperirritability, decreased attention span, vertigo, increased sleeping during day, difficulty in arousal. *Changes in neuromuscular activity:* hyperreflexia, twitching. *Changes in breath sounds:* rales not cleared by a cough, rhonchi, decreased or absence of breath sounds, friction rub, stridor, wheezing. *Cough*—persistent nonproductive, or productive of secretions that may be mucoid or purulent. *Barrel chest,* hunched shoulders, sitting positions that support arms away from the chest. Increased complaints of *severe fatigue,* picked up in children by their voluntary limitation of activity, squatting to catch their breath. *History of repeated respiratory infections:* family history of chronic obstructive pulmonary disease (COPD).

11.2 BLOOD GASES

11.2.1 Carbon Dioxide, Venous, Serum

Synonyms: plasma carbon dioxide; CO_2, venous; total CO_2; CO_2 combining power

Normal Range: 23–30 mEq/L

Explanation of the Test. Most often this test is done as part of a routine screening of serum electrolytes. It provides a reflection of overall acid-base balance, and is useful in checking and corroborating arterial blood gases, such as those of pCO_2 and pH. Venous CO_2 is actually an indirect measurement of blood base, specifically bicarbonate (HCO_3). All of the test titles given above are measurements of this value. Although venous HCO_3 can be measured more directly, most commonly it is measured as total CO_2, that is, with the other combined and dissolved CO_2 in the blood. The value reached approximates serum HCO_3 very closely since 89 to 90% of all CO_2 in serum is in the form of HCO_3. Levels of total CO_2 (measured as HCO_3) are slightly lower in arterial blood.

CO_2 combining power is used less frequently than total CO_2 because the process is more difficult, it excludes the respiratory contribution to the acid-base status, and it is more subject to error (Henry, 1979) (see also Section 1.2).

INCREASED IN:

1. *Metabolic alkalosis.*
2. *Compensation of respiratory acidosis.*

DECREASED IN·

1. *Metabolic acidosis.*
2. *Compensation of respiratory alkalosis.*

11.2.2 Total Arterial/Venous Blood Gases

Synonyms: arterial blood gases: ABG; venous blood gases: VBG

Normal Ranges

	Arterial	Venous
pH[a]	7.35–7.45	7.31–7.42
pCO_2	35–45 mmHg	39–55 mmHg
pO_2	80–100 mmHg	30–50 mmHg
HCO_3	22–29 mEq/L	22–28 mEq/L
O_2 saturation	95–100% (SaO_2)	75% (SvO_2)
Base excess/deficit	0 ± 2.3 mEq/L	
O_2 content	15.0–23.0 vol %	11–16 vol %
Hbg		
Female	12–15 g/dL	
Male	13–17 g/dL	

[a]pH range compatible with life: 6.8–7.8.

Explanation of the Tests. The "routine" blood gas test usually includes only the pH, pCO_2, pO_2, and HCO_3, but some laboratories routinely include one or more of the other determinations as well—for example, base excess/deficit (see Table 11.1). The combination

TABLE 11.1 *Individual arterial blood gases*

Substance tested	Definition	Significance in interpretation	Compensatory mechanism and discussion
pH	From a chemical point of view, it is the expression of the ratio between bicarbonate and carbonic acid: 20:1 = pH of 7.4; an expression of the hydrogen ion (H^+) in the blood	Low values indicate acid state (less than 7.35); high values indicate an alkalotic state (more than 7.45); the body adjusts (compensates) better with slow changes in pH than with rapid ones, which can be fatal; the body cannot tolerate values beyond the normal range, but still compatible with life, for prolonged periods	(See pCO_2 and HCO_3 for compensatory mechanism) pH measurement is unreliable in blood drawn more than ½ hr before testing and not refrigerated, or in blood allowed to contact ambient air
pCO_2	A measurement of dissolved carbon dioxide's tension (partial pressure[a]) in the blood	CO_2 unites with water in the ECF, forming carbonic acid (H_2CO_3); measurement of CO_2 tension is, in effect, measuring the H_2CO_3, its level is directly proportional to H_2CO_3 and is thus considered an acid (volatile), which indicates lung status; thus pCO_2 is a volatile acid and is excreted in water vapor and air from the lungs Increased pCO_2 = respiratory acidosis Decreased pCO_2 = respiratory alkalosis	The rate and depth of respirations affect the increase or decrease of pCO_2 but are not useful for compensation since the *problem* is respiratory in primary respiratory acidosis or alkalosis; increased renal secretion and/or reabsorption of H^+ or HCO_3 is the primary compensatory mechanism (see Table 11.2 for relationship between pH and pCO_2 in primary respiratory disease)
pO_2	A measurement of dissolved oxygen tension in the blood	The partial pressure (pp) of a gas is what determines the force it exerts; the pp of O_2 determines how rapidly, and to what extent, it can diffuse from the alveoli into the blood and from the blood to body cells; changes in pp can be due to decreased available oxygen and/or decreased available hemoglobin	Oxygen lack is compensated for, to some extent, by increased rate and depth of breathing; in chronic O_2 lack, RBC production increases, causing a secondary polycythemia; usually, O_2 pp is decreased to some degree in all restrictive or obstructive pulmonary disease, depending on the extent and severity of the disease process

TABLE 11.1 *Individual arterial blood gases (cont.)*

Substance tested	Definition	Significance in interpretation	Compensatory mechanism and discussion
HCO_3	Bicarbonate; the principal buffer substance in the plasma; calculated from known values of pH and pCO_2 using the Henderson-Hasselback equation, or a nomogram based on it	Decrease in HCO_3 levels usually indicates primary base deficit, called metabolic acidosis; increase in HCO_3 levels is usually due to a base excess (metabolic alkalosis) in ratio to H^+ available; HCO_3 also increases or decreases as a compensatory response to other imbalances, especially pCO_2	Primary mechanism is respiratory with excess H^+ being blown off by increased respiratory rate and depth, thereby usually restoring the 20:1 ratio; if not, and given adequate kidney function, compensation for severe A-B imbalances can usually be achieved by increased kidney tubule secretion or reabsorption of both H^+ and HCO_3
O_2 saturation	A measurement of the amount of O_2 being carried by the hemoglobin; O_2 saturation is the value used when plotting the oxyhemoglobin dissociation curve (see "Physiology," Section 2.1.2)	Decreased values indicate the lack of available O_2 or the lack of hemoglobin; the percent of saturation is limited by the capacity of the blood to bind O_2; thus increased administration of O_2 is useless in the face of inadequate hemoglobin stores	(See pO_2 above)
Base excess or deficit	A measurement of all buffers available in the blood, including both volatile (HCO_3) and nonvolatile (hemoglobin, Cl^-, PO_4, SO_4, protein), which are usually not measured (see Appendix A)	Base excess or deficit provides a more complete picture of the individual's acid–base status than does just the information available from the pH, pCO_2 and HCO_3	The compensatory mechanisms depend on the basic dysfunction causing the excess or deficit (see pCO_2 and HCO_3 above); base excess or deficit is calculated by plating measurements of pH, pCO_2, and hematocrit on a nomogram
O_2 content	A measurement of the total amount of O_2 in the blood, including that bound to hemoglobin (O_2 sat.) and that dissolved or "free" in the plasma	O_2 content varies directly with pO_2, but not in a linear relationship; its measurement helps explain differences which can occur between pO_2 and O_2 sat.	(See pO_2 above)

[a]Partial pressure is defined as the pressure exerted by one of the gases in a mixture of gases in a liquid. Each partial pressure is exerted independently of the other gases.

of blood gases (arterial) and spirometry are considered adequate for the assessment of most problems in clinical medicine involving the lungs. Arterial blood gas measurements are the most accurate, but venous blood is much more readily attainable. Arterial capillary blood from the finger can be used for pH and pCO_2 when conditions make acquisition of arterial blood too difficult. Such a sample is not acceptable for pO_2 measurement, but in some cases, arterialized capillary blood from an earlobe can be used for pO_2 values. Although arterial blood gases are much preferred for diagnosis and management of acute disease, venous blood gas samples are often used in conjunction with serum electrolytes in the management of chronic conditions that can be followed on an outpatient basis (Gump, 1980).

It is important to remember that all factors involved in acid-base balance are in dynamic interchange, attempting to maintain equilibrium. Therefore, the more factors that are known, the better the basis for health care. This includes not only the blood gases, but also the clinical history and present signs and symptoms.

Expected Changes in Arterial Acid-Base Factors in Given Conditions

Primary respiratory acidosis. Due to airway obstruction (severe COPD, severe asthma); neuromuscular disorders (myasthenia gravis, poliomyelitis, amyotrophic lateral sclerosis); respiratory center depression (trauma, narcotics, sedatives).

	pH	pCO_2	HCO_3	Base excess/deficit
Acute uncompensated*	D	I	N	N
Early compensation	D	I	I	I (excess)
Chronic compensated	N	I	I	I (excess)

*D, decreased from lower limits of norm; I, increased from upper limits of norm; N, within normal limits.

Primary respiratory alkalosis. Due to hyperventilation (anxiety, fever, artificial ventilation); hypoxemia (high altitudes, moderate COPD, moderate asthma, pulmonary embolism); early salicylate poisoning.

	pH	pCO_2	HCO_3	Base excess/deficit
Acute uncompensated	I	D	N	N
Early compensation	I	D	D	D (deficit)
Chronic compensated	N	D	D	D (deficit)

Primary metabolic acidosis. Due to increase in nonvolatile H^+ (ingestion of ammonium chloride, diabetic ketoacidosis, lactic acidosis, renal failure); exogenous poisoning (salicylates, late); loss of HCO_3 (diarrhea, renal tubular acidosis, prolonged intestinal suctioning, use of carbonic anhydrase inhibitors).

	pH	pCO_2	HCO_3	Base excess/deficit
Acute uncompensated	D	N	D	D (deficit)
Early compensation	D	D	D	D (deficit)
Chronic compensated	N	D	D	D or N

Primary metabolic alkalosis. Due to loss of H^+ (prolonged vomiting, prolonged nasogastric suctioning, diuretic therapy, hyper-adrenocorticism–Cushing's disease/syndrome, adrenal steroid therapy, aldosteronism); increased bicarbonate (excessive intake).

	pH	pCO_2	HCO_3	Base excess/deficit
Acute uncompensated	I	N	I	I (excess)
Early compensating	I	I	I	I (excess)
Chronic compensated	N	I	I	I or N

Mixed Acid-Base Imbalances. The older the individual or the more seriously ill he or she is, the less likely it is that the "pure" imbalances described above are to be found. Besides being under attack with the primary problem, most persons found in hospital settings are also doing battle to maintain A-B equilibrium in other areas, due to chronic or superimposed illnesses. For example, a respiratory and metabolic acidosis can coexist (COPD-DKA). To discover whether the respiratory problem is primary in origin, the relative change of relationships betwen pCO_2 and pH (see Table 11.2) can be plotted over a series of ABG measurements to see if the changes follow the "rule." Nothing is of more value, however, than a thorough understanding of the patient's past and present history and general status.

TABLE 11.2 *Changes in pH relative to pCO_2 in primary acute respiratory acid-base imbalances*[a]

pCO_2 (mmHg)	pH
10	7.7
20	7.6
30	7.5
40	*7.4 normal*
60	7.3
80	7.2
100	7.1

[a]There is an inverse relationship between pH and pCO_2 in acid–base imbalances due to primary (pure) acute respiratory problems. For each 0.1 decrease in pH below 7.4, a 20-mmHg increase in pCO_2 occurs. For each 0.1 increase in pH above 7.4, a 10-mmHg decrease in pCO_2 should occur (Milthorn, 1980).

Special Pediatric Procedures

Transcutaneous pO_2 *monitoring*

Normal Range: 50–110 mmHg

A miniature oxygen measuring electrode with a built-in warmer, which is placed on the infant's chest or thigh. As the skin warms, O_2 diffuses out of the capillaries. The electrode measures the amount of oxygen at the skin surface, which is proportional to the pO_2 of the blood. The amount of heat necessary to keep the infant's skin at 43°C is also recorded, which is said to correlate with blood tissue perfusion.

Scalp pH (*blood sample from a scalp vein*)

Normal Range: 7.25-7.40

Used, together with other clinical data, to help determine the need for a Caesarian section in some situations. A fetal scalp pH of less than 7.15 in the face of a normal arterial pH in the maternal blood indicates serious fetal acidosis and the need for immediate Cacsarian. A scalp pH of 7.15 to 7.24 is considered ambiguous and requires further close monitoring (SHMC, 1978).

11.2.3 Other Respiratory Function and Diagnostic Tests

The reader may wish to explore other tests related to pulmonary function. The scope of this book does not allow for their inclusion, which does not minimize their importance. Such tests include spirometry, or flow volume loops (vital capacity–VC, forced vital capacity–FVC, residual volume–RV, functional residual volume–FRV, total lung capacity–TLC, expiratory reserve volume–ERV, forced expiratory volume–FEV, maximal midexpiratory flow–MMEF, peak inspiratory/ expiratory flow rate–PIFR/PEFR, inspiratory capacity–IC, maximal voluntary ventilation–MVV, maximal breathing capacity–MBCO); lung scan; lung biopsy; pulmonary angiography, thoracentesis, bronchoscopy, bronchography, fluoroscopy, flat and oblique plates of the chest by x-ray.

The Cardiovascular System

chapter 12

12.1 LABORATORY AND CLINICAL INDICATIONS OF CARDIOVASCULAR SYSTEM DYSFUNCTION†

Laboratory Findings. Blood: Increased SGOT (AST) and LDH. SGPT (ALT) may be elevated as well if there is liver involvement due to congestion. Increased serum cholesterol.* Increased serum glucose,* decrease in plasma potassium, and some change in sodium—may be increased or decreased. *Urine:* Increased uric acid,* increased BUN, proteinuria, WBC increase in gross examination with granular casts. Creatinine usually within normal limits except in badly decompensated cardiac conditions, or those with concomitant renal disease. Specific gravity may increase with a decreased circulating volume.

Clinical Findings. Presence of edema (dependent), increased fatigue (in children evidenced by voluntary limitation of activity and squatting to rest), and complaints of dyspnea or overt shortness of breath are hallmark signs. Clubbing of finger and toe nails; poor peri-

†Findings indicated by an asterisk have been identified as a known risk factor.

pheral perfusion with cold extremities, mottling of skin of extremities; xanthomas on skin*. Presence of heart murmurs, S_3 and S_4 heart sounds (except in children where they may be normal), increased strength of PMI—may be visible on the chest wall (myocardial hypertrophy), hepatomegaly, tender liver. Complaint of anginal pain; pain on exertion or after eating. Dizziness, fainting, premature vascular disease. History of hypertension*, heavy cigarette smoking*, diabetes mellitus in family*, and/or diagnosed in the patient*, obesity*, oral contraceptive use*, hypothyroidism, excessive intake of saturated fats, renal disease, or alcoholism*. More common with increased age*. Evidence of retinal lipemia. Family history of death from heart disease before age 60*.

12.2 CARDIOVASCULAR LIPID PROFILE

Synonyms: lipid profile; lipid fractionation; plasma lipoproteins; includes (varies with the laboratory) total cholesterol (see Section 1.11); total lipid; phospholipid; triglycerides; high-density cholesterol (HDL-cholesterol); low-density cholesterol (LDL-cholesterol); "standing" plasma test (lipid phenotyping may be included but generally has not proven useful)

Normal Ranges (plasma or serum may be used)

Total lipids	500–1000 mg/dL
Phospholipids	125– 300 mg/dL
Triglycerides	30– 175 mg/dL
Cholesterol—total	
Greater than 40 years	140– 170 mg/dL
Less than 40 years	150– 330 mg/dL
(For a more complete breakdown, see Section 1.11)	
HDL-cholesterol	
Female	Mean 55 mg/dL
Male	Mean 45 mg/dL
LDL-cholesterol	
Female	Mean 131.1 mg/dL
Male	Mean 135.5 mg/dL‡

‡Calculated from data from Burke (1980). LDL-cholesterol is calculated. One formula for this calculation is

$$\text{total cholesterol} - \left(\text{HDL-cholesterol} + \frac{\text{triglycerides}}{5}\right) = \text{LDL-cholesterol}$$

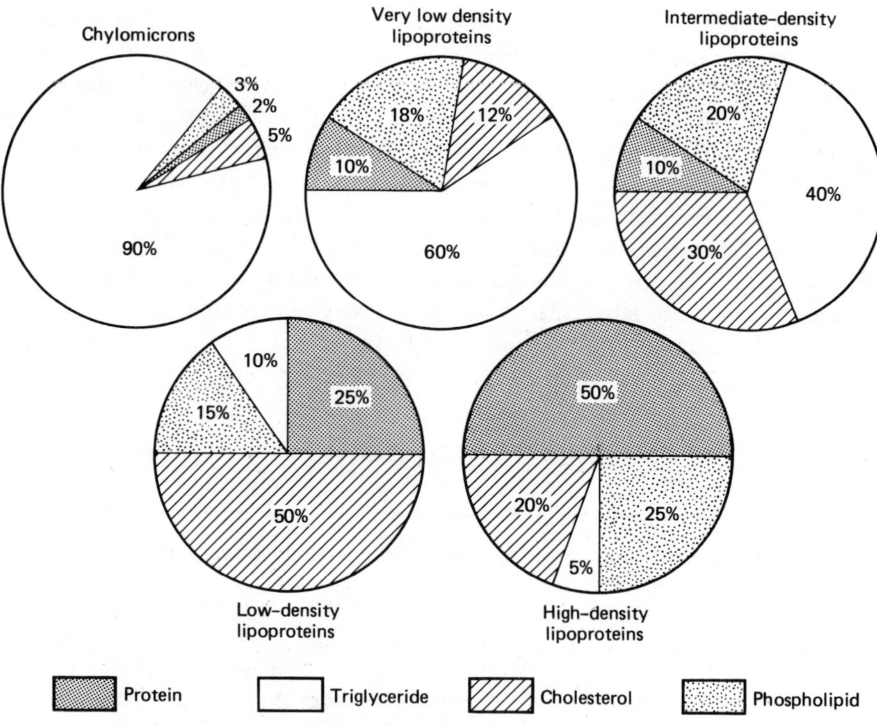

FIGURE 12.1 Compositions of the five lipoprotein classes. [From Robert I. Levy, "Hyperlipoproteinemia and Its Management," *Journal of Cardiovascular Medicine* (June 1980), 436.]

Explanation of the Test. Plasma lipids travel as complex molecules combined with several proteins, so that the lipid profile tests actually measure lipids and proteins. These lipoproteins appear in five classes in the plasma: chylomicrons—consisting almost entirely of *dietary* triglycerides; very low density lipoproteins (VLDL); intermediate-density lipoproteins (IDL); low-density lipoproteins (LDL)—also known as beta lipoproteins; and high-density lipoproteins (HDL)—also known as alpha lipoprotein. All five classes contain varying amounts of the different lipoproteins, as depicted in Fig. 12.1. The purpose of the lipid profile or fractionation is to more clearly characterize the various components that make up hyperlipidemic states and to identify the increased-risk patient.

Significance of the Tests

Total lipids. Increase when any fraction of the plasma lipids elevate (except triglycerides), in nephrotic syndrome, ketosis, and cardiovascular disease (atheroclerosis). Decreased total lipids may be found in malabsorption syndromes. Physiologic increase occurs after a fatty meal. Several drugs will elevate total lipids (e.g., oral contraceptives, estrogen).

Phospholipids. Increase with biliary obstruction, biliary cirrhosis. Decrease in ratio of phospholipid to cholesterol in atherosclerosis.

Triglycerides. Composed of glycerol and fatty acids. (Their concentration in the five classes of lipoproteins is shown in Fig. 12.1.) Conditions in which triglyceride lipids predominate can be derived from Tables 12.1, and 12.2, knowing that triglyceride content is greatest in chylomicrons, very low density lipoproteins, and intermediate-density lipoproteins. Increases of triglycerides with myocardial infarction may last as long as a year. Triglyceride levels by themselves have very little predictive value. Will increase after fat intake.

Cholesterol total. See Section 1.11.

HDL-cholesterol; LDL-cholesterol. Currently, is it thought that low-density lipoprotein, made up primarily of cholesterol, relates *directly* with the risk of coronary artery disease (high LDL = high risk; low LDL = low risk), and that high-density lipoprotein cholesterol relates *inversely* with that risk (high HDL = low risk; low HDL = high risk) (Burke, 1980). It is postulated that measurement of HDL and LDL-cholesterol is more important in the diagnosis of atherosclerosis development than is the measurement of total cholesterol. HDL increases with exercise training and is believed to be protective against atherosclerosis (Hartung and Squires, 1980).

"Standing" plasma test. Consists of observing a serum sample, which has been refrigerated overnight, for the presence of lactescence, or fatty turbidity, which indicates excess VLDL, primarily triglycerides, in the sample. Normally, the serum is clear. If a creamy layer appears on the top of the serum, it indicates either abnormality of VLDL content or that the sample taken was not a fasting sample. With excessive VLDL, the refrigerated sample will be uniformly turbid. Cholesterol and LDL levels cannot be demonstrated by this approach.

There are both primary (genetic) and secondary hyperlipoproteinemias. A classification was developed by Frederickson et al. to identify types of hyperlipoproteinemias (grouping of disorders that affect plasma lipid and lipoprotein concentrations in a similar manner) (see Table 12.2, page 427). The classification is limited in genetic analysis and the process of classification is elaborate. More recently, the use of the varying densities of the lipoproteins as organizational threads has been more widely accepted (Henry, 1979).

TABLE 12.1 *Biochemical and clinical features of the lipoprotein classes*

Class	Origin	Function	Catabolism	Plasma appearance in elevation	Clinical correlates of elevation
Chylomicrons	Intestine, from dietary fat	Transport dietary fat	Lipoprotein lipase at tissue sites chylomicron remnants cleared by liver	Creamy, supernate, clear infranate	Eruptive xanthoma, lipemia retinalis, organomegaly pancreatitis
VLDLs	Liver and small bowel, from carbohydrates, free fatty acids, medium-chain triglycerides	Transport endogenous triglycerides	Complex; probably requires lipoprotein lipase for degradation	Turbid	Glucose intolerance, hyperuricemia
IDLs	VLDLs	Unknown	(?) Degradation to LDL	Turbid	Glucose intolerance, hyperuricemia; premature atherosclerosis; tuboeruptive, tendinous, palmar planar xanthoma
LDLs	VLDL and IDL, (?) alternative source	Unknown	Primary site of removal unclear	Clear	Premature atherosclerosis, corneal arcus, tendinous and tuberous xanthoma, xanthelasma
HDLs	(?) intestine, liver	(?) Facilitate cholesterol ester and triglyceride metabolism	(?) Liver	Clear	No associated abnormality

Source: Robert I. Levy, "Hyperlipoproteinemia and Its Management." *Journal of Cardiovascular Medicine* (june 1980), 438.

TABLE 12.2 *Types of hyperlipoproteinemia*

Type	Features	Possible secondary causes
I	↑Chylomicrons	Insulinopenic diabetes mellitus, dysglobulinemia, lupus erythematosus
IIa	↑LDL	Nephrotic syndrome, hypothyroidism
IIb	↑LDL and VLDL	Obstructive liver disease, porphyria, multiple myeloma
III	↑IDL, sometimes with ↑chylomicrons	Hypothyroidism, dysgammaglobulinemia
IV	↑VLDL	Diabetes mellitus, nephrotic syndrome, pregnancy, hormone use, glycogen storage disease, alcoholism, Gaucher disease, Nieman-Pick disease
V	↑Chylomicrons and VLDL	Insulinopenic diabetes mellitus, nephrotic syndrome, alcoholism, myeloma, idiopathic hypercalcemia

Source: Robert I. Levy, "Hyperlipoproteinemia and Its Management," *The Journal of Cardiovascular Medicine* (June 1980), 439.

Patient Preparation for Lipid Profile Tests

1. *NPO other than water* for 12 to 14 hr prior to the test.
2. *The patient should be in a physiologic steady state* (no vigorous exercise) and on his or her usual diet the day prior to the test.

12.3 TESTS FOR CARDIAC MUSCLE CELL DAMAGE

12.3.1 Creatine Phosphokinase, Serum

Synonyms: CPK; creatine kinase; CK; creatine N-phosphotransferase

Normal Ranges

Female	8–150 IU/L
Male	10–190 IU/L

Explanation of the Test. CPK is primarily an intracellular enzyme that plays a major role in the energy-storing functions of cells. It is found primarily in cardiac, skeletal, and brain tissue. CPK is released from the cell in irreversible injury, which is the major source for the increase in serum levels of CPK following cardiac injury (MI, surgery). CPK is sensitive to, but not specific for, myocardial infarction. Prior to general availability of the CPK isoenzyme fractionation, the CPK measurement was considered an essential criterion to the diagnosis of MI, even though its lack of specificity was known. The duration of its elevation was felt to correlate with the extent and severity of the infarct (see Fig. 1.2). Serum CPK levels increase early—within 6 hr—in myocardial damage. Peaks occur at about 18 hr, and return to normal in 3 to 4 days if no further damage occurs (Grenadier and Palant, 1980).

CPK INCREASED IN:

1. *Muscle disorders* (skeletal), such as muscular dystrophy, polymyositis, alcoholic myopathies, dermatomyositis, due to the increased permeability of the cell membrane. Produces persistent remarkably high increases.
2. *Cardiac cell injury* or destruction as in angina, myocardial infarction.
3. *Conditions causing dysfunction of neural tissues,* such as meningitis, encephalitis, cerebral tumors, acute cerebral vascular accidents, convulsions, head trauma, and subarachnoid hemorrhage.
4. *Muscular trauma* such as with IM injections, vigorous exercise, surgical incisions through muscle (especially in heart surgery).
5. *Hypothyroidism,* believed to be due to skeletal muscle deterioration.

Patient Preparation. No special preparation is necessary.

12.3.2 CPK Isoenzyme M-B, Serum

Synonyms: creatine phosphokinase isoenzyme M-B; CPK-MB; CPK_2

Normal Range: Normally absent in serum; reported as negative; can be reported as a percentage of total CPK activity; greater than 4% is considered pathologically elevated

Explanation of the Test. CPK has been found to have three isoenzymes: CPK-BB (CPK_1), found primarily in the brain; CPK-MB (CPK_2), found primarily in cardiac cells (once thought to be contained exclusively in cardiac cells, but now known to also occur in some skeletal muscle, the tongue, and various viscera); and CPK-MM (CPK_3), found in both cardiac and skeletal muscle (Bauman, 1980).

When the CPK isoenzyme MB was first used as the "ideal MI marker," it was thought not only to be exclusive to cardiac cells, but also to be released only when there was irreversible destruction of the cell. However, increases in CPK-MB have been found with such conditions as unstable angina, sustained supraventricular arrythmias, and ischemia due to coronary insufficiency, with no evidence of MI. It has also been found to be present in differing concentrations in various parts of the myocardium, so that the locale of the infarct may influence the level of CPK-MB activity in the serum. Therefore, although the test is a useful adjunct to the diagnosis of MI, and it is probable that it will be elevated in most patients with cardiac cell necrosis within the first 48 hr, it can be elevated in the absence of an MI, or normal in the presence of one (Bauman, 1980).

The CPK-MB can be of particular use in many instances of differential diagnosis. Since it does not elevate secondary to muscular trauma, it can be used to assess chest pain in a person having received IM medications, or having had other muscular trauma. It has been found to be the most sensitive indicator of cardiac contusion after automobile accidents. It is more sensitive to myocardial infarct than is total CPK (Grenadier and Palant, 1980).

Patient Preparation. No special preparation is necessary.

12.3.3 Myoglobin, Serum and Urine

Synonyms: none

Normal Ranges

Serum	None detectable
Urine	0–4.0 mg/L

Explanation of the Test. Myoglobin is a globin complex similar to hemoglobin, but present in muscle tissue. It is excreted in the urine by way of glomerular filtration. Its excretion increases in circumstances involving any muscle cell damage. Serum and urine myoglobin measurements are used in the differential diagnosis of darkly pigmented urines, and to help substantiate or rule out a diagnosis of myocardial infarction (MI). In the presence of a normal total CPK, a normal serum and urine myoglobin, and ECG findings limited to short-lived ST and T wave changes, MI can usually be ruled out in patients with unstable angina (Grenadier, 1980).

Serum myoglobin peaks approximately 8 to 12 hr after an MI, and return to normal—or nondetectable levels—as early as 12 hr after rise. More frequently return to normal takes at least 24 hr. Serum myoglobin may appear intermittently in the first 6 to 18 hr after an MI, and serial determinations may be indicated.

Myoglobin increases can appear in the urine within 3 hr after an MI. Levels may return to high normal in 30 hr; usually, however, return to normal takes 72 hr or longer (Ravel, 1979).

MYOGLOBIN INCREASED IN:

1. *Cardiac muscle damage* (trauma, ischemia, inflammation, necrosis).
2. *Skeletal muscle damage,* most frequently in crushing injuries.
3. *Familial myoglobinuria* (Meyer-Betz disease).
4. *High fevers,* hyperthermia. In susceptible persons, fever causes muscle destruction (Henry, 1979).
5. *Uncommon occurrences with diabetic acidosis, hypokalemia,* or *barbiturate poisoning.*

12.3.4 LDH Isoenzymes, Serum

Synonyms: lactic dehydrogenase isoenzymes; LDH fractionation; isoenzymes, LDH; LDH electrophoresis

*Normal Ranges**

I	12– 81 IU
II	18–101 IU
III	8– 64 IU
IV	4– 25 IU
V	2– 25 IU

*Serum enzyme normal-range values are not comparable between laboratories. Use the reference ranges provided by the laboratory that does the test.

Explanation of the Test. The LDH isoenzymes are numbered sequentially, beginning with the most rapidly moving one and ending with the slowest moving. The individual LDH isoenzymes have different concentrations in different tissues, which provide a way of identifying the tissues responsible for an elevated total LDH. A separation, or fractionation, of the isoenzymes measures the individual concentrations of each isoenzyme. Measurement of the fractions is often done even if the total LDH is normal when a condition usually causing an increase of a given fraction is suspected. Because the range of normal for total LDH is quite broad, it is possible for the level of one or more isoenzymes to be increased, with a total LDH within normal limits.

General Interpretation of Isoenzyme Elevations

LDH_1 is found primarily in heart muscle and red blood cells and found in moderate amounts in the kidney. It increases long before a total LDH increase is seen in myocardial infarction (within 4 hr). By 24 hr there is a definite reversal of the normal LDH_1–LDH_2 ratio (normally LDH_2 has higher levels than LDH_1), often referred to as the *"LDH flip"* or "flipped LDH." This flip is of significant importance as evidence of myocardial infarct, renal infarct, or erythrocyte disease. The inverse ratio lasts longer in myocardial problems, but the initial increase of level is greater in hematological problems. It can be strikingly elevated in megoblastic anemia.

Because of its close correlation with myocardial infarction, new "mini" tests measuring LDH_1 only, and technically simple, are now on the market ("New Drugs," 1980).

Other conditions increasing LDH_1 include active myocarditis, following heart surgery [if the elevation persists more than 5 to 6 days postsurgery, a postoperative myocardial infarct (MI) should be suspected] (Widmann, 1979); megaloblastic anemia (pernicious anemia, folate deficiency anemia); hemolytic anemias; and muscular dystrophy (MD) (MD is a relative increase because $LDH_{4\text{-}5}$ are depressed).

LDH_2 is found primarily in kidney, heart, and in moderate amounts in brain tissue, in blood cells, both white and red, and probably in the cells of the reticuloendothelial system as well. Increased in myocardial infarction and other cardiac inflammatory conditions (LDH_2 does not increase as high as does LDH_1), granulocytic leukemia, pancreatitis, hemolytic and megoblastic anemias, some lymphomas, and MD (see note above regarding MD increase) (Henry, 1979).

LDH_3 is primarily of pulmonary origin, but is also found in moderate amounts in adrenal tissue, lymphocytes, skeletal muscles, brain, and kidney. Increased in pulmonary infarction and other pulmonary destruction, granulocytic leukemia, and pancreatitis. LDH_1 increase may confuse the picture in pulmonary infarct because of the frequency with which that condition is accompanied by hemorrhage (Widmann, 1979).

LDH_4 is found in about equal, but moderate, concentrations in liver, skeletal muscle, brain, and kidney. Increased in pulmonary infarct (may be due to subsequent circulatory collapse), congestive heart failure (CHF), viral and toxic hepatitis, and cirrhosis (Henry, 1979).

LDH_5 is found primarily in the liver. As LDH_1 is the "heart" enzyme, LDH_5 is the "liver" enzyme. It is found in significant amounts in skeletal muscle as well as in moderate amounts in kidney tissue. Increased in cirrhosis, toxic and viral hepatitis, CHF, and pulmonary infarct (as with LDH_4, probably due to circulatory collapse). Increases of LDH_5 in viral and drug associated hepatitis can be enormous. Increases usually precede jaundice and decreases occur before bilirubin or SGPT (ALT) levels fall. Moderate rises are found in LDH_5 in hepatitis associated with infectious mononucleosis, but total LDH increases are often very high in that disease.

FALSE INCREASES IN:

$LDH_{1\text{-}2}$ if the blood sample is allowed to hemolyze.

Patient Preparation. No special preparation is required.

Collagen-Vascular Disease or Syndromes

chapter 13

As indicated in the chapter title, collagen-vascular disease/syndromes are not considered a body system per se. They are, instead, an ill-defined collection of syndromes, involving many systems (Ravel, 1979), which share certain points in common. One of these common points is the tendency of the disorders included in this group to involve collagenous tissue in a fibrinoid necrosis, so that the disorders could be considered diseases of the connective tissue. A second shared trait is their collective tendency to involve various subdivisions of arteries in an inflammatory process, so that the disorders can be properly considered vascular disorders: hence the title "collagen-vascular." More recently, another major connection among these dissimilar conditions has been identified. The probability is that the group of disorders share an etiology based on immunologic hypersensitivity (Ravel, 1979). Therefore, in many texts the diseases, and/or syndromes, will be found in the discussion of immunologic problems. For the purposes of this text it seems less confusing to use the older designation, collagen-vascular, as immunologic testing can be mistaken for a discussion of immunologic disorders.

The most common disorders included in this group are rheumatoid arthritis (RA), systemic lupus erythematosus (SLE), polyarteritis nodosa

(PAN), and systemic sclerosis (SS; also known as scleroderma). Tests rather specific for acute rheumatic fever are included as well, as the disease demonstrates some similarity with the rheumatoid collagen-vascular group and may well be one of them.

13.1 LABORATORY AND CLINICAL INDICATIONS OF COLLAGEN-VASCULAR SYNDROMES OR DISEASES†

The major clues indicating possible collagen-vascular syndrome or disease are the presence of otherwise unexplained skin manifestations (rash, nodules), proteinuria or other abnormality of urine, polyarthralgia or arthritis, and less frequently, unexplained pleural effusion.

Laboratory Findings (General). *SLE:* the following may or may not be found; false-positive test for syphilis (VDRL or PRP)*, profuse proteinuria–greater than 3.5 g/day*, cellular casts in urine*, hemolytic anemia*, leukopenia, thrombocytopenia*, normocytic anemia*. *PAN:* anemia with very low hemoglobin, leukocytosis, eosinophilia, increased ESR, proteinuria–0.5 to 2.5 g/day, and hematuria. *SS:* hypergammaglobulinemia–abnormal urine sediment and renal involvement. *Juvenile rheumatoid arthritis (JRA):* anemia, at times profound. *Rheumatoid arthritis, acute (RA):* hypergammaglobulinemia, increased ESR; mild anemia, possible leukopenia and thrombocytopenia.

Clinical Findings. *SLE:* skin rash–butterfly distribution over cheeks and nose, sensitive to sunlight (photosensitivity), also known as focal erythema*, occurs in greatest frequency in females between ages 12 and 45 and in the black race; Raynaud's syndrome or phenomenon* (arterial vasoconstriction causing blanching of the fingers and hands, loss of sensation and pain–syndrome usually triggered by contact with cold); oral or nasopharyngeal ulceration*; polyarthritis without deformity*; evidence of pleuritis (pleural effusion) or pericarditis*; psychosis*, convulsions*; alopecia*; discoid lupus* (cutaneous lesions–sharply circumscribed erythematous macules and plaques–disc-shaped); urticaria; purpura. *PAN:* polyarthralgias, hypertension, abnormal urine in middle-aged person are cardinal signs. Other: skin manifestations: subcutaneous nodules, peripheral gangrene of fingers and toes; gastrointestinal manifestations, cramping, abdominal bleeding, bleeding ulcer; renal manifestations; flank pain and abnormal

†Findings indicated by an asterisk are criteria for the diagnosis of SLE. The patient must have at least four of the findings marked with an asterisk present serially, or simultaneously, over any period of observation (Conn and Conn, 1979).

urine; respiratory manifestations; bronchitis, possible pleural effusions. *SS:* skin manifestations; purplish indurated plaques that become waxy, smooth, shiny, and devoid of hair, linear on extremities—possibly on trunk; if muscle or bone involved—growth disturbances occur, or muscular atrophy, flexion contractions; if systemic—initial symptom usually Raynaud's phenomenon, swelling and sclerosis of distal extremities, pain, stiffness, weakness of joints and muscles. *JRA:* rheumatoid rash anywhere on body, myalgia, arthralgia, polyarthritis, fever, possible pleural effusion, growth retardation. *RA:* polyarthritis and persistent, prolonged morning stiffness (Conn and Conn, 1980).

13.2 ANTINUCLEAR ACTIVITY TESTS

Altered nuclear antibodies are antibodies against cell nuclear constituents which act as antigens. These antibodies are produced as common findings in systemic rheumatic diseases, many of which are collagen-vascular in type. They can also be seen occasionally in otherwise seemingly healthy persons.

ANA-positive diseases include rheumatoid arthritis (RA), Sjögren syndrome (keratoconjunctivitis sicca—dry eyes, xerostomia—dry mouth, and a connective tissue disease—usually rheumatoid arthritis), polymyositis, scleroderma, mixed connective tissue disease (MCTD), and lupus erythematosus (LE). These diseases may present with similar symptoms, although they vary greatly in both treatment and prognosis. Determination of the presence of certain antinuclear antibodies can be useful in the differential diagnosis of these conditions.

Antibodies to DNA and to the soluble nucleoproteins were determined some time ago. The antibody to a soluble nucleoprotein is that identified in the LE preparation. A more recently discovered area of antibody testing is that of antibodies against the nonhistone acidic nucleoproteins (Sumida and Mullarkey, 1979). [Histone proteins provide the base, or core, around which DNA is wound; nonhistone nucleoproteins serve more specific regulatory and catalytic roles in genetic expression (Sodeman and Sodeman, 1979).]

13.2.1 Screening Tests—Antinuclear Antibodies

A. Lupus erythematosus cell preparation

Synonyms: LE cell preparation; LE prep; LE, test for

Normal Reaction: negative

Explanation of the Test. This is the earliest and the traditional test used in the diagnosis of systemic lupus erythematosus (SLE). It is a screening test for antinuclear antibodies (ANA) and is positive in up to 90% of patients with untreated SLE if retested often enough. A positive test depends on the presence of LE factors or lupus factors (which are serum immunoglobulins, IgG), complement and leukocytes. LE cells are neutrophils which have phagocytized the nuclei of other neutrophils, which have been altered by interaction with the LE factor and complement. The test is relatively insensitive compared to the fluorescent antinuclear antibody tests, assays of complement, or tests of anti-native DNA activity (Horwitz, 1980).

It is possible, but not usual, for LE cell preps to be positive one day and negative the next; or several preps done the same day may have both positive and negative results. The test is usually repeated a specified number of times to overcome this aberration.

A positive LE test, combined with decreased complement (C′3, C′4) and a positive anti-DNA (double-strand) test, are considered definitive diagnosis of SLE (Henry, 1979).

LE PREP POSITIVE IN:

1. *60 to 90% of all cases of SLE.*
2. *9% of individuals with rheumatoid arthritis.*
3. *Uncommon but occasional cases of other collagen-vascular syndromes,* such as systemic sclerosis, periarteritis nodosa, and dermatomyositis.
4. *Occasional cases of patients with chronic active liver disease* (hepatitis), or lymphomas.
5. *Response to the administration of certain drugs* [e.g., hydralazine (Apresoline), procainamide at dosage of over 1.5 g/day, hydantoin derivatives].
6. *Some healthy, elderly individuals,* or some healthy relatives of patients with SLE.

Patient Preparation. No special preparation is necessary.

B. Indirect immunofluorescence test

Synonym: autoantibody screen

Reactions Reported

Normal	Negative
Presence of ANA	Positive

Explanation of the Test. This test is the most sensitive and practical one for use in screening. It is done when a systemic rheumatic disease is suspected. If present, ANA antibodies in the patient's serum will attach to nuclear antigens fixed to a glass slide in the laboratory. When fluorescent dye, conjugated with anti-human gamma globulin, is added to the slide, it binds to the antibody and allows the agglutination of antibody and antigen to be visualized. The fluorescent stain also takes on certain patterns with a positive reaction. Three patterns have been identified and associated with various disease states. Although no single pattern has been found to be truly diagnostic of any one disease, these patterns can be helpful in diagnosis.

Patterns and Relationships to Disease

1. *Homogenous* (H). The most common pattern, it occurs with antibodies to DNA or soluble nuclear proteins. High titers found in SLE. Occurs occasionally in RA and nonrheumatoid diseases.
2. *Nucleolar* (N). Occurrence is rare. Found with antibodies to low-molecular-weight RNA. Most frequently accompanies scleroderma (SS) and Sjögren syndrome. Occurs, but infrequently, in SLE and RA.
3. *Speckle* (S). Occurs with antibodies against acidic nucleoproteins. Seen in SLE, RA, Sjögren syndrome, scleroderma, and MCTD (Sumida and Mullarkey, 1979).

FALSE-NEGATIVE REACTIONS IN:

50% of patients with Sjögren syndrome, scleroderma (SS), polymyositis. If any of these are suspected, specific antibody tests should be carried out despite negative indirect immunofluorescent test.

A negative test rules out SLE.

Patient Preparation. No special preparation is required.

C. Latex agglutination test

Synonyms: ANA agglutination test; antinuclear antibody agglutination test

Reactions Reported

Normal	Negative
Presence of ANA	Positive

Explanation of the Test. As the name implies, this test involves nuclear antigen, attached to latex, being mixed with a patient's serum. If ANA is present in the serum, clumping occurs. The test gives virtually the same information as the LE prep but is simpler and faster. It has been thought by some authorities (Ravel, 1979) to be more sensitive than the LE test and therefore a more efficient screening test, but this point has been discredited by other investigators (Sumida and Mullarkey, 1979).

The test is highly nonspecific, occurring in many collagen-vascular and some liver disease. The use of the test is indicated in acute synovitis or other evidence of systemic rheumatic disease.

ANA POSITIVE IN:

See Section 13.2.1A.

13.2.2 Specific Antibody Tests

These tests are done to identify specific antibodies once the presence of ANA has been established by the screening tests. Specific antibodies or "serum markers" include, among others, anti-DNA. There are, however, two antibody-antigen responses against DNA, the single-stranded DNA and the double-stranded, or native DNA. The assay of double-stranded, or native DNA, is of clinical importance.

A. Anti-DNA binding antibody (Double-stranded DNA; DS-DNA; Native DNA)

Synonyms: DNAB; DNA binding; anti-DS-DNA; anti-native DNA

Normal Range: 0–15%

Explanation of the Test. This test is the most frequently used secondary study for patients with clinical and/or laboratory findings suggestive of SLE. Except in SLE, antibodies to native DNA are so rare as to be considered almost nonexistent. Therefore, high titers of anti-DNA antibody are highly specific for SLE. There are several laboratory processes to determine anti-DNA antibody. All such tests can be used not only to confirm SLE as a diagnosis, but also to indicate exacerbations and remissions of the disease, or to monitor long-term therapy. The test may be negative in clinically inactive disease;

therefore, the anti-native DNA should never be the only test used for diagnosis of SLE, despite its specificity (Sumida and Mullarkey, 1979).

INCREASED ANTIBODY LEVELS IN:

1. *SLE.* Considered diagnostic at levels greater than 30%. Rarely absent in persons with active disease.
2. *Very rare occurrences with other collagen vascular disease* (e.g., RA, Sjögren's syndrome).
3. *Lupus nephritis.* Serum level seems to correlate with disease activity (Martinez-Lavin et al., 1979).

Patient Preparation. No special preparation is necessary.

B. Antibodies to nonhistone acidic nucleoproteins

Antiextractable nuclear antigen (synonyms: anti-ENA; ENA). One of the earliest, more specific antibody tests, the anti-ENA is actually a composite of the two following antibody tests: anti-RNP and anti-Sm. Although it is more specific and sensitive than the tests given as screening tests, it is not as useful as are the tests of its component antibodies, as its response is more general. Found in high titers in mixed connective tissue disease (MCTD) and in over half of the patients with SLE, it is rarely found in other rheumatic disorders (Sharpe, 1980).

Anti-RNP. An antibody sensitive to an extractable nucleoprotein known as ribonucleoprotein (RNP). It is found in a variety of rheumatic diseases to include SLE, rheumatoid arthritis, Sjögren syndrome, scleroderma (SS), and discoid (cutaneous) lupus. Of greatest clinical import, it shows high titers in MCTD (1:1000) with no other antinuclear antibodies present (Sumida and Mullarkey, 1979).

Anti-Sm. Sometimes referred to as anti-smooth muscle antigen, but actually named for the person in whom the antibody was first identified, anti-Sm is highly specific for SLE. It has *not* been found in RA, Sjögren syndrome, scleroderma, dermatomyositis, discoid lupus, MCTD, or in normal individuals. It may be present in chronic active hepatitis—the "lupoid" hepatitis, which is often accompanied by other autoimmune phenomena (Widmann, 1979).

Anti-SS-A; *anti*-SS-B. These two autoantibodies are frequently identified in patients with Sjögren and Sicca syndromes, infrequently found in SLE, and not present in other rheumatoid diseases. Being newly available, their specificity for Sjögren syndrome is not absolutely proven (Sumida and Mullarkey, 1979).

Scl-l *antibody.* There is good correlation with this antibody and the presence of clinical scleroderma.

Rheumatoid arthritis precipitin (RAP). Newly discovered, the clinical value of RAP is as yet uncertain. Found in a relatively high percentage (two-thirds) of patients with rheumatoid arthritis and a small number of those with Sjögren's syndrome.

Explanation of Nonhistone Acidic Nucleoprotein Antibody Tests. The antibodies given above have been identified as more specific, or even highly specific, in some collagen diseases. This is particularly true in the case of MCTD, a fairly newly identified syndrome. A major reason for the need to identify MCTD in particular is its relatively low incidence of renal and central nervous system complications and its remarkable responsiveness to treatment with corticosteroids. Not all cases of SLE, scleroderma, or dermatomyositis are as responsive as MCTD, yet MCTD demonstrates symptoms of each of these disorders.

Specific antibody identification by means of one, or all, of the above tests is undertaken when the immunofluorescent test screen is positive and when there is need to support a clinical diagnosis. Because individual assays take time and are costly, a counter-immunoelectrophoresis screening test for anti-Sm, anti-RNP, and anti-SS-B can be done. (Technology to include anti-SS-A is not available at this writing.) Given a positive outcome, the assays can then be performed only on those few patients likely to have positive findings (Sumida and Mullarkey, 1979).

Patient Preparation. No special preparation is required.

13.3 RHEUMATOID ARTHRITIS FACTOR

Synonyms: rheumatoid arthritis (RA) latex; latex fixation; RA factor; RAF; RF

Reactions Reported

Normal	Negative
Positive reaction	Titer of 80 or greater

Explanation of the Test. A rheumatoid factor (a true auto-antibody) is an immunoglobin of the G, A, or M type (IgG, IgA, IgM). It is produced against a crystalized fragment of an IgG molecule. This test, a latex fixation test, measures only IgM factor, which appears to be the only important factor clinically (Wenig, 1980). Rheumatoid factors (RF) occur in the blood, tissues, and spinal (60%) and joint fluid of approximately 85% of individuals with the disease. They are thought to be secondary manifestations of RA, which is believed to be an autoimmune disease or to have an immune-based etiology.

The titer of RF does not necessarily change with disease activity, but will decrease with certain types of therapy (e.g., penicillamine) and can, therefore, be used to follow the success of that treatment.

RF appear in the serum of a variety of chronic inflammatory diseases other than RA, but the titers in RA tend to run higher. There are also a number of other tests for RF that differ mainly in the type of indicator system used to visually demonstrate the results [e.g., Rose-Waaler (the original test), Protz-Singer latex test, eosin slide]. The latex fixation method is a slide test, as opposed to a tube test, and, as such, is considered to be more sensitive but less specific than the tube tests. Its greatest use is as a screening test (Ravel, 1979).

FALSE POSITIVES IN:

14 to 67% of other collagen-vascular diseases, as well as in sarcoidosis, syphilis, various liver diseases (cirrhosis, hepatitis), and old age (8%).

13.4 HUMAN LYMPHOCYTE ANTIGEN B-27

Synonyms: HLA-B27; HLA-W27; human leucocyte antigen; histocompatibility locus A

Reaction Reported: Positive or negative (reaction does not apply as a "normal" since either positive or negative can be normal)

Explanation of the Test. The HL-A system is a complex antigen group of the white blood cells and found in nucleated cells of tissues other than WBCs as well. It makes up the major antigens of both leukocytes and platelets (Sodeman and Sodeman, 1979). The system has been closely identified with histocompatibility (tissue transplant compatibility), and has been found to have a relationship with various diseases. Testing of the HL-A system is of prime importance for skin and organ transplantation and for platelet and leukocyte transfusions in matching donor and recipient. HLA-B is one of the four major subgroups of HL-A and has been identified to have eight antigens, HLA-B27 being one of the eight.

The presence of HLA-B27 is frequently checked to diagnose, or, more important, to rule out, ankylosing spondylitis. It is associated with variants of rheumatoid arthritis (RA) and demonstrates the best association between disease and the HL-A system (Widmann, 1979). Much research is currently under way in subclassification of rheumatic syndromes using the HL-A system (Christian, 1980).

POSITIVE REACTIONS OCCUR IN:

1. *Ankylosing spondylitis* (Marie-Strumpell disease), in over 90% of the cases. A negative reaction virtually rules out the disease.
2. *Juvenile RA* in over 50% of patients.
3. *The arthritis associated with Reiter's syndrome.*
4. *Arthritis associated with psoriasis.*
5. *Enteropathic arthritis* (associated with ulcerative colitis, Crohn's disease, or *Yersinia enterocolitica*).

POSITIVE REACTIONS OCCUR MORE FREQUENTLY IN:

1. *The Caucasian race.*
2. *Men rather than women,* although recent investigation indicates ankylosing spondylitis may be more frequent in women than previously thought, with milder symptoms and less rapid progression (Goodman et al., 1980).

Patient Preparation. *No special preparations* are required.

13.5 TESTS TO RULE OUT RHEUMATOID OR MUSCULAR DISEASE (DIFFERENTIAL DIAGNOSIS)

13.5.1 Serum Aldolase

Synonyms: ALS; aldolase assay

Normal Range: 0-6.0 units/L

Explanation of the Test. Aldolase is a glycolytic enzyme (converts sugar to energy) found in almost all tissues. It is particularly sensitive to detection in early skeletal muscle disease, reaching strikingly high levels. It is less specific than is creatine phosphokinase (CPK). It should be measured, together with CPK, in the diagnosis of inflammatory muscle disease or progressive muscular dystrophies (Henry, 1979). It is also useful in differential diagnosis among muscular disorders, as serum levels of aldolase are normal in patients with neurogenic muscle disease.

SERUM ALDOLASE INCREASED IN:

1. *Physiologic conditions* such as those following strenuous exercise in untrained individuals.
2. *Conditions causing increased cell membrane permeability,* such as progressive muscular dystrophy, trichinosis, dermatomyositis, polymyositis, scleroderma with associated myositis, delirium tremens, and alcoholic myopathy.
3. *Conditions causing increased production of the enzyme,* such as extensive carcinoma [such elevations can be used as a guide to the effectiveness of chemotherapy (e.g., cancer of the breast or prostate)], megaloblastic anemia, acute granulocytic leukemia, infectious mononucleosis, and myocardial infarction.
4. *Other conditions with muscle involvement,* such as myotonic dystrophy, myotonia congenita, crush syndrome, and McArdle's disease (a glycogen storage disease).

Patient Preparation. No special preparation is necessary.

13.5.2 Synovial Fluid Analysis

Synonyms: synovial analysis; joint fluid exam; joint tap

Normal Range: see specific test in Table 13.1

Includes:

Routine	Cell count (WBC, differential—if WBC greater than 5, and RBC)
	Gross appearance—clarity/color/viscosity
	Mucin clot formation
	Polarized light microscopy
Special	Complement level
	Rheumatoid factors (RF)
	Glucose
	Total protein
	Culture and gram stain

TABLE 13.1 *General interpretation of joint tap tests*

Test	Normal	Deviations from normal —possible significance
Cell count		
WBC	Less than 5 cells/ml (or 200/ μL; usually flattened, lining cells and lymphocytes	See differential
RBC	None formed	Presence indicates hemorrhage or traumatic tap
Differential	Granulocytes less than 25% of nucleated cells	Polys: inflammation-septic arthritis; increased lymph or monos: tuberculosis, foreign body reaction
Other	Lining cells: mesothelial	With any injury, these cells react by becoming stratified, and change from flat to cuboidal; usually accompanied by a protective effusion Can mimic benign or malignant cells Malignancy involving serosal surfaces usually metastatic except for rare primary mesothelioma and a few sarcomas *In RA:* superficial synovial cells proliferate; marked villous hypertrophy; marked infiltration of chronic inflammatory cells (lymphocytes/plasma cells) tending to form "lymphoid nodules"; compact fibrin deposited on surface or interstitially; necrosis
Gross appearance	Crystal clear; straw color (pale yellow); transparent; turbidity reported as 1+ to 4+[a]	Turbid yellow: increased leukocytes secondary to infection–inflammation Milky (pseudochylous); tuberculous arthritis, chronic arthritis, acute gouty arthritis, or SLE Grossly purulent: acute septic arthritis, late stages Greenish tinged: influenza septic arthritis; chronic RA; in some instances of gout or pseudogout
String test[b] (viscosity)	Viscosity reported as normal or "high"; normal string test = formation of a string 4–6 cm in length; if string breaks before 3-cm length is reached, viscosity is below normal	Viscosity is decreased in a wide variety of inflammatory conditions (e.g., septic, gouty, or rheumatoid arthritis); decreased viscosity can also occur following trauma, or with fever
Mucin clot test (Rope's test)	A firm clot forms rapidly after a drop of synovial fluid (SF) is placed in an acetic acid solution Reported as: Good or abundant Fair: soft clot in slightly turbid solution Poor: friable clot in turbid solution; shreds on agitation Very poor: no clot formation; flakes in cloudy suspension	Generally as for viscosity above, with exceptions of acute effusions (e.g., rheumatic fever, sepsis, trauma, overuse); while viscosity is decreased by fever, clot formation remains normal

TABLE 13.1 *General interpretation of joint tap tests (cont.)*

Test	Normal	Deviations from normal —possible significance
Polarized light microscopy	No crystals	Simple, precise, definitive test; aids in differential diagnosis of gout and pseudo-gout by demonstrating urate (gout) and phosphate (pseudo-gout) crystals. Phosphate: calcium pyrophosphate dihydrate (CPPD) Urate: monosodium urate (MSU) Apatite crystals: rare form of arthritis Talcum crystals: rare form of arthritis secondary to joint surgery Crystalline: secondary to therapeutic injection of corticosteroids Osteo- or traumatic arthritis: fragments of cartilage and collagen fibrils
Complement	Varies with the concentration of synovial fluid (SF) protein; expressed in relationship to total protein	Decreased in RA and SLE Occasionally decreased in rheumatic fever, bacterial arthritis, gout, pseudo-gout, and other types of inflammatory arthritis Total hemolytic complement increased in arthritis of Reiter's syndrome
Rheumatoid factors (RF)	Absent	Present in about 60% of patients with RA; may be present before becoming measurable in serum; high incidence of false positives
Glucose	70–110 mg/dL: concentration identical or slightly less than plasma glucose (usually within 10 mg/dL)	If patient not fasting 6–12 hr before test, synovial fluid (SF) glucose may be lower than plasma; under 40 mg/dL suggests decreased SF glucose in this instance Noninflammatory arthritis: SF glucose decreased 10 mg/dL Inflammatory arthritis: SF glucose decreased more than 25 mg/dL or 50 mg/dL
Total protein	1–3 g/dL; often expressed as SF/plasma ratio	Levels of individual proteins in SF change with changes in plasma proteins Increased SF/plasma TP ratio occurs with inflammation due to increased permeability of synovial membrane Therefore, increased SF/plasma TP = evidence of inflammation

[a]0, crystal clear fluid; 1+, faintly "cloudy," "smoky," "hazy" with slight (barely visible) turbidity; 2+, turbidity clearly present—newsprint easily read through the tube; 3+, newsprint not easily read through tube; 4+, newsprint cannot be seen through tube.

[b]A string test is an estimate of viscosity done by allowing synovial fluid to form a string by dropping from a syringe into a beaker (Henry, 1979).

Source: Data from SHMC, 1978; Wenig, 1980; Henry, 1979; and Bienenstock, 1980.

Explanation of the Test. Since there is little fluid in any joint (0.1 to 2.0 mL), a "dry" tap is common unless an effusion is present. For this test, joint fluid is aspirated from an involved joint by a process known as *arthrocentesis,* that is, withdrawal of fluid by way of a sterile needle and syringe. The area to be aspirated is generally prepped as for orthopedic surgery, and strict sterile technique is employed to prevent infection of the joint. The test is a fairly simple one, it provides substantial information, and the cost is relatively low. Therefore, it is often used for initial evaluation, or differential diagnosis of possible arthritis, suspected infection, or other inflammatory rheumatoid conditions (Christian, 1980); see Table 13.1.

Patient Preparation

1. *Fasting* for at least 6 to 8 hr if glucose is to be measured.
2. *If infectious arthritis is suspected,* a Gram stain and culture are usually carried out as well.

Hematologic System

chapter 14

Disorders of the red blood cells (RBCs), hemoglobin (Hgb), or white blood cells (WBCs) are usually diagnosed in a step-wise fashion. The basic screening tests are done first (see Part I), as well as a thorough history and physical examination. If anemia is evident but a definitive diagnosis is still lacking, a reticulocyte count is usually done to determine marrow function roughly. At this point most anemias can be identified. Only after a tentative diagnosis is arrived at are further tests usually ordered, since the tests tend to be specific to given foci or etiology, and are more expensive.

14.1 LABORATORY OR CLINICAL INDICATIONS OF HEMATOLOGIC SYSTEM DYSFUNCTION

Laboratory Findings. Evidence of anemia that is persistent and/or nonresponsive to therapy; decreased number of reticulocytes present, given the severity of the anemia (percent may increase but not to appropriate levels); pancytopenia; poikilocytosis, anisocytosis, stippling, or polychromatophilia in RBCs; presence of target cells; WBC–increased above 25,000 per mm^3, or decreased below 1000 per

mm^3, decreased neutrophils, wide shift to the left with large numbers of blast cells. In urine, persistent hemoglobinuria or hemosiderinuria.

Clinical Findings. Chronic, progressive fatigue, pallor, weakness; dyspnea; bleeding such as petachiae in lower extremities, small retinal hemorrhages, oozing from mucous membrane; lemon yellow jaundice; splenomegaly; decreased resistance to infection with recurrent infections, especially of mucous membrane (e.g., oral cavity, anorectal area, genitourinary tract, and respiratory tract); neurologic symptoms such as headache, vertigo, tinnitus; joint pain, acute with disability, swelling of hands and feet otherwise unexplained.

14.2 TESTS OF HEMATOLOGIC PRODUCTION

14.2.1 Bone Marrow Examination

Synonyms: None

Includes: Bone marrow aspiration, bone marrow biopsy

Normal Range: see Table 14.1

Explanation of the Test. Bone marrow aspiration is one of the nine basic tests of hematology, not in the sense of a screening test, but rather as a keystone of diagnosis. Marrow cells are either aspirated or removed by biopsy (percutaneous needle biopsy is the most common method). If the marrow cannot be aspirated (dry tap), biopsy is required. There is a technique that permits both aspiration and biopsy, which provides more information and is endorsed by many practitioners (Harvey, 1979). A biopsy includes both bone and marrow. An aspiration provides marrow only. The most accessible marrow-containing bone is the sternum, but in adults the iliac crest is used primarily. Marrow cellularity (the ratio of volume of hematopoietic cells to total marrow space volume) decreases with age and varies with the site. Marrow-containing bones in the adult, in decreasing order of marrow cellularity, are the vertebrae, sternum, iliac crest, and the ribs. Once the specimen is obtained, smears are made and examined or a clot section (clotted marrow) is processed like an ordinary histologic specimen. The specimens are examined for the presence, number, and developmental, or maturational stage of each type of cell. A differential count of the cells may be done and the myeloid (leukocytes of the myeloid or nucleated series)/erythroid (nucleated erythrocytic cells) ratio (M/E) determined. Iron stores can also be determined by a staining process when requested.

Normal values for the differential count vary widely depending on the source used. Variation occurs because of differing cell classification, type of process used, the wide range of normal values, and the fact that reliable data regarding normal bone marrow are scarce (Widmann, 1979).

TABLE 14.1 *Differential cell counts of bone marrow (percent of total nucleated cells)*

	Rosse (1977) Birth	Rosse (1977) 1 month	Mauer (1969) Over 4 months		Wintrobe et al. (1974) Adult	
	Mean±S.D.	Mean±S.D.	Mean	Range	Mean	Range
Normoblasts, total	14.5 ±7.2	8.0 ±5.0	23.1		25.6	(18.4–33.8)
Pronormoblasts	0.02±0.06	0.10±0.14	0.5	(0–1.5)		(0.2–1.3)
Basophilic normoblasts	0.24±0.24	0.34±0.33	1.7	(0.2–4.8)		(0.5–2.4)
Polychromatophilic normoblasts	13.1 ±6.8	6.9 ±4.4	18.2	(4.8–34.0)		(17.9–29.2)
Orthochromatic normoblasts	0.69±0.73	0.54±1.88	2.7	(0–7.8)		(0.4–4.6)
Neutrophils, total	60.4 ±8.7	32.4 ±7.7	57.1		53.6	(49.2–65.0)
Myeloblasts	0.31±0.31	0.62±0.50	1.2	(0–3.2)		(0.2–1.5)
Promyelocytes	0.79±0.91	0.76±0.65	1.4	(0–4.0)		(2.1–4.4)
Myelocytes	3.9 ±2.9	2.5 ±1.5	18.3	(8.5–29.7)		(8.2–15.7)
Metamyelocytes	19.4 ±4.8	11.3 ±3.6	23.3	(14.0–34.2)		(9.5–24.6)
Bands	28.4 ±7.6	14.1 ±4.6				(9.5–15.3)
Semented	7.4 ±4.6	3.6 ±3.0	12.9	(4.5–29.0)		(6.0–12.0)
Eosinophils	2.7 ±1.3	2.6 ±1.4	3.6	(1.0–9.0)	3.1	(1.2–5.3)
Basophils	0.12±0.20	0.07±0.16	0.06	(0–0.8)	0.1	(0–0.2)
Lymphocytes, total	15.6	49.0	16.0	(4.8–35.8)	16.2	(11.1–23.2)
Transitional	1.2 ±1.1	2.0 ±0.9				
Small (mature)	14.4 ±5.5	47.0 ±9.2				
Plasma cells	0.00±0.02	0.02±0.06	0.4	(0.2–0.6)	1.3	(0.4–3.9)
Monocytes	0.88±0.85	1.01±0.89			0.3	(0–0.8)
Megakaryocytes	0.06±0.15	0.05±0.09			0.1	(0–0.4)
Reticulum cells					0.3	(0.–0.9)
M/E ratio	4.4	4.4	2.9	(1.2–5.2)	2.3	(1.5–2.3)

Gross appearance: dark blood with greater viscosity than blood.

From Douglas A. Nelson, "Hematopoiesis," in John Bernard Henry, ed., *Clinical Diagnosis and Management by Laboratory Methods,* 16th ed. (Philadelphia: W. B. Saunders Company, 1969), p. 958.

Source: Data from C. Rosse, M. J. Kraemer, T. L. Dillon, R. McFarland, and N. J. Smith, "Bone Marrow Cell Populations of Normal Infants: The Predominance of Lymphocytes," *J. Lab. Clin. Med.* (v. 89, 1977), p. 1225. A. M. Mauer, *Pediatric Hematology* (New York, McGraw-Hill Book Company, 1969); and M. M. Wintrobe et al., *Clinical Hematology,* 7th ed. (Philadelphia: Lea & Febiger, 1974).

INDICATIONS FOR USE:

1. *Diagnosis of megaloblastic anemias,* leukemia, or multiple myeloma.
2. *Demonstration of bone marrow cellular precursor deficiency* (hypoplasia) as the cause of decreased levels of one or more cellular elements of the blood.
3. *To document a decrease in body iron stores* in certain iron-deficiency anemias.
4. *To demonstrate metastatic neoplasm.*
5. *To demonstrate certain types of infectious disease* (tuberculosis, histoplasmosis).
6. *To determine the existence of diseases that affect macrophages* (e.g., lipid or glycogen storage diseases).

CHANGES IN BONE MARROW (INTERPRETATION IS ORDINARILY DONE BY A HEMOTOLOGIST OR A CLINICAL PATHOLOGIST):

1. *Hypoplasia* (decreased cellular production) due to:
   a. Chronic infection.
   b. Hypothyroidism (present in one-third of patients with macrocytic anemia).
   c. Chronic renal failure, due to decreased erythropoietin production.
   d. Advanced liver disease, such as far advanced cirrhosis.
   e. Marrow replacement, due to fibrosis (myelofibrosis) or neoplasm.
   f. Aplastic anemia, due to toxic destruction or idiosyncratic reaction (Ravel, 1979).
2. *Hyperplasia* (increased cellular production) due to:
   a. Anemias such as iron deficiency or pernicious: other folate and vitamin B_{12} metabolic disease with peculiar RBC appearance as well as megaloblastic maturation; thalassemias as a compensatory response to inadequate or ineffective peripheral blood cells.
   b. Hemoglobinopathies.
   c. Hypersplenism, due to increased cell sequestration or destruction.
   d. Enzyme deficiencies (e.g., G-6-P) due to ineffective cellular activity.
   e. Red cell membrane abnormalities [e.g., hereditary spherocytosis (as for d above)].

f. Destructive processes (e.g., antibody-mediated, bacterial or chemical hemolysis), due to increased cell loss.

3. *Appearance of abnormal or rare cell types* in marrow, found in:

Cell	Associated disorder	Comment
Tissue mast cells	Increase in number in aplastic or refractory anemias and macroglobinemia	Occur frequently
Osteoblasts, osteoclasts	Occur in adult marrow with hyperparathyroidism, Paget's disease, metastatic tumor, or after a recent biopsy at the same site	Occur normally in small numbers in infants and children
Metastatic neoplastic cells	Metastatic tumor at site of biopsy sample; resemble primitive blast cells	Usually appear in clusters or clumps

Source: Data from Henry, 1979.)

4. *Increases and decreases in M/E ratio* (normal range = 2:1 to 4:1)
   a. Increases in (increased number of myeloid cells or decreased number of nucleated red cells):
      (1) Normal newborns and infants, only slightly higher than the norm, and less than 4:1.
      (2) Infection, chronic myelogenous leukemia, and erythroid hypoplasia.
   b. Decreased in (less than 2:1; greater than normal proportion of nucleated red cells due to depression of leukopoiesis, or increased number of nucleated red blood cells) polycythemia vera.

5. *Iron stain for siderocytes* (synonyms: siderocyte stain; sideroblast stain);
   a. Explanation of the test: normoblasts (marrow RBC's) in the bone marrow—containing iron granules can be demonstrated by special staining. The stained cells, called sideroblasts, are a normal and expected inhabitant of bone marrow.
   b. Deviations from normal:
      (1) Sideroblasts are totally absent or greatly reduced in patients with iron-deficiency anemias.
      (2) The number of granules per cell (sideroblast) if greatly increased in sideroblastic anemias and form a ring around the nucleus.

See also Section 14.2.3.

Patient Preparation. Except for the skin preparation and psychological support, no special preparation is necessary. Iliac crest taps are painful and the patient will need advance warning and instruction in methods of coping (e.g., instructions and assistance in placement to maintain position during the tap so that a second puncture will not be necessary; pain control by way of arranging for availability of sedatives prior to the procedure and analgesics after).

14.2.2 Schilling Test

Synonym: vitamin B_{12} uptake

Normal Value: values are dose dependent; 7% excretion/24 hr with 0.5-μg dose

Range: 8–40%/24 hr

Explanation of the Test. This test is used to further define the cause of a macrocytic or megaloblastic anemia—for differential diagnosis of pernicious anemia and various other malabsorption syndromes. The person with pernicious anemia does not absorb vitamin B_{12}, due to the lack of intrinsic factor in the gastric secretions. Intrinsic factor is essential to vitamin B_{12} absorption from the terminal end of the ileum. The Schilling test is the most convenient method for determining the ability of the patient to absorb an oral dose (0.5 to 2.0 μg) of radioactive vitamin B_{12}. This is done by measuring the radioactivity in a 24-hr urine sample. To assure that the labeled vitamin B_{12} absorbed will be excreted into the urine and not bound to protein in the body, a parenteral dose of unlabeled vitamin B_{12} is given as a large flushing dose. It is given parenterally for quicker absorption and will saturate tissue binding sites, allowing the labeled vitamin B_{12} to be excreted into the urine. The timing of this dose varies with the facility using the test. It has been given prior to the labeled dose of vitamin B_{12}, at the same time, or 1 or 2 hr after.

If the test is abnormal, that is, less than 7% excretion in 24 hr, it is repeated, usually after 3 days. The test is then identical except that hog intrinsic factor is given in adequate amounts, together with the oral labeled vitamin B_{12}. If excretion is within normal limits on the second test, the diagnosis of pernicious anemia is made since supplying the missing factor normalized response. If the 24-hr excretion is still below, or at the lower limit of normal, something other than intrinsic factor lack is the cause (e.g., folate deficiency or malabsorption), and further tests are indicated.

BELOW-NORMAL REACTIONS OCCUR IN:

Conditions other than pernicious anemia, such as in:

1. *Individuals with poor renal function.* The test is usually prolonged to 48- or 72-hr collection in known cases of reduced urine production, or when a BUN is elevated.
2. *A considerable number of patients with sprue,* due to malabsorption.
3. *The elderly.* This is a physiologic and normal finding usually.
4. *Incomplete urine collection for the test*—a false low value. Measurement of urine creatinine may be helpful in checking on completeness of urine collection.

Patient preparation

1. *NPO except for water* 12 hr before the test and maintained until the "flushing dose" of nonlabeled vitamin B_{12} has been given.
2. *Thorough patient instruction* with follow-up observation and reminders are indicated when the patient is responsible for collecting the urine.
3. *If a bone marrow examination* is planned, it should precede this test because the large dose of vitamin B_{12} given in the second step of the test can quickly convert the megaloblastic changes to a normal picture.
4. *The test may be done* even though treatment for pernicious anemia has already begun, as long as intrinsic factor itself is not given.

14.2.3 Iron Studies

A. Total iron

Synonyms: Serum iron concentration; serum iron; SI

Normal Ranges

Adult	65–175 μg/dL
Senior adult	As for adult
Pediatric	
Newborn	100–200 μg/dL
4 months–2 years	40–100 μg/dL
Thereafter	85–150 μg/dL

Explanation of the Test. Iron studies, in general, are undertaken when a microcytic, hypochromic anemia has been discovered and blood loss cannot be documented. Iron deficiency is the most common cause of that type of anemia (MCV less than 80 fL; MCHC less than 32%—on Coulter counter may be within normal limits or only slightly hypochromic). Knowledge of serum iron levels and the total iron-binding capacity usually permits discrimination between iron-deficiency anemia and the second most commonly occurring anemia, that associated with chronic disorders.

Iron-deficiency anemia due to dietary lack is very rare in adults, but not uncommon in infants and the elderly. The anemia of chronic illness is not uncommon in the adult with a slow, gradual onset.

Serum iron is often decreased in anemias other than pure iron deficiency. Iron-deficiency anemia is almost always due to one of three factors, or a combination of the three factors: inadequate dietary iron intake, poor absorption of iron from the intestine, and chronic blood loss—probably in reverse order of occurrence.

Other tests of importance in diagnosis and follow-up of iron deficiency anemia are: MCV (see above); total iron-binding capacity (TIBC); ESR; serum bilirubin [helpful in patients with liver disease: bilirubin is a normal end product of RBC destruction and when cells are lost from the body before the end of their life span, serum bilirubin levels will decrease and can be totally absent (Sirridge, 1980)].

SERUM IRON DECREASED IN
(SEE ALSO THE TABLE IN SECTION 14.2.3B):

1. *Physiologic diurnal variation* with a decrease of as much as 100 mg% in evening levels over morning levels.
2. *The nephrotic syndrome* due to urinary loss of protein, to include transferrin, the transport plasma protein for iron. Transferrin is also sometimes called siderophilin.
3. *Response to long-term chronic blood loss.* In the adult over 40 years of age, gastrointestinal cancer should be ruled out. Other causes include heavy menstrual flow, peptic ulcer, ulcerative colitis, Crohn's disease, diverticulitis, and hemorrhoids.
4. *Periods of rapid growth,* such as the infant aged 6 months to 2 years—particularly the premature and/or the infant on a prolonged milk-only diet.
5. *Decreased intake at any age* over a prolonged period of time—2 to 3 months.
6. *Some malabsorption syndromes* or other disorders of the digestive tract, such as achlorhydria (acid environment is necessary for iron absorption).

7. *Repeated pregnancies,* especially when coexisting with a marginal intake. Each pregnancy causes 600 to 900 mg of iron loss, due in part to fetal demand for iron.
8. *Conditions leading to chronic slight hematuria,* such as tumors, stones, or inflammatory disease. Rarely, large amounts of iron are lost in the urine of patients with a chronic hemolytic disorder.
9. *Infection.* Occurs rarely in adults, frequently in children who have repeated infections, such as upper respiratory or chronic inflammatory processes (e.g., rheumatic fever). Other factors are also instrumental in the occurrence of iron-deficiency anemia in children with rheumatic fever.
10. *Individuals receiving certain drugs therapeutically* (e.g., ACTH, steroids, hydroxyurea).

SERUM IRON INCREASED IN:

1. *Sideroblastic anemias*[a] such as thalassemia due to decreased synthesis of available iron in hemoglobin (Miale, 1972).
2. *Increased intake.*
3. *Increased hemoglobin breakdown,* as in the hemolysis of sickle-cell anemia.
4. *Individuals who are being treated with a number of drugs* (e.g., estrogen, oral contraceptives, Chloramphenical).
5. *Hemochromatosis* due to a highly increased rate of iron absorption by the intestinal mucosal cell.

Patient Preparation. No special preparation is necessary; however, a fasting specimen is preferred.

B. Total iron-binding capacity

Synonyms: Iron-binding capacity; IBC; TIBC; human transferrin test

Normal Ranges

Adults	250–450 μg/dL
Senior adults	As for adults
Pediatric	
Newborn	60–175 μg/dL
4 months–2 years	100–400 μg/dL
Thereafter	350–450 μg/dL

[a][conditions in which the body is unable to incorporate iron into hemoglobin and in which iron granules are found ringing the nucleus of marrow RBCs (normoblasts), in peripheral erythrocytes, and in diffuse body tissues].

Explanation of the Test. Iron enters the body in a ferrous state. Once absorbed it is transported by a plasma protein called transferrin, or siderophilin, which combines avidly with the iron. Once combined, the iron is converted to its ferric state. The capacity of transferrin to combine with iron is measured as iron-binding capacity and its concentration is markedly consistent. Generally, but not always, conditions that decrease serum iron increase iron binding, that is, the less iron available to be bound, the greater the number of empty binding sites. The capacity of transferrin to bind iron is about three times as great as the normal serum concentration of iron.

Usually the *percent saturation of TIBC* is calculated when the TIBC is done. Percent saturation represents the ratio of serum iron to the TIBC concentration. It follows a diurnal pattern much as serum iron does, being highest in the morning and lowest in later afternoon and early evening. Values below 15% indicate an iron-deficiency anemia, or iron-deficient erythropoiesis (Henry, 1979).

COMPARISON OF CHANGES OF TIBC, SERUM IRON, AND PERCENT SATURATION IN SELECTED DISORDERS:

Pathology	TIBC	Serum iron	Percent saturation
Iron-deficiency anemia	Inc.	Dec.	Dec.
Thalassemia, trait	Normal (N)	N or inc.	
Thalassemia	Dec.	Inc.	Inc.
Anemia of chronic disease	N or dec.	Dec.	
Sideroblastic anemia	Dec.	Inc.	
Nephrosis	Dec.	Inc.	Inc.
Chronic infections	Dec.	Dec.	Dec.
Menses—heavy	N	Dec.	Dec.
Hemolytic anemia	N or dec.	Inc.	Inc.
Hemochromatosis	N or dec.	Inc.	Inc.
Oral contraceptives, use of	Inc.	N or inc.	N
Acute hepatitis, viral	Inc.	Inc.	N or inc.
Chronic renal disease	Dec.	Dec.	N or dec.

Source: Data from Henry, 1979; Miale, 1972; and Widmann, 1979.

Patient Preparation. No special preparation is necessary.

C. Serum ferritin concentration

Synonym: Iron stores

Normal Range

12 to 300 μg/L—RIA

Male mean 123 ng/mL

Female mean 56 ng/mL radiometric assay

Iron depletion at less than 30 ng/mL

Absent iron stores at less than 10 ng/mL

Explanation of the Test. Ferritin is the body's major iron storage protein, a high-molecular-weight protein. It is found in almost all body tissue but is located primarily in reticuloendothelial cells and liver cytoplasm. Its measurement (quantitation) accurately reflects intracellular iron stores. When done together with serum iron and TIBC measurements, a more complete diagnostic picture is available and may eliminate the need for bone marrow examination for the diagnosis of iron deficiency.

The test is used mainly for differentiating iron-deficiency anemia from other microcytic, hypochromic anemias, as it is a more specific indicator than the other standard tests. It can also be used for monitoring iron stores in patients with chronic renal failure on hemodialysis, or for monitoring therapy for patients with iron deficiency or overload. Another use proposed, the value of which is not fully assessed at this time, is to evaluate malignancy in certain patients and their response to treatment, or as an indicator of liver damage (Henry, 1979).

DECREASED IN:

1. *Iron-deficiency anemia.*

NORMAL OR INCREASED IN:

1. *Other forms of anemia.*
2. *Conditions that disturb erythropoiesis,* such as liver disease (e.g., infectious hepatitis, cirrhosis, cancer, Hodgkin's disease with liver involvement) and leukemia.

14.3 TESTS OF HEMOGLOBIN

14.3.1 Hemoglobin Electrophoresis

Synonyms: None

Normal Ranges

Hemoglobin A + F	96.5–98.2%
Hemoglobin A_2	1.8– 3.5%
Hemoglobin F (fetal hemoglobin, alkali-resistant hemoglobin):	
Adult	0% of total
Adolescent	0– 2% of total
Newborn	40–70% of total
Neonatal	20–40% of total
Infant	2–10% of total

Abnormal Hemoglobins	
Hemoglobin S adult (sickle-cell test)	0% of total
Methemoglobin adult (hemoglobin M-Hgb M)	2% of total
Carboxyhemoglobin	
adult	0 – 2.3% of total
Smoker	2.1– 4.2% of total
Hemoglobin C adult	0%

Explanation of the Test. Electrophoresis is the movement of charged particles suspended in a liquid on a specific medium (starch, agar, paper) under the influence of an electric field and a controlled pH. In this test the differing molecular structure of the various hemoglobins is identified by the rate and direction in which they travel. Although there are many different methods of electrophoretic separation, none are able to separate *all* the hemoglobins. The methods most frequently used for routine hemoglobin electrophoresis separate hemoglobins S, F, C, A, and A_2, which identifies normal hemoglobins and those hemoglobins most commonly abnormal in humans as well as most important in the western hemisphere (Ravel, 1979).

Hemoglobin electrophoresis is used as a screening test for patients believed to have one of the many hemoglobinopathies. By characterizing the presence of an abnormal hemoglobin(s), or the presence of abnormally large or small amounts of normal hemoglobin(s), the specific disorder(s) can be diagnosed. Most abnormal hemoglobins result from the substitution of a single amino acid for another one on the four globin polypeptide chains of the hemoglobin molecule, but do not always result in hemolytic anemias. Hemoglobinopathies can also be due to a deficient synthesis of normal hemoglobin, such as thalassemia (Miale, 1972). See also Section 1.14.3.

Table 14.2 lists the clinical syndromes associated with hemoglobinopathies.

TABLE 14.2 *Clinical syndromes in hemoglobinopathies*

Syndrome	Abnormal hemoglobin	Comments
Sickle cell anemia	Hbg-S present (60%); SS—homozygote; Hbg-F (10%)	Infants protected by presence of Hbg-F; can become anemic, however; causes crises due to intravascular sickling of RBC and decreased blood flow to the part (see Section I.14.3)
Sickle cell trait	Hbg-S present; AS—heterozygote	Usually no clinical disease; provides protection against malarial infection (*Plasmodium flaciparum*)

TABLE 14.2 (*cont.*)

Syndrome	Abnormal hemoglobin	Comments
Hemoglobin-C disease	Hgb-C present; CC–homozygote	Rare; mild chronic anemia usually but can be quite severe; large number of target cells present
Hemoglobin-C trait	Hbg-C present; AC-heterozygote	Usually asymptomatic; occurs in 2–5% of black Americans; target cells present
Sickle cell–hemoglobin-C disease	SC; both Hbg-C and -S present	Causes moderate to severe hemolytic disease; many target cells; hematuria, splenomegaly (contrasts with pure sickle cell anemia), necrosis of bone even more common than in pure sickle cell disease
Beta thalassemia major (Cooley's anemia; Mediterranean anemia)	No abnormal hemoglobin in any pure thalassemias; beta-chain defect with decreased synthesis rate; two patterns: increased % Hbg-F + Hgb-A_2 normal or decreased; Hgb-F normal, Hgb-A_2 greater than normal	Usually detected in childhood, thus the normal Hgb-F; found primarily in Mediterranean races; most severe of the thalassemias; Howell-Jolly bodies often present in RBCs; severe anemia; often increased WBCs; splenomegaly
Beta thalassemia minor	Hgb-F decreased or normal or may even be higher than normal; increased Hbg-A_2	Usually asymptomatic; mild anemia of iron-deficient type but nonresponsive to iron; serum iron concentration is high normal or above normal; decreased total iron binding capacity
Alpha thalassemia major and minor	Alpha-chain defect causing slowed synthesis	Homozygous, or major, incompatible with life; heterozygous: may be asymptomatic or have a mild hemolytic anemia
Hbg-C thalassemia	Presence of Hbg-C; Hbg-F may be increased (severe cases); Hgb-A_2 cannot be measured —moves in same pattern as Hgb-C	Mild in American blacks; more severe in Mediterranean races; target cells present in peripheral smear; RBC crystals
Sickle-cell thalassemia	Presence of Hbg-S with beta-chain defect, and decrease in Hbg-A_1; % of Hbg-S greater than that of Hbg-A_1	Can occur as a severe sickling disease or a mild hemolytic anemia; target cells present; since Hbg-A may be entirely absent, requires measurement of Hbg-F and -S for diagnosis; easily misdiagnosed as sickle-cell disease without such tests
Hereditary persistence of fetal hemoglobin (HPFH)	Defect in "switching mechanism" High levels of Hbg-F persist into adult life: 15–35%; Homozygous: only Hbg-F; no Hbg-A present	Usually heterozygous and usually occurs in the black race; Hbg-F found equally in all body cells, which helps distinguish it from beta thalassemia

Source: Compiled from data taken from Conn and Conn, 1977; Frolich, 1976; Groer and Shekleton, 1979; Luckmann and Sorensen, 1974; and Miale, 1972.

Patient Preparation. No special preparation is necessary.

14.3.2 Serum Haptoglobin

> *Synonyms:* none
>
> *Reactions Reported*
>
> Normal
> Abnormal (increased/decreased)

Explanation of the Test. Haptoglobins are $alpha_2$ globulins that bind any free hemoglobin in the plasma to the amount of 100 mg/dL. Once its binding capacity is exceeded, the free hemoglobin is excreted into the urine (hemoglobinuria). The complex formed by hemoglobin and haptoglobin is cleared from the plasma by the liver. The presence of free hemoglobin in plasma is a sure indicator of pathologic red cell destruction (Widman, 1979) and decreases in serum haptoglobin are a fairly sensitive indicator of that hemolysis. However, in cases where haptoglobin levels are increased, hemolysis cannot be ruled out by a normal haptoglobin finding.

Haptoglobins can be estimated by haptoglobin binding capacity (electrophoresis or chemical methods) or measured directly as total haptoglobin (immunologic antibody test). The binding capacity is more sensitive to decreases of haptoglobin, as it responds more rapidly than does the assay.

SERUM HAPTOGLOBIN INCREASED IN:

1. *Any inflammatory disease.*
2. *Patients on steroid therapy.*

SERUM HAPTOGLOBIN DECREASED, OR ABSENT, IN:

1. *Hemolysis,* regardless of cause.
2. *Severe liver disease,* due to decreased production of haptoglobin.
3. *Infectious mononucleosis.*
4. *Congenital absence* (ahaptoglobinemia), which occurs in approximately 3% of the black race, rare in other races.

Patient Preparation. No special preparation is necessary.

14.4 TESTS FOR HEMOLYTIC DISEASE

14.4.1 Coombs' Test—Direct, Indirect, and Quantitative

Synonyms	
Direct	Direct antiglobulin Test; DAGT
Indirect	Indirect antiglobulin test; IAGT; antibody screening test
Coombs' test	Antiglobulin test; AGT
Quantitative test	RBC antibody, quantitative; RBC antibody assay
Reactions Reported	
Direct	Normal/negative
Indirect	Normal/negative
Quantitative	Normal range: 0–35 molecules/RBC

Explanation of the Tests. This antiglobulin testing (AGT) is known as the Coombs' test to honor one of the men who produced the first anti-human serum antibody used as a laboratory reagent for the test. AGT is based on the principle that anti-human globulin antibodies will cause agglutination of RBCs that have been coated with globulin antibodies (sensitized). Globulin antibodies often attach themselves to RBCs without causing RBC agglutination. Complement-activating antibodies will also attach a complement component to a RBC at times without adhering to the RBC themselves. Since RBC attached globulin, or complement fragments, are difficult to visualize, and their presence indicates unexpected, or abnormal, antibodies, antiglobulin testing is used for visualization by causing agglutination of previously dispersed RBCs. The anti-human serum antibody reagents (or Coombs' serum) used for testing vary in makeup depending on what is suspected or what is to be identified. There is a broad-spectrum antiserum globulin (ASG) used for screening, as well as single antibody serums, or various combinations [e.g., anti-IgG, anti-Rh_0(D), anti-Ig + anti-C_3d]. The tests then can be used to diagnose causes of hemolytic disease, determine blood types, or investigate causes of transfusion reactions.

The *direct test* is so-called because it is a one-step process done directly on the patient's cells. Anti-human serum antibody is mixed with the patient's washed RBCs. (The washing is an important step as the Coombs' serum will react, even reacts preferentially, with any unbound globulin present.) If agglutination of the patient's RBCs occurs, this indicates the presence of an antibody on the cells, but does not identify the antibody.

The *indirect test,* or antibody screening test, is a two-step process in which RBCs with known antigenic makeup are exposed to the patient's serum. The outcomes of that combination are then visualized by the second stage of the test in which Coombs' serum is added to the known-antigen RBCs and patient's serum mixture, after careful washing of the RBCs to remove free globulin. If the patient's serum contains the antibody to the RBCs' specific antigen, agglutination takes place, and the antibody is identified. The first stage of the indirect test can also be done by using a known specific antibody serum which is exposed to washed RBCs from the patient. The indirect test can then detect and identify either the free antibody in a patient's serum, or specific red cell antigens (Ravel, 1979 Widman, 1979).

It is estimated that 100 to 500 IgG molecules bound on RBCs are required for detection by the routine (direct–indirect) Coombs' tests. Any smaller number will produce a negative reaction. When immunohemolytic anemia is suspected and routine Coombs' testing produces negative results, a *quantitative test* may be done. It is also useful for following the response to treatment in immunohemolytic anemias, as the amount of antibody decreases. The qualitative test can be done as a complement-fixation assay of the patient's serum incubated with antihuman antibody from rabbits (Coombs' serum), in which the amount of lysis is compared to a control.

INDICATIONS FOR USE (EXPECTED POSITIVE REACTIONS):

1. *Direct test:*
   a. Diagnosis of hemolytic disease of the newborn.
   b. Diagnosis of acquired autoimmune hemolytic anemias, both idiopathic and secondary.
   c. Investigation of hemolytic transfusion reaction, incompatibility, within first hour following reaction.
2. *Indirect test:*
   a. Detection and/or identification of antibodies to the antigenic blood systems, such as Duffy (Fy), Kidd, (jk), Kell (K) or Rh.
   b. Detection of immunoglobulin antibodies against platelets and leukocytes.
   c. Demonstration of autoantibodies in patients with autoimmune hemolytic anemia.

Patient Preparation. No special preparation is necessary.

14.4.2 Glucose-6-Phosphate Dehydrogenase

Synonym: G-6-PD

Reaction Reported: Normal or abnormal

Explanation of the Test. Glucose-6-phosphate dehydrogenase (G-6-PD) is a red cell enzyme. It controls one of the glucose metabolic pathways in the RBC. Deficiency of G-6-PD is the most common of the rather uncommon RBC enzyme defects (Miale, 1972). The defect is a sex-linked genetic one, determined by a gene on the X chromosome. The disease is most severe in males, although some females who have abnormal genes on both X chromosomes are equally affected. Females with only one abnormal gene are carriers and may be asymptomatic or moderately affected. The G-6-PD defect is found mainly in blacks and to a lesser degree in other Mediterranean races (e.g., Italian, Greek, Sephardic Jews).

When the defective RBCs are exposed to certain chemicals in sufficient concentrations, they are destroyed, causing a drug-induced hemolysis. The older RBCs are destroyed preferentially, since they have lost much of their G-6-PD activity in the process of aging. If the chemical (drug) is discontinued, hemolysis will stop within 48 to 72 hr. The few whites affected are likely to have a more intense hemolysis and thus more likely to be anemic. Not all persons with the defect develop hemolytic anemia, and there are many molecular variants of the disease.

The test is specific to G-6-PD and is used as a screening test for the enzyme defect. It is based on the length of time needed for an oxidative reduction to occur. The greater the time required, the less G-6-PD present. Other tests, such as the Heinz body preparations (stain)—an old test rarely used—have been used to detect this defect, but are less specific. For example, Heinz bodies appear in some normal newborns and postsplenectomy patients, as well as in thalassemia major.

EPISODES OF HEMOLYSIS OCCUR IN:

1. *Individuals with G-6-PD defect after exposure to certain drugs,* such as antimalarials (Primaquine, Quinacrine); sulfonamides and sulfones (many but not all varieties); analgesics (Acetanilid, phenacetin—not in all variants), nonsulfa antibacterials agents (chloramphenicol—not in all variants, nitrofurantoid) (Prchal, 1980).

2. *Individuals with G-6-PD defect after ingestion of fava beans* (favism) and may be seen in patients with the defect being treated for Parkinsonism with *l*-dopa. *L*-Dopa may be the precursor of the active hemolytic principle in fava beans.

FALSE NORMAL MAY OCCUR IN:

1. *Individuals with very elevated reticulocyte counts,* as in a patient with the defect 3 to 10 days after a severe hemolysis. Because reticulocytes are young cells, their enzyme level is proportionately greater.
2. *Heterozygote females* (only one X chromosomal defect).

Patient Preparation. No special preparation is necessary.

14.4.3 Pyruvate Kinase Deficiency

Synonym: PKD

Reaction Reported

Normal	Decreased or no fluorescence
Abnormal	Persistence of fluorescence

Explanation of the Text. Defect of PK, a rare condition, is an autosomal recessive trait causing severe, chronic, nonspherocytic hemolysis, brought on, or made worse, by stresses, such as infection. Despite the rarity, PKD is the second most frequent deficiency of RBC enzymes. Screening tests for PKD are not as yet adequate (Prchal, 1980).

This test is based upon the known activity of PK in the RBC. It catalyzes the reaction producing ATP from ADP, forming pyruvate. Pyruvate is required to oxidize NADH to NAD, forming lactate. NADH fluoresces; NAD and lactate do not. Therefore, the loss of fluorescence indicates the presence of active PK, and vice versa. For this test any white blood cells must be carefully removed from the blood sample, as they normally contain about 300 times as much PK as do RBCs, and do not share the defect when it is present (Miale, 1972).

Patient Preparation. No special preparation is necessary.

14.5 BLOOD TYPING AND CROSS MATCHING

14.5.1 Type and Rh Factor

Synonyms: ABO and Rh; Rh factor and type; blood groups

Reactions Reported:

ABO blood group: A–B–AB–O (no abnormals)

Rh = normal = positive or negative

Explanation of the Test. These tests are required to determine compatibility before any whole blood, or most blood components, can be given. A, B, AB, O, and Rh are designations of red cell antigens, chemical structures that cause the surface of the RBCs to have differing properties, depending on the antigen. Blood typing to determine the blood group is the identification of the antigen present on an individual's RBC surface. Antigens are identified by their agglutination properties. Within the body they cause antibody production. The blood types serve as antigens. The O phenotype is a very weak antigen, so that for all practical purposes it can be considered nonantigenic. Each blood type produces antibodies to the other blood types but not to its own. Type O therefore has antibodies to both types A and B (see Table 14.3). Type A has the strongest antigenic properties.

Blood typing is also used to collaborate parentage and for definition of medicolegal problems, such as inheritance (Miale, 1972).

Patients needing transfusions are given blood of their own type whenever possible. In cases of real emergency the secondarily acceptable blood types can be given, but only in dire need and only until truly compatible blood is available. Whole blood transfusions are rarely given. Blood components are given instead—a specific part of the blood to treat a specific deficiency. This approach has been found safer and more effective. It also allows better utilization of available blood stores (McGowan, 1980) (see Table 14.4 for a quick overview of the blood components and their uses).

Rh Factor. Many blood groups or systems exist, which makes the process of cross-matching essential whenever blood or blood components are given. The best known blood group after ABO, is the Rh system. There are eight subgroups of agglutinogens in the Rh system. The factors produced are known by two classifications and generally identified by both. One, the American or Wiener classification, uses hr′, hr″, rh′, rh″, RH_0, and various combinations of the designations. The

TABLE 14.3 *ABO blood types and compatibility*

Blood group and phenotype	Can accept from:	Can donate to:	Antigen present on red blood cell	Antibodies present in serum	Frequency of occurrence (%) in U.S.: rank ordered	
O OO	O	A, B AB and O[a]	None	Anti-A Anti-B	1	46
A AA AO	A O	A AB	A Has strongest antigenic activity	Anti-B	2	42
B BB BO	B O	B AB	B	Anti-A	3	9
AB AB	AB A, B, O[b]	AB	A and B	None	4	2

[a]Known as the universal donor. Depends on antibody titer. If more than 1:100, not used for replacement.

[b]Known as the universal recipient. Not necessarily true. Dependent on the titers of anti-A or -B in the donor's blood (Miale, 1972).

Source: Data from Miale, 1972; Watson, 1979; Whaley and Wong, 1979; and Widman, 1979.

English, or Fisher-Race classification is based on a theory of three genes per chromosome and has, therefore, three major designations, in both capital and lowercase letters, (i.e., Cc, Dd, and Ee). Each gene contains one of each letter in combinations of lowercase and capital letters (e.g., Cde, cdE, CDe).

The most important of the Rh antigens is Rh_0 (D). When present, the person is considered Rh positive; 20% of the white population lack Rh_0 (D) and are therefore negative Rh. [The percentage of Rh-negative persons is much less in the black race (5-7%) as well as in the American Indian or Mongoloid races (1%).] Rh_0 (D) is often the only subtype tested for, but further testing is done if Rh_0 (D) is not present. Frequently, Rh_0 variant (D^u) will be tested for, as it often fails to give a strong positive reaction in general screening tests, and a false Rh-negative reaction can occur. The other sub-types are checked when necessary.

All blood groups (antigens) are present on each person's RBCs and the need to screen for the presence of antibodies to groups other than ABO and Rh increases as the number of persons in the population who have been transfused increases. Usually, these systems produce reaction only with prior sensitization, as is true with the Rh group. These other groups include the Kell system (K), Duffy system (Fy), the Kidd system (jk), the M N, P, Lewis (Le), and Lutheran (Lu) systems, as well as subgroups of A (A_1, A_2, A_i, etc.) (Ravel, 1979; Miale, 1972).

TABLE 14.4 *Blood components and their uses*

Component	Indicated in	Comments
Whole blood	Hypovolemia, hypovolemic shock due to acute hemorrhage	
Red blood cells (packed cells)	Nonhypovolemic deficits of RBC mass	Use of cells without serum reduces the possibility of antigen–antibody reactions to plasma constituents and volume overload
Frozen–thawed–washed RBCs	As for RBCs above, plus in the presence of leukocyte antibodies (multiple transfusions/ or pregnancies); history of febrile transfusion reactions; patients on hemodialysis; possible candidates for organ transplantation	Makes available rare blood by storing it; can be used as a mechanism for storage in advance when autogenous/(self) transfusion is necessary (transplantation); washing removes any unbound globulin—a potential antigen
Platelet concentrate	Thrombocytopenia	Most effective with thrombocytopenia due to decreased platelet production or increased platelet loss; least effective with platelet destruction
Leukocyte concentrate (buffy coat)	Severe granulocytepenia; infection refractory to intensive antibiotic treatment	Experimental use at present; usually given daily until clinical evidence of improvement; concentrate collected and given as closely together as possible
Fresh frozen plasma	Multiple or single coagulation deficiencies (e.g., severe liver disease, massive transfusion reaction treatment)	Can be stored for a year, thus immediately available; provides coagulation factors
Normal serum albumin (25% solution)	Treatment of conditions causing protein loss (nephrosis) or hypoproteinemia Both used in conditions requiring blood volume expansion	Prepared from pooled plasma and treated to inactivate hepatitis virus; a purified preparation of albumin only
Plasma protein fraction	Initial treatment of shock due to hemorrhage, plasma loss (burns), or dehydration	Contains albumin and alpha and beta globulins; long storage life even without refrigeration
Cryoprecipitate	Hemophillia	Prepared from frozen plasma. Contains factor VIII concentrated 15 to 40 times normal; also rich in factors VII and I (fibrinogen); must be kept frozen.
Immune serum globulin	Conditions with reduced naturally occurring antibody content: hypogammaglobulinemia, agammaglobulinemia; prophylaxis or attenuation of certain infectious diseases: hepatitis B, tetanus, pertussis, mumps, vaccinia, etc.	Prepared from pooled plasma Specific immune globulin solutions can be prepared from individuals with high titers of specific antibodies

Source: Data from McGowan, 1980 and Phipps, et al. (1979).

14.5.2 Blood Cross-Match

Synonym: compatibility testing

Reactions Reported

Compatible	No agglutination or hemolysis
Incompatible	Clumping (agglutination) and/or hemolysis occur

Explanation of the Test. Not only must the ABO and the Rh blood types of patient and donor blood or constituents be known before introducing alien blood into a body system, but a pretest for match is done between the two supposedly compatible sets of blood to eliminate the chance of any other blood group incompatibility. The recipient's serum is also screened routinely for the presence of antibodies. Transfusion reactions occur with incompatible blood and can be fatal. A transfusion reaction is the body's response to alien antigens by way of antibody production, with subsequent agglutination and hemolysis. The ABO blood types react immediately. The others usually require presensitization.

Cross-matching can be done by mixing the transfusion recipient's serum (which would contain antibodies if sensitized) with the donor's cells and examining the mixture for agglutination. It is possible that antibodies in donor serum could cause problems with specific antigens on the recipient's cells, but this is not ordinarily a major concern, as the donor blood component will be greatly diluted when in the recipient's plasma.

There are three techniques used to detect as many incompatibilities as possible: antiglobulin, albumin media, and enzyme-treated cells. At least one procedure is done at room temperature in serum or saline to detect any cold agglutinins (antigens). The use of indirect antiglobulin testing is done at 37°C to detect nonagglutinating antibodies.

Antibodies do not appear spontaneously to antigens except to the ABO system. A transfusion of Rh-positive blood in an Rh-negative person will cause antibodies to form slowly. Only with a second transfusion, again with Rh-positivie blood, will agglutination and hemolysis of RBCs occur. The same principle applies when an Rh-negative mother carries an Rh-positive fetus. The first child has usually no ill effects unless the mother has been previously sensitized by an Rh-positive transfusion. Subsequent pregnancies with Rh-positive fetuses will be threatened, however. In the instance of an Rh-positive mother or recipient and an Rh-negative child or donor, there is usually no difficulty for the pregnant mother or the transfused individual.

Types of Transfusion Reactions. (data from Miale, 1972)

Hemolytic. Most important because it is the most dangerous. **Cause**: Incompatibility between donor and recipient blood. **Signs and symptoms**: Variable but classically these are: pain in lumbar region; rapid increase of temperature and pulse; chills; flushing of skin; nausea, vomiting; precordial pain; blood pressure may drop. **Action**: Stop transfusion (see "Implications for Nursing" in Section 4.10, item 4). Save remainder of blood and all equipment for examination.

Pyrogenic. Not seen as much with use of disposable IV equipment. **Cause**: Contamination of transfusion substances, usually bacterial, or contamination in process of IV puncture. **Signs and symptoms**: Fever shortly after transfusion begins; may be accompained by chills, mild or severe. **Action**: Stop transfusion. Save remainder of blood and all equipment for examination. Treat symptomatically.

Allergic. **Cause**: Usually presence of an allergen–often derived from food–in the blood to which the recipient is sensitive (Miale, 1972) **Signs and symptoms**: May have only urticaria, or may have acute bronchial asthma, angioneurotic edema, or anaphylactic shock. **Action**: Give antihistamines; depending on severity, blood administration may be stopped. To prevent: All donors should be fasting; all donors with active allergies should be eliminated; premedication with antihistamine with history of allergic reaction to transfusion.

Hemoclastic (reaction to unidentified plasma component). Occurs with plasma transfusions. **Cause**: Nonspecific? Leukoagglutinin reaction? **Signs and symptoms**: Chills; fever; backache; leg pain. **Action**: Stop transfusion.

Circulatory overload. Occurs most often in children, the elderly, and/or persons with heart disease. **Cause**: Too large a quantity of blood given, or blood given at too rapid at rate. **Signs and symptoms**: Those of heart failure: dyspnea, cough, cyanosis. **Action**: Discontinue blood stat; IV TKO only; medical measures to remove fluid rapidly (e.g., diuretics); with pulmonary edema appropriate steps to decrease cardiac return (e.g., rotating tourniquets, sitting position–legs dependent).

Hemorrhagic reaction. Infrequent occurrence. **Cause**: DIC? Washing out of platelets and other coagulation factors in exchange transfusions with inadequate replacement. **Signs and symptoms**: petechial hemorrhages; ecchymosis; hematuria; gastrointestinal hemorrhage (tarry stool); uncontrollable bleeding from operative site.

Patient Preparation. No special preparation is necessary.

The Neurologic System

chapter 15

15.1 LABORATORY AND CLINICAL INDICATIONS OF NEUROLOGIC SYSTEM DYSFUNCTION

Laboratory Findings. Findings may be specific for an infectious causative disorder or of the general physical state of the individual. In general, laboratory findings from screening tests are nonspecific and not useful as clues to neurological problems.

Clinical Findings. Indication of risk groups include: history of vascular disease (arteriosclerosis), plus any condition that significantly reduces cardiac output and/or blood pressure, plus age over 40 (TIA with potential for stroke; history of persistent headache longer than 1 year in previously uncomplaining person should have neurological consultation, as should history of head injury plus any of the following signs or symptoms. *Children:* (exclusive to, or more frequent in) projectile vomiting, increase in head circumference, tight or bulging fontanels with history of URI or otitis media; poor feeding; increased restlessness, irritability. *Adults:* alterations in level of consciousness (LOC); impaired mentation (orientation, cognition, memory); muscular changes—weakness (palsy), spasticity, rigidity, particularly nuchal (inability to press chin on chest), tremors (intention and nonintention), changes in handwriting; changes in reflex response: presence of pathologic reflexes (e.g., Babinski), increased deep tendon reflexes, absence of reflexes, hyperreflexia, clonus; changes in gait, movement, and posture; changes in sensation: numbness, hyperesthesia (increased or altered response to superficial sensation), parasthesias ("funny feelings"), "trigger points" for pain sensation; visual changes: acuity/blurring, photophobia, diminution, total vision loss, field/visual cuts (contralateral to muscular changes indicate stroke), diplopia; dizziness, lightheadedness, dizziness with postural change; changes in personality/behavior (inappropriate); changes in speech: slurring, dysphasia, aphasia; abnormal sleep patterns (data from Conn and Conn, 1979, and Conway, 1978.)

15.2 LUMBAR PUNCTURE

Synonyms: LP; spinal tap; examination of cerebral spinal fluid (CSF)

Normal Ranges: see Table 15.1

Explanation of the Test. Examination of the aspirated cerebral spinal fluid (CSF) is composed of many separate tests, not all having to do with visualizing fluid contents (e.g., measurement of CSF pressure). Some observations, or tests, are not done routinely, but for the "routine" spinal or lumbar puncture, if such a thing exists, the tests include measurement of pressure, examination of gross appearance (consistency, turbidity, viscosity, tendency to clot), measurement of protein and glucose concentrations and a cell count, with a differential count when indicated.

Brief Physiology Review. Cerebral spinal fluid is formed in the ventricles of the brain, circulates over and bathes the surface of the brain, spinal cord, and nerve roots, and is reabsorbed by the arachnoid villa (the arachnoid is the delicate membrane between the dura and the pia mater covering the brain and spinal cord). There is no direct communication between the cerebral blood supply, or the CNS interstitial fluid, and the CSF (blood/CSF barrier and CSF/brain barrier) in the normal healthy person. Substances can cross these barriers by way of active transport (chemical ions such as K^+, H^+, Mg^+, Ca^+), and, in some instances, substances will diffuse rather rapidly across the barrier (e.g., water, chloride). Several pathologic mechanisms open the barrier (e.g., acute hypertension, hypercapnea) as do nonpathologic, but intrusive procedures, such as the injection of radiographic dyes. The lumbar puncture is carried out at the L_3 - L_4 space or lower in adults to avoid the spinal cord. The cord persists lower in children and the tap must be done at L_4 - L_5 space or lower (Henry, 1979).

TABLE 15.1 *Reference values for lumbar cerebrospinal fluid in adults*

	CNS	Serum
Protein (total)	15–45 mg/dL	6.0–7.8 g/dL
Pediatric		
Neonatal	20–170 mg/dL	
Infant	10–30 mg/dL	
Senior adult	30–60 mg/dL	
Prealbumin	2–5%	—
Albumin	56–76%	52–67%
$Alpha_1$ globulin	2–7%	2– 5%
$Alpha_2$ globulin	4–12%	6–14%
Beta globulin	8–18%	8–16%
Gamma globulin	3–12%	10–22%
Electrolytes		
Sodium	136–150 mEq/L	136–150 mEq/L
Potassium		
Lumbar CSF	2.6–3.0 mEq/L	3.0–4.5 mEq/L
Cisternal CSF	2.3–2.7 mEq/L	—
Chloride	118–130 mEq/L	96–104 mEq/L
Bicarbonate	20– 25 mEq/L	21– 26 mEq/L
Calcium	2.1–2.7 mEq/L	4.6–5.4 mEq/L
Magnesium	2.4–3.0 mEq/L	1.5–2.4 mEq/L
Lactate	10– 22 mg/dL	3–7 mg/dL
Osmolality	280–295 mOsm/L	280–295 mOsm/L
Acid Base		
pH		
Lumbar CSF	7.28–7.32	7.38–7.42
Cisternal CSF	7.32–7.34	(arterial)
pCO_2		
Lumbar CSF	44–50 mmHg	36–40 mmHg
Cisternal CSF	40–44 mmHg	(arterial)
pCO_2	40–44 mHg	45–100 mmHg
Special chemistry		
Ammonia	0.5–1.0 μg/mL	1.0–2.0 μg/mL (arterial)
Creatinine	0.5–1.2 mg/dL	0.5–1.2 mg/dL
Glucose	50–80 mg/dL	70–100 mg/dL
Iron	1–2 μg/dL	50–150 μg/dL
Phosphorus	1.2–2.0 mg/dL	3.0–4.5 mg/dL
Urea	6–16 mg/dL	8– 20 mg/dL
Uric acid	0.5–3.0 mg/dL	2.0–8.0 mg/dL
Zinc	2.6 μg/dL	50–150 μg/dL
Pressure	50–180 mm of CSF (lateral recumbent position)	

Source: Adapted from Arthur Kreig, "Cerebral Spinal Fluid and Other Body Fluids," in John Bernard Henry, *Clinical Diagnosis and Management by Laboratory Methods* (Philadelphia: W. B. Saunders Company, 1979), pp. 636, 638, 647.

Indications for Lumbar Puncture

1. *Suspected meningitis,* encephalitis, brain abcess, subarachnoid hemorrhage, leukemia involving the central nervous system (CNS), multiple sclerosis (MS), Guillain-Barré syndrome, and spinal cord tumor (*not* intracranial tumors).
2. *To document impairment of CSF flow.*
3. *Differential diagnosis of hemorrhagic versus ischemic syndromes* in cerebral-vascular disease [transient ischemic attacks (TIA)–stroke], or the differential diagnosis of cerebral infarct versus intracerebral hemorrhage.
4. *Introduction of anesthetics, radiographic contrast media, or certain medication* [e.g., methotrexate (meningeal leukemia), amphotericin (fungal meningitis)].
5. *The treatment of selected patients with benign intracranial hypertension* (the effectiveness of such treatment has not been determined) (Widmann, 1979).

Contraindications for Lumbar Puncture

1. *Presence of, or suspected presence of, intracranial tumors,* because of the potential for tentorial hernation with pressure shifts.
2. *In most cases when increased intracranial pressure* (IICP) *and papilledema* (edema and hyperemia of the optic disc–choked disc) are present, for the reason given with item 1. The criteria necessary for a physician to go ahead with an LP when the foregoing situation is present are generally that:
   a. Necessary information is not available by any means other than LP.
   b. The probability is high that the CSF findings will have a significant impact on *both* treatment and outcome.
   c. Neurosurgical consultation is available (Henry, 1979).
3. In most patients with *primary clotting defects* (thrombocytopenia) or those defects secondary to anticoagulant drug use because of the possibility of the formation of extradural, or subdural hematoma, and resultant paralysis.
4. *In the presence of systemic sepsis* as well as infection or severe dermatologic disease in the lumbar area, because of the potential for meningitis.
5. *Some spinal deformities and in extreme age* in some cases because of the difficulty in the procedure.
6. *In some cases of severe personality problems* in the patient, as the trauma can become the basis of further personality disruption.

Routine Tests with Lumbar Puncture (Tables 15.2 to 15.8)

Patient Preparation

1. *If an accurate determination of CNS sugar* is particularly important, the test should be done in the fasting patient (NPO except for water for 8 to 12 hr prior to the test). All "routine" lumbar taps—as opposed to emergency taps—are best done on a fasting patient.
2. *Lumbar tap is one of the more fear-producing diagnostic tests.* Any measures that will reduce patient anxiety and increase cooperation during the procedure should be undertaken. Infants and children are usually restrained.
3. *Inform the laboratory* of any suspected infective organisms when requesting stain and/or culture on the CSF.

Other Tests Done on CSF

1. *Organism stain*—slide stain (see Section 6.1.1 for more detailed information). Gram stain, Wright's stain, India ink stains are used to assist in the identification of infective organisms or the presence of malignant cells.
2. *Organism culture* is usually done to help isolate an infective organism (see Sections 6.1.2 and 6.1.3).
3. *Serology*—specifically the Venereal Disease Research Laboratory Test (VDRL) and/or the Fluorescent Treponemal Antibody Absorption Test (FTA-ABS) are often done on both blood and CSF when syphilis is suspected, or must be ruled out (see Section 6.2.1).

Tests Not Covered in This Book

1. *Angiography* is used for definitive diagnosis in strokes and is also used to determine the extent of subdural hematomas or cerebral aneurysm.
2. *Skull x-ray,* computerized axial tomography (CAT scan, CT scan, or EMI scan), and radioisotope brain scan (technetium) are very frequently used for diagnosis and/or location of CNS lesions. CT scans are especially useful and noninvasive.
3. *Electroencephalograms* (EEG) are done in seizure disorders as well as in cerebral-vascular disease.
4. *Further tests* include echoencephalogram, pneumoencephalogram, and ventriculogram.

TABLE 15.2 *Gross appearance*

Normal	Variations from normal and significance
Clear	Changes causing turbidity may be due to increased presence of leukocytes—at least 200 cell/μL of CSF necessary to cause slight turbidity (see also Table 13.1, footnote a, for numerical identification of degree of turbidity); increase in turbidity also due to increased erythrocytes—at least 400 cells/μL CSF; presence of microorganisms (bacteria, fungi, amebas), or contrast media; also due to aspiration of epidural fat with spinal puncture
No clot formation	Clots often due to increased protein in CSF; always occurs when protein levels are 1000 mg/dL or greater; very fine clotting occurring with lower levels can be seen if specimen is refrigerated 12–24 hr; occurs with increased fibrinogen, due to traumatic tap and certain types of meningitis or neurosyphilis
Viscosity of water	Increased viscosity reported with metastatic mucinous adenocarcinoma of the the meninges
Colorless	White or cloudy due to high WBC (over 500 WBC/mm^3) or increased protein Xanthochromia: yellowish discoloration, can actually range from pale pink to orange and yellow; change in color indicates presence of RBCs, usually, and their age—the younger the cell the pinker the color; specimen must be examined within 1 hr after tap to prevent false positive due to lysis; RBC increase and presence of xanthochromia most often due to subarachnoid hemorrhage; color change can also be due to presence of bilirubin with increased serum bilirubin, presence of carotenoids with increased serum carotene, or presence of melanin due to meningeal melanosarcoma; xanthochromia expected in premature infants due to increased bilirubin, increased CSF protein and immaturity of blood–brain barrier

Source: Data taken from Henry, 1979, and Ravel, 1979.

TABLE 15.3 *Pressure*

Normal and comments	Increased in:	Decreased in:
50–180 mm of CSF (lateral recumbent position) Minor variations occur with respiration If initial pressure is over 200 mm Hg, only 1–2 mL CSF should be removed A 25–50% drop in ICP after removal of 1–2 mL CSF indicates cerebral herniation or spinal cord compression Normal pressure, sitting position: over 300 mm H_20	Anxiety: if over 180 at start of tap check for breath holding, muscle tightening, jugular compression Infections: high with bacteria or TB; lesser increase with encephalitis, neurosyphilis Meningeal inflammation Congestive heart failure Acute obstruction of the superior vena cava—early Thrombosis and obstruction of intracranial venous sinuses Acute hypoosmolality due to hemodialysis Increased CSF protein, or hemorrhage (subarachnoid) impairing CSF reabsorption Mass lesions (tumor, abscess, IC hemorrhage) Cerebral edema	Actually a rare occurrence Circulatory collapse Severe dehydration Acute hyperosmolality Loss of CSF with leakage (dural tear, CSF rhinorrhea, previous puncture) Complete spinal subarachnoid block (noncommunication) With no initial increase in pressure, CSF pressure should not drop more than 5–10 mm for each mL CSF fluid removed If final pressure drop is less than the 5–10 mm/mL after fluid is removed, an increased CSF pool is indicated (e.g., hydrocephalus) If final pressure drop is greater than the norm a decreased CSF pool is indicated (e.g., tumor, spinal block)

Source: Data taken from Henry, 1979, and Widmann, 1979.

TABLE 15.4 *Queckenstedt test*

Procedure	Normal response and comments	Variations from normal
Bilateral jugular compression for 10 sec Indications for use: suspicion of subarachnoid block or spinal cord tumor *Not* a routine test	CSF pressure increases rapidly to 300 mm and rapidly returns to normal when compression ceases Principle: CSF space is a closed system; pressure exerted in one part of a closed system should be reflected in all other parts	CSF pressure decreased or delayed (more than 20 sec) = a 'positive' test; occurs in: Sinus thrombosis Obstruction at foramen magnum Mass spinal canal lesion With abnormal or positive test, the normal variation of pressure with respiration is absent

Source: Data from Henry, 1979, and Clark, 1975.

TABLE 15.5 *Glucose (see Table 15.1 for Normal Range)*

Increased in	Decreased in	Comments
Some cases of aseptic or viral meningitis False increase with serum hyperglycemia	50% of patients with bacterial meningitis 25% of patients with mumps meningoencephalitis Variable decrease in meningitis (due to Tbc, fungus, virus). Subarachnoid hemorrhage (4–8 days after onset) Some cases of neurosyphilis; false decrease secondary to hypoglycemia	Normal level is usually about one-half to two-thirds that of serum glucose Must be compared to serum concentration to detect false increase or decrease (CSF glucose rises or falls approximately 2 hr after plasma levels change) Major pathologic significance found in decreased levels Decrease usually due to impairment of active transport or increased utilization

Source: Data from Conn, 1979, and Henry, 1979.

TABLE 15.6 *Protein, total (see Table 15.1 for normal range)*

Increased in	Decreased in	Comments
Normally in neonate and older adult Presence of blood (traumatic tap) 1 mL blood can increase protein to 400 mg/dL Increased permeability of blood/CSF barrier; common cause of pathologic increases, as in: Bacterial, fungal, Tbc meningitis Subarachnoid hemorrhage Cerebral thrombosis Intracerebral hemorrhage	CSF loss from leakage, as in: Dural tear with trauma Rhinorrhea Otorrhea IICP due to increased filtration through the the arachnoid Hyperthydroidism, mechanism unknown	Increased CSF protein is roughly proportional to the degree of leukocytosis; thus cell count usually increases as well Protein from plasma diffuses into CSF Concentration varies slightly with age Protein can also be fractionated by electrophoresis (See Table 15.1 for normals); increases in gamma globulin most important in detection of multiple sclerosis (MS)

TABLE 15.6 (*cont.*)

Increased in	Decreased in	Comments
Obstruction of CSF circulation, as in: Tumor Herniated disc Increased CNS synthesis of IgG, as in: Guillain-Barré syndrome Collagen diseases Tissue degeneration as in amyotrophic lateral sclerosis (ALS)		

Source: Data from Ravel, 1979, and Henry, 1979.

TABLE 15.7 *Lactate (lactic acid) (see Table 15.1 for normal range)*

Increased in	Decreased in	Comments
Any condition with a decreased cerebral blood flow, decreased oxygenation of the brain, or IICP, as in: Traumatic brain injury Seizures Respiratory alkalosis Intracranial hemorrhage Hydrocephalus TIA Multiple sclerosis (MS) Bacterial meningitis	Decreases are of little clinical importance	Lactate concentrations may be of assistance in the differential diagnosis between bacterial meningitis (lactate increased to over 25 mg/dL) and aseptic meningitis (most cases have no increase in lactate) Also may be useful as a screening test to detect CNS disease; becoming a more routine test because of this

Source: Data from Henry, 1979.

TABLE 15.8 *Cell count (CSF cell count; spinal fluid cell count)*[a]

Cell type (normal cells)	Normal range adults	Normal range neonates	Increased in:
Lymphocytes	62% ± 34%	20% ± 18%	Increased in many infections, and in partially treated bacterial meningitis; in parasitic disease (toxiplasmosis), subacute sclerosing panencephalitis (SSPE) secondary to measles virus, MS, drug abuse encephalitis, Guillain-Barré syndrome, polyneuritis, periarteritis
PAM[b] cells and monocytes	36% ± 20%	72% ± 22%	Increased in mixed reactions, with many other cells increased, such as Tbc, fungal, chronic bacterial, and leptospiral meningitis; amebic encephalomyelitis; rupture of brain abcess
Neutrophils	2% ± 5%	3% ± 5%	When increased with monocytes, may indicate Tbc meningitis; some authorities consider even one neutrophil abnormal; numbers increase with

TABLE 15.8 (*cont.*)

Cell type (normal cells)	Normal range adults	Normal range neonates	Increased in:
			traumatic tap, bacterial infections, early in viral infections, and other infectious processes; also increased in CNS hemorrhage, injections of foreign materials into subarachnoid space, in metastatic tumor, and infarct
Histiocytes	Rare	5% ± 4%	
Ependymal cells	Rare	Rare	Ependymal cells are cells from the ventricular and central canal of the spinal membrane lining; increased following pneumoencephalograms, with hydrocephalus, after cisternal or ventricular puncture, or after administration of chemotherapeutic agents intrathecally
Eosinophils	Rare	Rare	Increased over 5% in some cases of pneumococcal meningitis, Tbc meningitis, fungal meningitis (coccidiodomycosis) and syphilis meningoencephalitis; in parasitic infection and after foreign protein injections (radioactive serum albumin); after rabies vaccination, intracranial shunts; with allergic or hypersensitive reactions to food or drugs; in allergic asthma; in CNS lymphocytic leukemia
			Found in:
Plasma cells	0	0	Often associated with lymphocytic reactions; may be the only abnormality in multiple sclerosis (MS); lymphocytes may undergo transformation to plasma cells in CNS.
Basophils	0	0	Found with CNS granulocytic leukemia
Macrophages (includes giant cells)	0	0	Found in Tbc, mycotic meningitis; after brain surgery; after trauma; after subarachnoid hemorrhage
Leukemic cells	0	0	Uncommon initially in leukemias; occur with long-established disease after severe illness, usually during remissions; most common in lymphoblastic leukemia and acute myeloblastic leukemia
Tumor cells	0	0	From primary or metastatic cancer

[a]*Normal Range:* Just what cells can appear normally, and in what amount, is somewhat controversial. Each laboratory provides their own "normal," which is usually given as a count of cells rather than a percent. When more than the accepted normal number are seen, a WBC differential is performed and all cells noted are identified. The counts given above are in percentage of total cells usually seen, including some rather controversial "usuals."

[b]Pia-arachnoid mesothelial cells.

Source: Data from Henry, 1979.

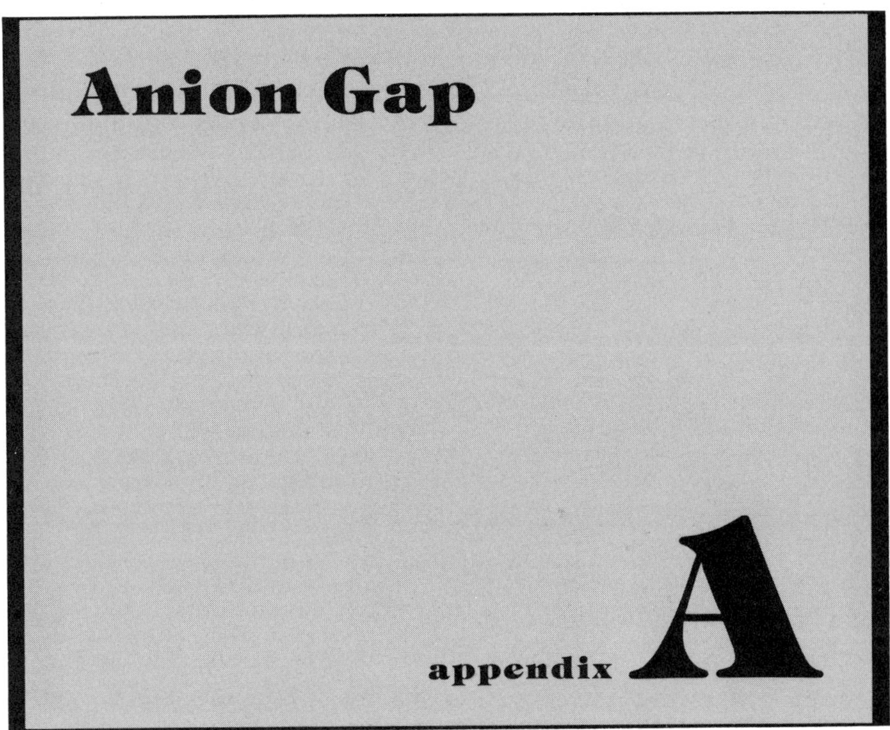

A true discrepancy always occurs in metabolic acidosis between the sum of the cations measured in the plasma and the sum of the anions (Harper, 1971). This discrepancy, called the anion gap, or in some instances the "R" factor, is composed of increased amounts of unmeasured anions (phosphates, sulfates, proteinates, organic acids such as ketone bodies, lactic acid) produced in the acidotic state. Determination of these unmeasured anions is not a routinely available clinical procedure. But it is possible to get helpful laboratory data about the existence of these unmeasured anions by looking at the difference between the sum of the serum cations and the sum of the serum anions:

$$([Na^+] + [K^+]) - ([Cl^-] + [HCO_3^-])$$

Values in excess of 20 are associated with some increase in nonvolatile anions. Volatile anions are not useful in the calculation because when the unmeasured anions initially increase, bicarbonate is displaced (decreased venous CO_2 values) and pH drops. This stimulates the respiratory compensation with an increase in respiratory rate and depth, which results in the volatile acid, carbonic acid (pCO_2), being blown off. A slight increase in the pH results though the concentration of non-volatile anions remains unchanged.

If the sum of the anions is greater than that of the cations, the probability is that a laboratory error has been made.

Physiologic Response to Stress and Related Laboratory Changes

appendix B

Besides the mechanisms specifically related to providing extra glucose in times of stress, the following physiologic changes occur which cause variation in laboratory findings.

1. *The spleen contracts,* forcing increased numbers of RBCs into circulation (hemoconcentration with increased RBC count, increased hemoglobin and hematocrit).
2. *Bronchi dilate* so that air can be moved more easily in and out of the lung (hyperventilation—respiratory alkalosis, decreased pCO_2).
3. *The hypothalamus produces corticotropin releasing factor* (CRF), stimulating release of stored ACTH, which in turn stimulates release of glucocorticoids (increased plasma cortisol) (Frolich, 1976).
4. *Glucocorticoids foster the fat mobilization* [increased free fatty acids (FAAs)] as well as glucagon production and release, which accounts for the increased serum glucose.
5. *During stress, there is a reduction in lymphatic tissue,* including the spleen noted above, and the thymus: this means fewer lymphocytes in circulation.

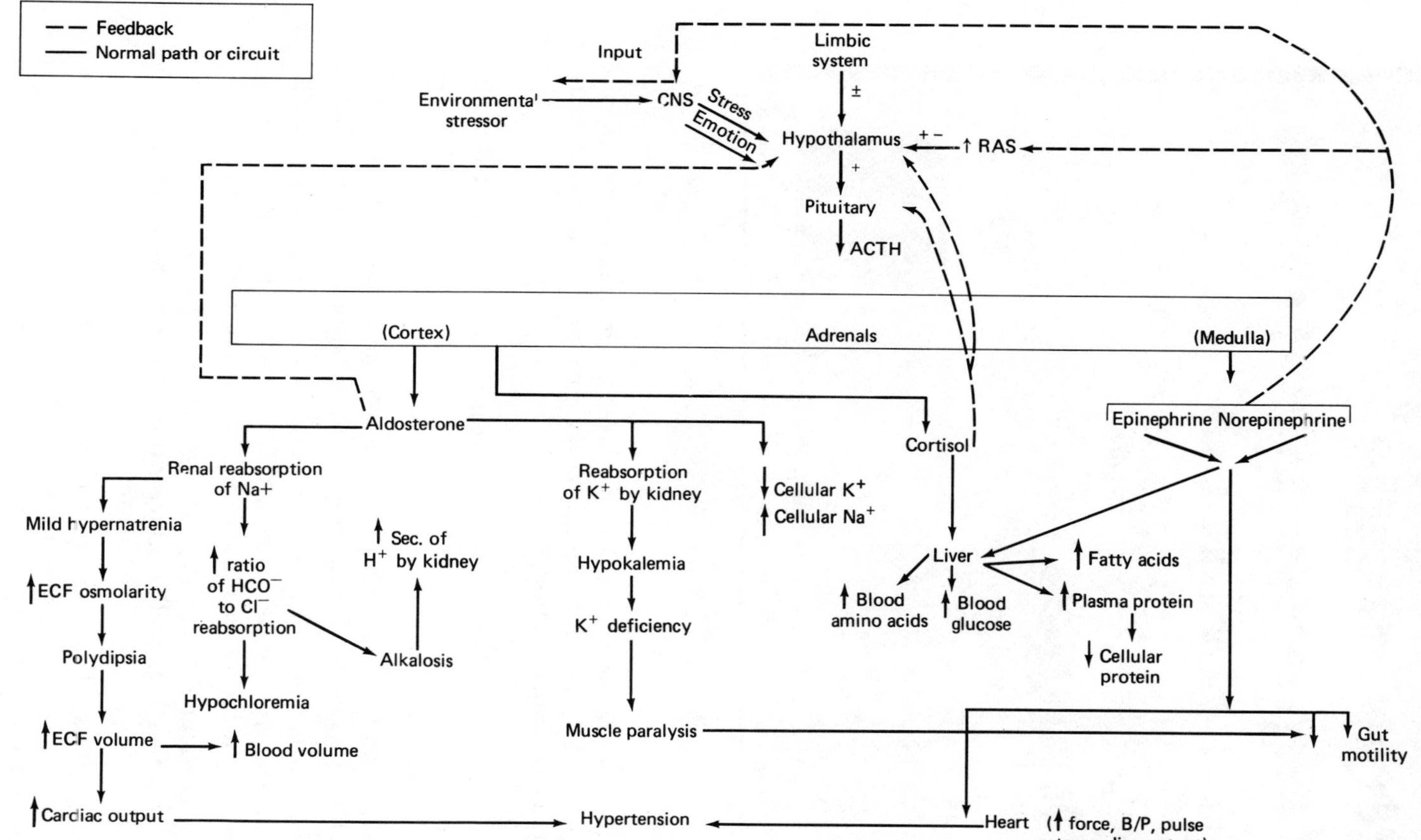

FIGURE B.1 Environmental stress and the physiologic response of the adrenal system with feedback channels. [Reprinted with permission from Mary E. Hazzard, *Critical Care Nursing—Nursing Outline Series* (Garden City, N.Y.: Medical Examination Publishing Company, Inc., an Excerpta Medical Company, copyright 1978), p. 39.]

6. *Eosinophils are also reduced* in the circulating blood, for reasons that are not yet clear (see Fig. B.1).
7. *ADH is released by the pituitary* retaining fluid, and if the ECV is decreased, aldosterone is released and sodium reabsorbed, causing further water conservation (potential dilutional hyponatremia, potassium loss, increased serum bicarbanate, decreased sodium and chloride, potential metabolic alkalosis).
8. *Urinary output is decreased* during and following stress (concentrated urine).
9. *There is a net catabolic effect* from these hormonal responses, causing muscle loss, weight loss, and an increased serum urea nitrogen (BUN) (Harvey et al., 1976).
10. *The generalized response to stress* may be less effective if called upon during the night. The diurnal rhythm of adrenocorticosteroid output is diminished during the night (MacBryde and Blacklow, 1970).
11. *Since cholesterol is a precursor in the formation of adrenocorticol hormones,* cholesterol increases in the blood (cholesteremia).
12. *White blood count increases* due to an increase of polymorphonuclear cells, despite the decrease in lymphocytes and eosinophils.

Dialysis Disequilibrium Syndrome

appendix C

The cause of the disequilibrium syndrome is thought to be due to the rapid removal of urea from the bloodstream, with its accompanying removal from the brain being at a slower rate. This leads to a reverse osmotic gradient that pulls water into the brain, causing cerebral edema —hence the signs and symptoms of headache, nausea, vomiting, and rise of blood pressure. The coil dialyzer removes urea more rapidly than do other types of dialyzers, and the use of this machine has been linked with the occurrence of the syndrome. It is also found to occur most frequently in acutely ill individuals with excessively increased serum urea nitrogen levels. Only occasionally has this syndrome been observed in patients who have undergone previous prolonged periods of uneventful dialysis. Thus, at risk is the person first starting hemodialysis.

Treatment of the condition is primarily in the field of the physician with a change in dialysate [increased glucose concentration in the dialysate has been found helpful in preventing the syndrome (Czaczkes and De-Nour, 1978, pp. 56-58)], or a change in the length or frequency of dialysis. Change in the type of dialyzer is indicated if a coil machine has been used. Frequently, the use of anticonvulsants prior to dialysis is felt to prevent the syndrome (Harrington and Brener, 1973, pp. 140-141).

Information on Laboratory Reporting Units

appendix **D**

Units of measurement

Term	Definition	Abbreviation
decaliter	10 liters	Not used in reporting laboratory values
deciliter	1/10 liter or 100 milliliters	dL
femtoliter	10^{-15} liter	fL
International unit	Number of moles of substrate converted per second under defined conditions (Henry, 1979)	IU
milligram	1/1000 (10^{-3}) gram or 0.015432 grain	mg
gram	Basic weight unit of metric scale—15,432 grains	Gm, gm, G, or g[a]
microgram	One-millionth (10^{-6}) of a gram or 1/1000 (10^{-3}) milligram	μg[a] or mcg
micromicrogram or picogram	10^{-12} gram	pg[a] or μμg
milli International unit	1/1000 IU (International unit)	mIU
millimicrogram	1/1000 (10^{-3}) microgram or 10^{-9} gram	mμg
micrometer or micron	10^{-6} meter	μm
nanogram	10^{-9} gram	ng[a] or nμg

[a]Used in this text.

Unit conversion

1 dL	=	100 mL
1 mg/dL	=	1 mg/100 mL = 1 mg%
g/L	=	g% × 10
1 IU/mL	=	83.3 ng/mL
1 mIU/mL	=	0.08 ng/mL
1 ng/mL	=	12 MIU/mL

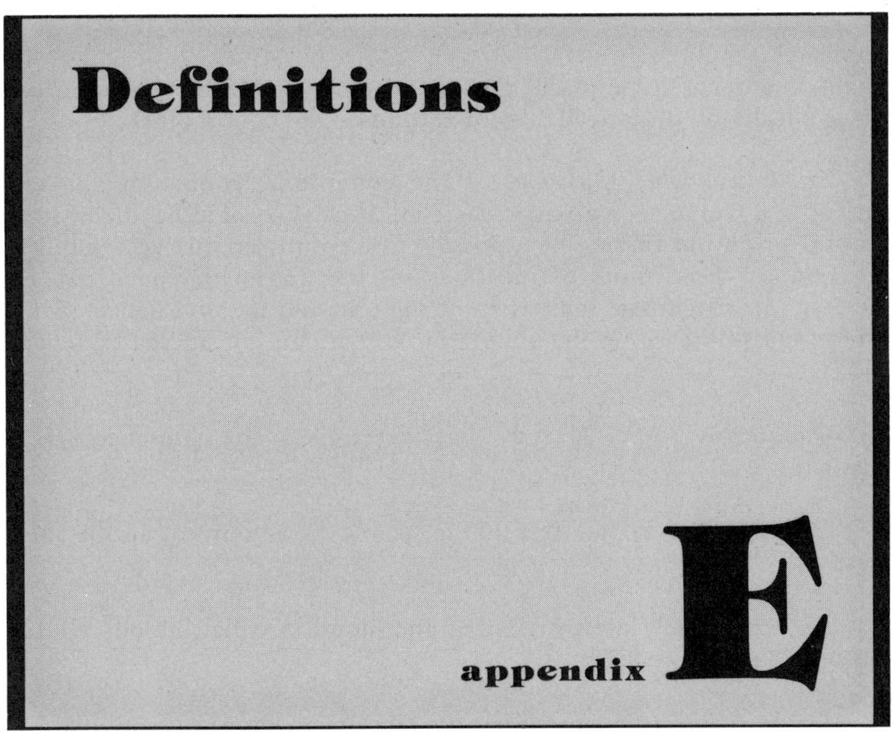

Assay. Is the analysis of a substance to define its nature and proportions. "The fundamental principle on which all assays (radio, competitive binding, radioimmuno) are based depends on the use of a limited amount of specific binding reagent which is held constant in the system. The binder may be an antibody (insulin assay), specific binding proteins (thyroxine assay); cellular receptor; or even an enzyme (renin assay). The requirement of the technique is that there must be a means of separating or identifying the bound and free components" (Henry, 1979).

Cushing's disease. A condition caused by pituitary dependent overproduction of glucocorticoids from the adrenal cortex, due to pituitary basophilism (tumor of basophil cells of the pituitary), causing increased ACTH secretion and adrenal hyperplasia–bilateral (Krueger, 1976).

Cushing's syndrome. A condition due to the hypersecretion of cortisol caused by overproduction of the adrenal cortex, which may affect only one of the adrenal glands. The condition may be due to multiple etiologies [e.g., benign or malignant tumors of the adrenal gland(s), adrenal hyperplasia due to an ectopic ACTH syndrome, or iatrogenically by prolonged administration of glucocorticoids].

Predictive value, positive. "The conditional probability that a patient is a member of a particular clinical class (read as having a given disease) given the finding of a positive test result. Predictive value is a function of three units of information: the diagnostic specificity of the test, the diagnostic sensitivity of the test, and the prevalence of the clinical class (disease) in the population of patients considered" (Henry, 1979).

Qualitative test. A test that determines the presence of a substance.

Quantitative test. A test that measures the amount of a substance present.

Plasma. The fluid portion of the blood in which blood cellular substances are suspended.

Serum. Plasma from which the fibrinogen has been separated by the process of clotting.

Test sensitivity. "A measure of frequency of positive test results in patients with a certain disease. If most patients with a disease have positive test results, the test is said to be highly sensitive" (Harrington and Brener, 1973).

Test specificity. "A measure of the frequency of negative test results in persons who do not have the disease. If most persons without the disease do not have positive test results, the test is said to be hightly specific for that disorder" (Harrington and Brener, 1973).

Normal Flora and Unusual or Abnormal Flora by Site

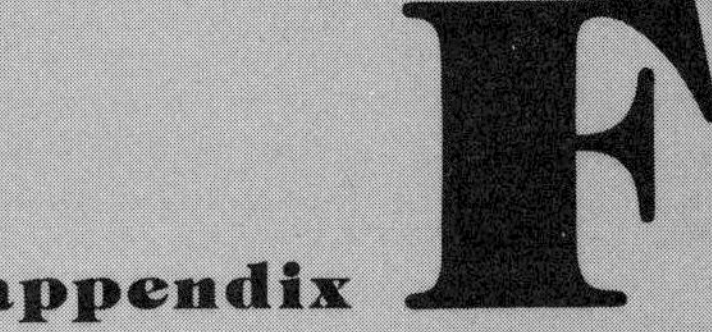

appendix F

Site	Normal	Abnormal or unusual
Body fluids and blood (i.e., pleural, synovial, bile, etc.)	Sterile (rarely contaminated with a few diphtheroid or *Staphylococcus epidermidis*)	Potentially any organism
Cerebral spinal fluid	Sterile	Any organism
Ear Outer	*Staphylococcus epidermidis* Diphtheroids Micrococci *Bacillus* species	*Pseudomonas aeruginosa* *Staphylococcus aureus* *Beta hemolytic streptococci* *Hemophilus influenzae* *Escherichia coli* Coliforms[a]
Inner	Sterile	As above
Eye	Small numbers of *Staphylococcus epidermidis* Viridans streptococci group Diphtheroids	*Staphylococcus epidermidis* *Streptococcus pneumoniae* *Hemophilus influenzae* (*H. aegyptius*) *Pseudomonas aeruginosa* Viridans streptococci group Beta hemolytic streptococci *Neisseria gonorrheae* *Acinetobacter* species *Chlamydia* group

Site	Normal	Abnormal or unusual
Lung (brushings, needle aspirates)	Scant oral flora (Viridans streptococci, plus diphtheroids, *Staphylococcus epidermidis)*	*Staphylococcus aureus* Beta hemolytic streptococci *Pseudomonas* species Coliforms (particularly *Klebsiella, Enterobacter*) *Hemophilus influenzae* Acid-fast bacilli Fungus (*Coccidioides, Aspergillus, Penicillium*) Yeast (*Cryptococcus,* diphasic fungi) *Pneumocystis carinii* *Legionella pneumophila* and other Legionnaires'-like organisms (TexKL, WIGA) Anerobic bacteria
Lower respiratory tract (expectorated sputum, endotracheal suction)	See Upper respiratory tract	As listed below
Upper respiratory tract: throat, nasopharynx, mouth	Viridans streptococci Staphylococcus epidermidis Scant to occasional *Staphylococcus aureus* Some beta hemolytic streptococci Micrococci Diphtheroids *Neisseria* species Occasional coliforms Anerobic gram-negative and gram-positive bacilli and cocci	Beta hemolytic streptococci especially Group A, occasionally Groups C, F, G *Staphylococcus aureus* *Corynebacterium diptheriae* *Hemophilus influenzae* and occasionally *H. parainfluenzae* *Candida albicans* (if heavy) Fusiforms and spirochetes in synergy (Vincent's disease) *Neisseria meningitidis* *Neisseria gonorrheae* *Bordatella pertussis* *Pasteurella multocida* *Branhamella catarrhalis*
Skin	Staphylococcus epidermidis Diphtheroids (other than *Corynebacterium diptheriae*) *Bacillus* species Viridans streptococci Coliforms Saprophytic yeast and fungi Micrococci	Beta hemolytic streptococci *Staphylococcus aureus* *Corynebacterium diptheriae* Some fungi Heavy *Candida albicans* *Staphylococcus epidermidis* (in stitch abscess) *Pasteurella multocida* (in cat or dog bites) Anerobic streptococci plus aerobic or facultative organisms in decubiti
Urogenital sites; bladder urine (clean voided)	Occasional to scant lower urethral contaminants (*Staphylococcus epidermidis,* diphtheroids, other skin microflora)	Greater than 100,000 organisms per milliliter of urine; usually a single type, but occasionally mixed infection *Escherichia coli* *Klebsiella* species *Enterobacter* species *Proteus mirabilis* Indole positive *Proteus* Enterococci (fecal streptococci)

Site	Normal	Abnormal or unusual
Urogenital sites; bladder urine (clean voided) (*cont.*)		*Staphylococcus saprophyticus* and other *Staphylococcus epidermidis* *Ureaplasma urealyticum* *Cytomegalovirus* *Chlamydia* group Rarely, *Salmonella* species, pneumococc Yeasts (*Candida, Torulopsis*)
Catheterized urine	Sterile	Same as above, but counts of 10,000/ml or less may be significant
Urethra	As noted with clean voided urine	*Neisseria gonorrheae* *Hemophilus influenzae* *Gardinerella vaginalis* *Ureaplasma urealyticum* *Trichomonas vaginalis* *Candida albicans* Others from clean voided list
Vagina	Lactobacilli *Staphylococcus epidermidis* Micrococci Coliforms Occasional Group B beta hemolytic streptococci Mixed anerobic gram-negative and positive bacilli and cocci Enterococci Occasional *Candida*	*Neisseria gonorrheae* *Hemophilus influenzae* *Gardinerella vaginalis* (when associated with "clue" cells) Herpes virus *Chlamydia* *Mycoplasma* species *Ureaplasma urealyticum* *Staphylococcus aureus* Heavy growth of Group B beta hemolytic streptococci *Trichomonas vaginalis* *Candida albicans*
Cervix	Scant amounts of normal vaginal organisms	*Neisseria gonorrheae* *Hemophilus influenzae* *Streptococcus pneumoniae* All others listed above for vagina (Significant anerobic gram negative bacilli such as *Bacteroides bivius, B. disiens, B. fragilis,* and *B. melaninogenicus* as well as anerobic gram positive cocci; anerobic flora may reflect P.I.D., may be assessed only if cervical culture is taken with special procedures to decontaminate cervical os; best ruled in as pathogens through culdocentesis procedure)
Wounds, abscesses	Surface wounds (i.e., decubiti) as for skin	As for skin
	Deep wounds: sterile	Many organisms, including but not limited to: *Staphylococcus aureus* Beta hemolytic streptococci *Pasteurella multocida* Occasionally *P. multocida* and non-cholera vibrios

Site	Normal	Abnormal or unusual
Wounds, abscesses (*cont.*)		Coliforms of all types Viridans streptococci groups Anerobic gram-negative bacilli and cocci, especially *Bacteriodes fragilis, B. melaninogenicus* *Clostridium perfringens* *Clostridium tetani* Other *Clostridium* species *Actinomyces* species Parasites from liver and bowel abscesses
Stool	Coliforms such as most strains of *Escherichia coli* *Klebsiella, Enterobacter, Proteus,* etc. Fecal streptococci Many different anerobic and microaerophilic organisms Yeasts Some types of parasites (*Endamoeba coli*) Occasional *Pseudomonas* and *Acinetobacter* species	*Campylobacter fetus* sp. *jejuni* *Salmonella* species *Shigella* species *Arizona* species Some strains of *Escherichia coli* Some strains of *Proteus mirabilis* *Yersinia enterocolitica* *Yersinia pseudotuberculosis* *Clostridium difficile* with cytotoxin *Staphylococcus aureus* (enterotoxic) Enterotoxin producing *Escherichia coli* *Clostridium perfringens* Enteroviruses (e.g., rota virus, Norwalk agent) Parasites such as *Giardia lamblia, Endamoeba histolytica, Trichuris, Ascaris*

[a]"Coliforms": a term to describe a group of gram-negative bacteria which are non-spore-forming, facultative anerobes, such as *Escherichia coli, Klebsiella-Enterobacter* group, *Proteus, Morganella, Hafnia,* etc., which are found ubiquitously in human and animal environs, occasionally occurring in water, on vegetation. etc.

Source: Prepared by Patricia C. Harris, M.S., S.M. (AAM) Chief Microbiologist, General Hospital of Everett, Everett, Washington.

Somogyi Reaction

appendix G

The Somogyi reaction is the name applied to a situation in which a diabetic demonstrates glycosuria in response to an *overdosage* of insulin rather than a lack of insulin. This paradox is understandable when the pathophysiology is explained.

Briefly the pathophysiology is as follows. Hypoglycemia, due to insulin overdosage, occurs during sleep—often around 2 A.M. The individual is unaware of the early subjective symptoms. Hormonal response to the hypoglycemia occurs, stimulating those hormones that counter hypoglycemia (epinephrine, cortisol, and perhaps growth hormone). In response, the blood glucose rises at a rapid rate as the level of plasma insulin falls, leading to an 8 A.M. glycosuria. Despite the administration of too much insulin, the interpretation is often insufficient insulin and a cycle is produced.

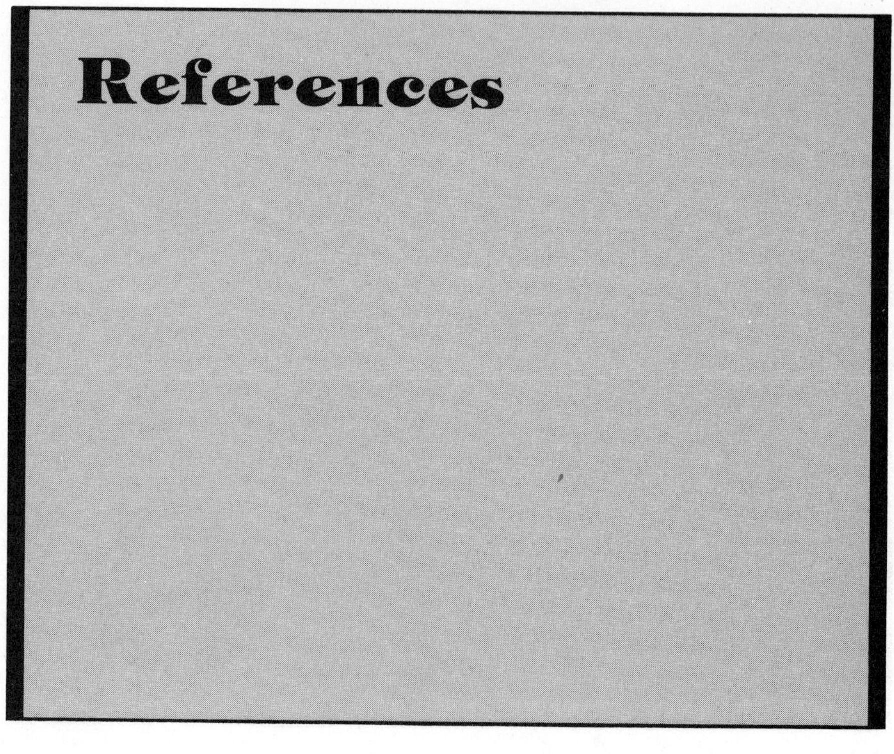

References

ACKLEY, ALEXANDER, and DAVID J. GOCKE. "Viral Hepatitis." *American Family Physician* (May 1980), 156–162.

BAUMAN, DENNIS J. "Creatine Phosphokinase Isoenzymes and the Diagnosis of Myocardial Infarction." *Postgraduate Medicine* (January 1980), 103–106, 109–112, 115–116.

BECK, WILLIAM S. *Human Design.* New York; Harcourt Brace Jovanovich, Inc., 1971.

BERMAN, LEONARD B., and VICTOR VERTES. "The Pathophysiology of Renin." *Clinical Symposia,* 25, No. 5 (1973), 1-35.

BIENENSTOCK, HARRY. "Arthritis: Diagnostic Guide." *Hospital Medicine* (April 1980), 27–28, 35.

BIGLIERI, EDWARD G., and JAN STOCKIGT. "Primary Aldosteronism" *Clinician –1: The Adrenal Gland* (1971), 59–67.

BLEVINS, DOROTHY R. *The Diabetic and Nursing Care.* New York: McGraw-Hill Book Company, 1979.

BONDY, PHILIP. "Adrenal Masculinizing and Feminizing Syndromes." *Clinician–1: The Adrenal Gland* (1971), 95–109.

BRAND, JANET C., and STEPHEN H. TOLINS. *The Nursing Students' Guide to Surgery*. Boston: Little, Brown and Company, 1979.

BRUNNER, LILLIAN, and DORIS SUDDARTH. *The Lippincott Manual of Nursing Practice*, 2nd ed. New York: J. B. Lippincott Company, 1978.

BURKE, M. DESMOND. "Low Sodium: Delusion, Depletion or Dilution?" *LAB 79*, 2 (June 1979), 40-44.

BURKE, M. DESMOND. "Cholesterol, Triglycerides, and Lipoprotein Studies: Strategies for Clinical Use." *Postgraduate Medicine* (March 1980), 263-66, 269, 273.

CAMERON, J. STEWART, ALISON RUSSELL, and DIANA SALE. *Nephrology for Nurses: A Modern Approach to the Kidney*, 2nd ed. Flushing, N.Y.: Medical Examination Publishing Company, Inc., 1976.

CAPRINI, JOSEPH A. *Bleeding Problems: Diagnosis and Treatment.* Hagerstown, Md.: Harper & Row, Publishers, 1973.

CARNEVALI, DORIS L., and MAXINE PATRICK, eds. *Nursing Management for the Elderly*. Philadelphia: J. B. Lippincott Company, 1979.

CHRISTIAN, CHARLES L. "Managing Arthritis: Three Guides to Differential Diagnosis (DDx), Lab, Tests, and Drugs." *Modern Medicine* (June 30-July 15, 1980), 18-23.

CLARK, RONALD G. *Manter and Gate's Essentials of Clinical Neuroanatomy and Neurophysiology*, 5th ed. Philadelphia: F. A. Davis Company, 1975.

COLLER, B. S., and others. "Plasma Cofactor of Platelet Function: Correlation with Diabetic Retinopathy and Hemoglobins $A_{1a\text{-}c}$, Studies in Diabetic Patients and Normal Persons." *Annals of Internal Medicine* (March 1978), 311-316.

COLLINS, R. DOUGLAS. *Illustrated Manual of Laboratory Diagnosis: Indications and Interpretations.* 2nd ed. Philadelphia: J. B. Lippincott Company, 1975.

CONN, HOWARD F., and REX B. CONN, eds. *Current Diagnosis 5*. Philadelphia: W. B. Saunders Company, 1979.

CONWAY, BARBARA LANG, ed. *Carini and Owens' Neurological and Neurosurgical Nursing*, 7th ed. St. Louis, Mo.: The C. V. Mosby Company, 1978.

CZACZKES, J. W., and A. KAPLAN DE-NOUR. *Chronic Hemodialysis as a Way of Life*. New York: Brunner/Mazel, 1978.

DANOVITCH, STUART, RALPH HARTWELL, JOHN LADUE, ELLIOTT MANCALL, and FRITZ STREULL. "When to Order Serum Enzyme Studies and Why." *Patient Care* (February 28, 1971), 69-81.

DAVIDSOHN, ISRAEL, and JOHN B. HENRY. *Todd-Sanford Clinical Diagnosis by Laboratory Methods*, 14th ed. Philadelphia: W. B. Saunders Company, 1969.

FARESE, ROBERT V. "How to Make Sense Out of the New Thyroid Tests." *Medical Times* (April 1980), 95-98, 103, 106.

FAULKNER, WILLIARD, JOHN W. KING, and HENRY DAMM, eds. *Handbook of Clinical Laboratory Data,* 2nd ed. Cleveland, Ohio: The Chemical Rubber Company, 1968.

FINCH, CLEMENT A. *A Patient Oriented Approach to General Medicine.* Seattle, Wash.: University of Washington Publications, 1972.

FRAWLEY, THOMAS F. "Cushing's Syndrome." *Clinician—1: The Adrenal Gland* (1971), 37-53.

FROHLICH, EDWARD, ed. *Pathophysiology: Altered Regulatory Mechanisms in Disease,* 2nd ed. Philadelphia: J. B. Lippincott Company, 1976.

GANONG, WILLIAM F. *Review of Medical Physiology,* 6th ed. Los Altos, Calif.: Lange Medical Publications, 1973.

GOODMAN, CAROL E., RICHARD L. LANGE, JACK WAXMAN, and THOMAS E. WEISS. "Ankylosing Spondylitis in Women." *Archives of Physical Medicine and Rehabilitation* (April 1980), 167-170.

GOVONI, LAURA, and JANICE HAYES. *Drugs and Nursing Implications,* 3rd ed. New York: Appleton-Century-Crofts, 1978.

GREISHEIMER, ESTHER M., and MARY P. WIEDEMAN. *Physiology and Anatomy,* 9th ed. Philadelphia: J. B. Lippincott Company, 1972.

GRENADIER, E., G. ALPAN, and A. PALANT. "CPK and CPK-MB in Myocardial Infarction and Ischemia." *Practical Cardiology* (March 1980), 107, 110-111, 113-116.

GROER, MAUREEN E., and MAUREEN E. SHEKLETON. *Basic Pathophysiology: A Conceptual Approach.* St. Louis, Mo.: The C. V. Mosby Company, 1979.

GUMP, FRANK. "Acid-Base Evaluations: Are Venous Samplings Still Useful?" *Diagnosis* (April 1980), 50-58, 62-63.

HALL, E. HAROLD. Class lecture. Seattle, Wash., May 1972.

HARPER, HAROLD. *Review of Physiological Chemistry,* 13th ed. Los Altos, Calif.: Lange Medical Publications, 1971.

HARRINGTON, JOAN, and ETTA BRENER. *Patient Care in Renal Failure.* Philadelphia: W. B. Saunders Company, 1973.

HARRIS, PATRICIA C., Chief Microbiologist, General Hospital of Everett, Wash., Written comments. Summer 1980.

HARTUNG, G. HARTLEY, and WILLIAM G. SQUIRES. "Exercise and HDL Cholesterol in Middle-aged Men." *The Physician and Sports-Medicine* (January 1980), 74-79.

HARVEY, A. MCGEHEE, RICHARD JOHNS, ALBERT OWENS, and RICHARD ROSS. *The Principles and Practice of Medicine,* 19th ed. New York: Appleton-Century-Crofts, 1976.

HARVEY, A., MCGEHEE, JAMES BORDLEY III, and JEREMIAH A. BARONDES. *Differential Diagnosis*, 3rd ed. Philadelphia: W. B. Saunders Company, 1979.

HAZZARD, MARY E. *Critical Care Nursing–Nursing Outline Series.* Garden City, N.Y.: Medical Examination Publishing Company, Inc., 1979.

HEKELMAN, FRANCINE, and CARL OSTENDARP. *Nephrology in Nursing: Perspectives of Care.* New York: McGraw-Hill Book Company, 1979.

HENRY, JOHN BERNARD, ed. *Todd-Sanford-Davidsohn. Clinical Diagnosis and Management by Laboratory Methods,* 16th ed., 2 vols. Philadelphia: W. B. Saunders Company, 1979.

HOLLOWAY, NANCY MEYER. *Nursing the Critically Ill Adult.* Menlo Park, Calif.: Addison-Wesley Publishing Company, 1979.

HORWITZ, CHARLES A. "Laboratory Diagnosis of Rheumatoid Disease." *Postgraduate Medicine* (May 1980), 193-195, 198-200, 203.

HOWARD, ROSANNE B., and NANCIE H. HERBOLD. *Nutrition in Clinical Care.* New York: McGraw-Hill Book Company. 1978.

JONES, DOROTHY, CLAIRE DUNBAR, and MARY JIROVEC. *Medical-Surgical Nursing: A Conceptual Approach.* New York: McGraw-Hill Book Company, 1978.

KAGAN, LYNN WENIG. *Renal Disease: A Manual of Patient Care.* New York: McGraw-Hill Book Company, 1979.

KASANOF, DAVID. "Blood Chemistries: Best Use of Those Multiple Test Profiles." *Patient Care* (December 15, 1972), 54-56, 60-69, 72-74, 77.

KEE, JOYCE LEFEVER. *Fluids and Electrolytes with Clinical Applications: A Programmed Approach,* 2nd ed. New York: John Wiley & Sons, Inc., 1978.

KINNEY, ANNA BELLE, and MARY BLOUNT. "Effect of Cranberry Juice on Urinary pH." *Nursing Research* (September-October 1979), 287-290.

KINTZEL, KAY C. ed. *Advanced Concepts in Clinical Nursing,* 2nd ed. New York: J. B. Lippincott Company, 1977.

KOENIG, RONALD J., and others. "Hemoglobin A_{1c} as an Indicator of the Degree of Glucose Intolerance in Diabetes." *Diabetes* (March 1976), 230-232.

KOENIG, RONALD J., STEVEN H. BLOBSTEIN, and ANTHONY CERAMI. "The Structure of Carbohydrate of Hemoglobin A_{1c}." *Journal of Biological Chemistry* (May 1977), 2992-2997.

KRUEGER, JUDITH, and JANIS RAY. *Endocrine Problems in Nursing; A Physiologic Approach.* St. Louis, Mo.: The C. V. Mosby Company, 1976.

KUNIN, CALVIN. *Detection, Prevention and Management of Urinary Tract Infections: A Manual for the Physician, Nurse and Allied Health Worker.* Philadelphia: Lea & Febiger, 1972.

The Lab, Drugs and Nursing Implications: Tapes I Thru XII. Chestnut Hill, Mass.: Health-Care Education Programs of America, 1978; course offered October-November 1979, Seattle, Wash.

The Lab, Drugs and Nursing Implications: Workbook. Chestnut Hill, Mass.: Health-Care Education Programs of America, 1978.

LEVINSKY, NORMAN G. "Hyperkalemia: The Clinical Spectrum." *Clinician: Potassium in Clinical Medicine* (1973), 58-64.

LEVY, ROBERT I. "Hyperlipoproteinemia and Its Management." *The Journal of Cardiovascular Medicine* (May 1980), 435-442, 447-449, 452.

"Lithium as a Granulopoietic Agent." *Current Prescribing* (September 1979), 25-32.

LUCKMANN, JOAN, and KAREN SORENSEN. *Medical Surgical Nursing: A Psychopathophysiologic Approach.* Philadelphia: W. B. Saunders Company, 1979.

LUTWICK, LARRY I. "Principles of Antiobiotic Use in the Elderly," *Geriatrics* (February 1980), 54-56, 58-60.

MACBRYDE, CYRIL MITCHELL, and ROBERT STANLEY BLACKLOW. *Signs and Symptoms: Applied Pathologic Physiology and Clinical Interpretation,* 5th ed. Philadelphia: J. B. Lippincott Company, 1970.

MCGOWAN, EOLINE. "Blood Component Transfusion Therapy." *Continuing Education for the Family Physician* (July 1980), 37-40.

MARKS, ROBERT G. "NIH Panel Urges Wider Use of Amantadine in Influenza A." *Current Prescribing* (February 1980), 55, 58.

MARTINEZ-LAVIN, M., J. H. VAUGHN, and E. M. TAN. "Autoantibodies and the Spectrum of Sjogren's Syndrome." *Annals of Internal Medicine* (August 1979), 185-190.

MECKLENBURG, ROBERT S., and PAUL N. FREDLUND. "Recognition and Treatment of Hypothyroidism." *Bulletin of the Mason Clinic* (Winter 1978-79), 129-138.

METHENY, NORMA M., and W. D. SNIVELY, JR. *Nurses' Handbook of Fluid Balance,* 3rd ed. Philadelphia: J. B. Lippincott Company, 1979.

MEUWISSEN, HILAIRE J. "Evaluating Patients with Suspected Immunodeficiency: Guideline for Clinical and Laboratory Diagnosis." *Postgraduate Medicine* (November 1979), 116-131.

MIALE, JOHN B. *Laboratory Medicine: Hematology,* 4th ed., St. Louis, Mo.: The C. V. Mosby Company, 1972.

MILLER, BENJAMIN, and CLAIRE B. KEANE. *Encyclopedia and Dictionary of Medicine and Nursing.* Philadelphia: W. B. Saunders Company, 1972.

MILTHORN, H. T., JR. "Understanding Arterial Blood Gases." *American Family Physician* (March 1980), 112-120.

MINSHAW, BARBARA H. "Assays and Antimicrobial Susceptibility." *Drug Therapy* (August 1979), 79-83, 87-88, 91, 95-96.

MOSS, GERALD. "Postsurgical Decompression and Immediate Elemental Feeding." *Hospital Practice* (May 1977), 73-82.

MOUNTCASTLE, VERNON, ed. *Medical Physiology,* 13th ed., 2 vols. St. Louis, Mo.: The C. V. Mosby Company, 1974.

MOWAD, JOSEPH J. "Pyuria: Guide to Management." *Hospital Medicine* (December 1979), 34-37.

NADOLNY, MARY DIANE. "Infection Control in the Hospital: What Does the Infection Control Nurse Do?" *American Journal of Nursing* (March 1980), 430-431.

"New Drugs/Drug News." *Drug Therapy* (June 1980), 21-23, 27.

NORDIN, DAVID, M.D. Written comments. Everett, Wash., Spring 1980.

NOTMAN, D. D., N. KURATA, and E. M. TAN. "Profiles of Antinuclear Antibodies in Systemic Rheumatic Diseases." *Annals of Internal Medicine* (October 1975), 464-469.

PERMUTT, M. ALAN. "Is It Really Hypoglycemia? If So, What Should You Do?" *Medical Times* (April 1980), 35-43.

PETERSON, CHARLES M., RONALD KOENIG, ROBERT JONES, CHRISTOPHER SAUDEK, and ANTHONY CERAMI. "Correlation of Serum Triglyceride Levels and Hemoglobin A_{1c} Concentrations in Diabetes Mellitus." *Diabetes* (1977), 507-509.

PHIPPS, WILMA J., BARBARA C. LONG, and NANCY F. WOODS, eds. *Medical-Surgical Nursing: Concepts and Clinical Practice.* St. Louis, Mo.: The C. V. Mosby Company, 1979.

PRCHAL, JOSEF T. "Red Cell Enzymes: An Overview." *Continuing Education for the Family Physician* (July 1980), 41-42, 44, 49-50.

PRICE, SYLVIA A., and LORRAINE M. WILSON. *Pathophysiology: Clinical Aspects of Disease Processes.* New York: McGraw-Hill Book Company, 1978.

PRITCHARD, JACK, and PAUL MACDONALD. *William's Obstetrics,* 15th ed. New York: Appleton-Century-Crofts, 1976.

RAVEL, RICHARD. *Clinical Laboratory Medicine: Application of Laboratory Data,* 2nd ed. Chicago: Year Book Medical Publishers, Inc., 1973.

RAVEL, RICHARD. *Clinical Laboratory Medicine: Clinical Application of Laboratory Data*, 3rd ed. Chicago: Year Book Medical Publishers, Inc., 1979.

RING, ALVIN M. *Laboratory Correlation Manual.* Springfield, Ill.: Charles C Thomas, Publisher, 1969.

SABISTON, DAVID C., ed. *Davis-Christopher's Textbook of Surgery: Biological Basis of Modern Surgical Practice,* 11th ed. Philadelphia: W. B. Saunders Company, 1977.

SAXON, SUE V., and MAY JEAN ETTEN. *Physical Change and Aging.* New York: The Tiresias Press, 1978.

SCIPIEN, GLADYS, MARTHA BARNARD, MARILYN CHARD, JEANNE HOWE, and PATRICIA PHILLIPS. *Comprehensive Pediatric Nursing.* New York: McGraw-Hill Book Company, 1975.

SCOGGIN, CHARLES H., and STEVEN A. SAHN. "The Common Cold—A Few New Tricks That Make the Going Easier." *Modern Medicine* (January 15-30, 1980), 28-33.

SEIGLER, PETER E., and GEORGINA FALUDI. "Immunologic Aspects of Thyroid Disease." *Today's Clinician* (June 1978), 26-29.

SERRIDGE, MARJORIE S. "The Anemic Patient." *Family Practice Recertification* (May 1980), 44-47, 50-52.

SHARPE, GORDON. "Mixed Connective Tissue Disease: Diagnosis and Treatment." *Continuing Education for the Family Physician* (May 1980), 33-40.

SHMC (Swedish Hospital Medical Center), Laboratory of Pathology. "Laboratory Procedure Manual." Seattle: SHMC, 1978 (mimeographed).

SILVER, HENRY, C. HENRY KEMPS, and HENRY BRUYN. *Handbook of Pediatrics,* 8th ed. Los Altos, Calif.: Lange Medical Publications, 1969.

SODEMAN, WILLIAM A., JR., and WILLIAM A. SODEMAN. *Pathologic Physiology: Mechanisms of Disease,* 4th ed. Philadelphia: W. B. Saunders Company, 1968.

SODEMAN, WILLIAM A., JR., and WILLIAM A. SODEMAN. *Pathologic Physiology: Mechanisms of Disease,* 5th ed. Philadelphia: W. B. Saunders Company, 1974.

SODEMAN, WILLIAM A., and THOMAS M. SODEMAN. *Pathologic Physiology: Mechanisms of Disease,* 6th ed. Philadelphia: W. B. Saunders Company, 1979.

SOLL, DAVID, and ELLIOT S. COHEN. "Ocular Manifestations of Thyroid Disease." *Today's Clinician* (June 1978), 22-25.

SORENSEN, KAREN, and JOAN LUCKMANN. *Basic Nursing: A Psychophysiologic Approach.* Philadelphia: W. B. Saunders Company, 1979.

SPENCER, ROBERTA T. *Patient Care in Endocrine Problems.* Philadelphia: W. B. Saunders Company, 1973.

STEFFES, MICHAEL. "Testing for Hyperthyroidism." *LAB 79* (January-February 1979), 18-22.

STREETEN, DAVID. "Secondary Aldosteronism." *Clinician—1: The Adrenal Gland* (1971), 76-93.

STROOT, VIOLET, CARLA LEE, and C. ANN SCHAPER. *Fluids and Electrolytes: A Practical Approach,* 2nd ed. Philadelphia: F. A. Davis Company, 1977.

SUMIDA, STANFORD E., and MICHAEL MULLARKEY. "Antinuclear Antibodies: Characterization and Clinical Applications." *Bulletin of The Mason Clinic* (Spring 1979), 25-32.

THORN, GEORGE W. "Adrenal Corticol Hypofunction." *Clinician—1: The Adrenal Gland* (1971), 23-34.

TIETZ, NORBERT W., ed. *Fundamentals of Clinical Chemistry.* Philadelphia: W. B. Saunders Company, 1970.

TROUTMAN, MONTE E., MICHAEL J. BLEND, JOHN L. KNIAZ, and MARK E. FRUSY. "Antigen and Antibody Testing in Viral Hepatitis A and B." *Osteopathic Physician* (March 1980), 35, 39-41.

TUCKER, ERNEST S., and ROBERT M. NAKAMURA. "Laboratory Studies for the Evaluation of Systemic Lupus Erythematosus and Related Disorders." *Laboratory Medicine* (November 1980), 717-726.

TURCK, MARVIN. "Urinary Tract Infections." *Hospital Practice* (January 1980), 49-58.

VINICOR, FRANK, and JAMES COOPER. "Early Recognition of Endocrine Disorders." *Hospital Medicine* (December 1979), 38-47.

WALLACH, JACQUES. *Interpretation of Diagnostic Tests: A Handbook and Synopsis of Laboratory Medicine.* Boston: Little, Brown and Company, 1970.

WATSON, JEANNETTE E. *Medical-Surgical Nursing and Related Physiology.* Philadelphia: W. B. Saunders Company, 1979.

WELT, LOUIS G., and WILLIAM BLYTHE. "A Primer on Potassium Metabolism." *Clinician: Potassium in Clinical Medicine* (1973), 13-24.

WENIG, PAUL. "Diagnosis and Treatment of Rheumatoid Arthritis." *Osteopathic Annals* (April 1980), 17-19, 22-25, 29, 33-35, 38-40.

WHALEY, LUCILLE F., and DONNA L. WONG. *Nursing Care of Infants and Children.* St. Louis, Mo.: The C. V. Mosby Company, 1979.

WHEELIS, ROGER F. "Making Sense of Coagulation Tests." *Bulletin of the Mason Clinic* (Spring 1979), 1-9.

WIDMANN, FRANCES. *Clinical Interpretation of Laboratory Tests,* 8th ed. Philadelphia: F. A. Davis Company, 1979.

ZIEGEL, ERNA, and CAROLYN VAN BLARCOM. *Obstetric Nursing,* 6th ed. New York: Macmillan Publishing Co., Inc., 1972.

Index

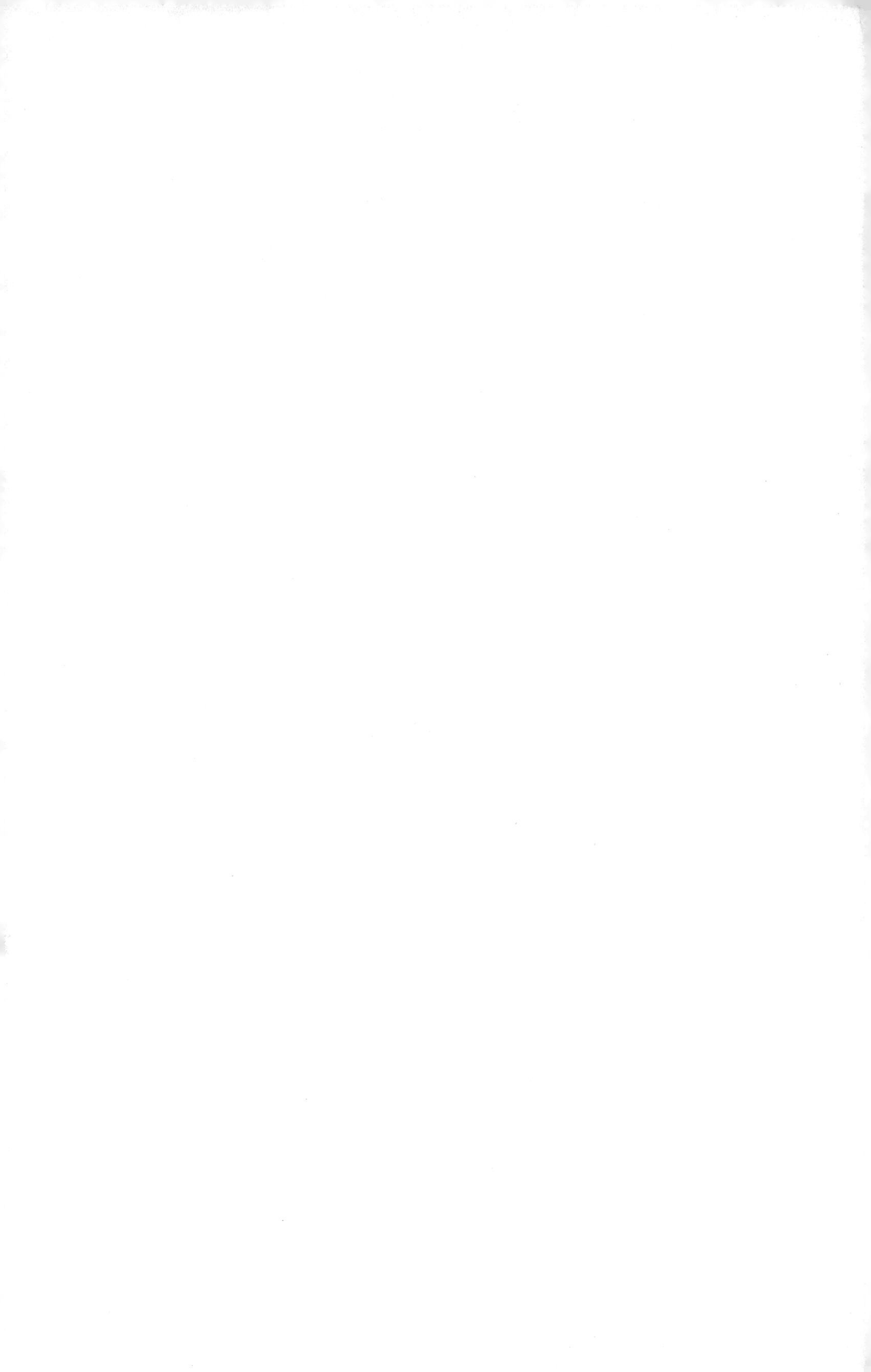